AN INTEGRATED APPROACH TO THERAPEUTIC EXERCISE

Theory and Clinical Application

Patricia E. Sullivan, MS, RPT
Clinical Assistant Professor
Sargent College of Allied Health Professions
Boston University

Prudence D. Markos, MS, RPT
Adjunct Assistant Professor
Sargent College of Allied Health Professions
Boston University

Mary Alice D. Minor, MS, RPT
Assistant Professor
College of Health Related Professions
Wichita State University

Photographs by:
Robert Littlefield, M.Ed.
Manager of Photography Services
Director, School of Biomedical Photography
Beth Israel Hospital, Boston

AN INTEGRATED APPROACH TO THERAPEUTIC EXERCISE

Theory and Clinical Application

Reston Publishing Company
A Prentice-Hall Company

Reston, Virginia

Library of Congress Cataloging in Publication Data

Sullivan, Patricia E., 1946–
An integrated approach to therapeutic exercise.

Bibliography: p.
Includes index.
1. Exercise therapy. 2. Physically handicapped—Rehabilitation. I. Markos, Prudence D., 1940– II. Minor, Mary Alice D., 1944– . III. Title.
RM725.S84 615.8′2 81-23380
ISBN 0-8359-3088-2 AACR2

Editorial/production supervision and interior design by Barbara J. Gardetto

10

Printed in the United States of America

The great thing in this world is not so much where we stand as in what direction we are moving. . . .

Oliver Wendell Holmes

To the professionals dedicated to the improvement of patient care

Contents

chapter 9
Spinal Cord Injury 258

PART III
TREATMENT OF PATIENTS WITH SELECTED ORTHOPEDIC DISABILITIES 293

Authors' Note

A basic knowledge of normal development, proprioceptive neuromuscular facilitation (PNF) and the function of exteroceptive and proprioceptive receptors such as pressure receptors and the muscle spindle, is desirable for a thorough understanding of this text. The reader will find some fundamental information in the glossary of terms. For additional background and supplementary material, the references cited below are recommended. When consulting these sources, however, the reader should bear in mind that recent investigations have used technology that was not available when many of the early studies were conducted. Although some concepts and hypotheses from that time have been corroborated, doubt has been cast on others. Current articles dealing with certain controversies and evolving theories can be found in the reference lists at the end of most chapters.

- Barnes MR, Crutchfield CA, Heriza CB: The Neurophysiological Basis of Patient Treatment. Atlanta, GA, Stokesville Publishing Co, 1978, vol 2
- Crutchfield CA, Barnes MR: The Neurophysiological Basis of Patient Treatment. Atlanta, GA, Stokesville Publishing Co, 1975, vol 1
- Exploratory and Analytical Survey of Therapeutic Exercise (NUSTEP). Baltimore, Waverly Press, 1966
- Knott M, Voss DE: Proprioceptive Neuromuscular Facilitation, ed 2. New York, Harper & Row, 1968

- McGraw MB: The Neuromuscular Maturation of the Human Infant. New York, Columbia University Press, 1948. Reprinted edition, New York, Hafner Publishing Co, 1962
- Payton OD, Hirt SH, Newton RA: Scientific Bases for Neurophysiologic Approaches to Therapeutic Exercise: an Anthology. Philadelphia, FA Davis, 1977

Acknowledgments

This book required a tremendous amount of cooperative effort from many people. We would like to thank our families and friends for their understanding and support.

Many physical therapists reviewed the manuscript at various stages of completion; for their cooperation and constructive comments we thank: Mary Lou Barns, Pauline Cerasoli, Suzanne Dean, Holly Herman, Carolyn Heriza, Linda Holland, Patricia Kammerer, Eugene Lambert, Anne Latham, Janet Muth, Suzanne Olsen, Anne Rinesmith, Carol Ritter, Thomas Schmitz, Patricia J. Sullivan, Lynn Troy, and Mary Watkins.

For their generosity in spending time posing for photographs we thank: Suzanne Dean, Holly Herman, Linda Holland, Jennifer Kelley, Bill Markos, Ken O'Neil, Mary Sullivan, Andrew Titcomb, and Lynn Troy.

We also thank the many people who typed the manuscript.

All progress is initiated by
challenging current conceptions. . . .
George Bernard Shaw

Preface

Therapeutic exercise has evolved as an integral part of physical therapy. As a result of increasing emphasis on research and improved technology, exercise has metamorphosed from an empirically based art to procedures with a developing scientific basis. Many people have promoted, assisted, and caused this evolution. Their contributions have been based on careful observations of patients, on empirical research, and on didactic research in physical therapy and related fields. We feel honored and fortunate to have had the opportunity to observe and learn directly from some of these contributors. Furthermore, we appreciate their efforts to share their expertise through publications and teaching.

Herman Kabot together with Margaret Knott and Dorothy Voss described functional patterns of movement that were used to improve muscle control of patients having both orthopedic and neurological problems. Many techniques were also developed by them to enhance relaxation or to increase strength by promoting irradiation from stronger to weaker muscle groups.

Our primary training in proprioceptive neuromuscular facilitation (PNF) forms the basis of the integrated approach to therapeutic exercise presented in this book. We are indebted to Margaret Knott, Dorothy Voss, and Marjorie Ionta for stimulating our interests in PNF and therapeutic exercise through their classroom and clinical teaching. All three therapists have contributed to the body of knowledge supporting therapeutic exercise treatments by publishing accounts of their clinical experience (1–11). In addition, Knott and Voss have authored a book on PNF (12). Through the efforts of

Dorothy Voss, the Northwestern University Special Therapeutic Exercise Project (NUSTEP) was implemented in 1966.

Margaret Rood's understanding of the importance of sensory stimulation and her descriptions of various types of facilitatory and inhibitory input have supported and broadened the use of afferent input in many PNF procedures. In addition to emphasizing and clarifying Rood's concepts, Shirley Stockmeyer at NUSTEP further broadened the Rood approach by adding and defining the stages of motor control necessary for the development of skill (13). The progression of motor control is essential, we believe, to proper treatment planning. This progression is fundamental to an integrated approach to therapeutic exercise.

Signe Brunnstrom's contribution to the evolution of therapeutic exercise goes beyond her development of evaluation procedures and treatment techniques for the hemiplegic patient. Her belief in the need to provide a rationale for our treatment procedures is evidenced, in part, by the number of abstracts from neurological and developmental literature provided in her book, *Movement Therapy in Hemiplegia* (14). By integrating biomechanical and kinesiological principles with information gleaned from classical studies, she developed a basis for the use of certain positions, movement combinations, and treatment procedures. One of Brunnstrom's special qualities was her obvious concern for the welfare of the patient as an individual.

The impetus to develop new approaches to therapeutic exercise arose in other countries as well. Karl and Berta Bobath were leaders in moving away from purely an orthopedic perspective to a neurological one in the treatment of patients with disorders of the central nervous system (CNS), especially cerebral palsy. Their description of postural reflex mechanisms and the relationship to normal function widened the spectrum of techniques that had previously been available for both children and adults with CNS dysfunction. The Bobaths have published several articles and books on their neurodevelopmental treatment theory that have fostered the growth of therapeutic exercise and the quality of patient care (15–27).

These people represent merely a few of the contributors who have promoted the advancement of therapeutic exercise. Without such efforts, most physical therapists would never have acquired their present competencies. Despite the encouraging strides made in our field in recent years, however, we must not be satisfied with or complacent about our present skills. Although some areas of therapeutic exercise have been well defined, others require further study and development. Research is needed to increase our understanding of normal functioning and variations that occur in pathological conditions. Continued scientific investigations in academic settings is important to increase our understanding of normal movement. Clinical research is the only valid way to determine the efficacy and efficiency of our treatments. Each patient treatment is considered a research project. Careful evaluation, establishment and implementation of a treatment plan, and accurate assessment of the results of that plan will make the therapist aware of the success or appropriateness of specific procedures. With precise documentation and sharing of information, a sound body of knowledge will continue to develop and expand. The therapists mentioned above have provided us with examples worth emulating.

Our interest is not to initiate a new approach, but rather by borrowing and blending to develop an integrated approach to therapeutic exercise. This book is organized so that the beginning chapters introduce the treatment planning process and provide the rationale underlying therapeutic procedures. The supporting rationale is based on our current body of knowledge. We recognize that results of future research will corroborate some of the present concepts and will prompt us to reevaluate others. New information is welcome, as it can only lead to a better understanding of our treatment methods and consequently to a higher quality of patient care.

Later chapters describe the implementation of these procedures for patients with both orthopedic and neurological disorders. The treatment regimens illustrate the information presented in Part I. Our intent was not to establish stereotyped programs for each disability, but rather to assist the therapist in treatment planning. Each patient is unique and requires procedures tailored to meet specific needs.

We hope that you will examine the information in the following chapters carefully and try out your new knowledge cautiously. In order to be comfortable with and successful in your application of the material in this book, we suggest beginning with a patient who is not the ultimate challenge. Remember, learning requires time, practice, and the positive feedback provided by success. Most importantly, we encourage you to be a critical reader and to research the concepts proposed in this text. The continuing maturation of therapeutic exercise depends on your efforts.

REFERENCES

1. Ionta MK: Facilitation technics in the treatment of early rheumatoid arthritis. Phys Ther Rev 40:119–120, 1960
2. Knott M: Avulsion of a finger with protracted disability. Phys Ther Rev 38:52, 1958
3. Knott M: Bulbar involvement with good recovery. J Amer Phys Ther Assoc 42(1):38–39, 1962
4. Knott M: Neuromuscular facilitation in the treatment of rheumatoid arthritis. J. Amer Phys Ther Assoc 44:737–739, 1964
5. Knott M: Report of a case of Parkinsonism treated with proprioceptive facilitation technics. Phys Ther Rev 37:229, 1957
6. Knott M, Barufaldi D: Treatment of whiplash injuries. Phys Ther Rev 41:573–577, 1961
7. Knott M, Mead S: Facilitation technics in lower extremity amputation. Phys Ther Rev 40:587–589, 1960

8. Mead S, Knott M: Question on immersion in ice water. Phys Ther 47:1149, 1967
9. Voss DE, Knott M: The application of neuromuscular facilitation in the treatment of shoulder disabilities. Phys Ther Rev 33:536–541, 1953
10. Voss DE: Proprioceptive neuromuscular facilitation: The PNF method. In Pearson PH, Williams CE(eds): Physical Therapy Services in the Developmental Disabilities. Springfield, IL, Charles C Thomas, 1972, pp 223–282
11. Voss DE: Proprioceptive neuromuscular facilitation. In Bouman HE(ed): An Exploratory and Analytical Survey of Therapeutic Exercise: Northwestern University Special Therapeutic Exercise Project. Baltimore, The Williams & Wilkins Co, 1966, pp 839–898
12. Knott M, Voss DE: Proprioceptive Neuromuscular Faciliation Patterns and Techniques, New York, Harper & Row, 1968
13. Stockmeyer SA: An Interpretation of the Approach of Rood to the Treatment of Neuromuscular Dysfunction. In Bouman HD(ed): An Exploratory and Analytical Survey of Therapeutic Exercise: Northwestern University Special Therapeutic Exercise Project. Baltimore, The Williams & Wilkins Co, 1966, pp 900–956
14. Brunnstrom S: Movement Therapy in Hemiplegia. New York, Harper & Row, 1970
15. Bobath B: Adult Hemiplegia: Evaluation and Treatment, ed 2. London, William Heinemann Medical Books Ltd, 1978
16. Bobath B, Bobath K: Motor Development in the Different Types of Cerebral Palsy. London, William Heinemann Medical Books Ltd, 1975
17. Bobath K: The neuropathology of cerebral palsy and its importance in treatment and diagnosis. Cerebral Palsy Bulletin 1:13–33, 1959
18. Bobath B: The treatment of neuromuscular disorders by imposing patterns of co-ordination. Physiotherapy 55:18–22, 1969
19. Bobath K: The prevention of mental retardation in patients with cerebral palsy. Acta Paedopsychiatrics 3:141–154, 1963
20. Bobath B: Treatment principles and planning in cerebral palsy. Physiotherapy 49:122, 1963
21. Bobath B: A neuro-developmental treatment of cerebral palsy. Physiotherapy 49:242–244, 1963
22. Bobath K, Bobath B: The facilitation of normal postural reactions and movements in the treatment of cerebral palsy. Physiotherapy 50:246–262, 1964
23. Bobath B: The very early treatment of cerebral palsy. Developmental Medicine and Child Neurology 9:373–390, 1967
24. Bobath K, Bobath B: The neuro-developmental treatment of cerebral palsy. Phys Ther 47:1039–1041, 1967

25. Bobath K, Bobath B: Cerebral palsy. In Pearson PH, Williams CE(eds): Physical Therapy Services in the Developmental Disabilities. Springfield, IL, Charles C Thomas, 1972, pp 31–185

26. Bobath B, Finnie NR: Problems of communication between parents and staff in the treatment and management of children with cerebral palsy. Developmental Medicine and Child Neurology 12:629–235, 1970

27. Bobath B: Motor development, its effect on general development and application to the treatment of cerebral palsy. Physiotherapy 56:11, 1971

Introduction

The main purpose of this book is to enable both physical therapy students and clinicians to recognize and evaluate the component parts of a therapeutic exercise procedure. A new use of terminology is presented in this book to define these component parts. A therapeutic exercise procedure is divided into three units:

Activity (A): A posture and any movements occurring in that posture.

Technique (T): The type(s) of muscle contraction(s)—concentric, eccentric, isometric.

Elements (E): Sensory input used either to facilitate or inhibit a response.

Because no consistent terminology existed, we developed these terms initially to assist students in establishing appropriate treatment procedures and a system for the progression of treatment. The terms provided not only a mechanism for consistency but also a means of organizing and defining basic concepts.

This terminology has proved to be of value in converting evaluative findings into a meaningful treatment plan, and, when necessary, in developing rational alternatives. If all procedures were constructed on the basis of a sound rationale, implementation of an exercise regimen purely on the basis of trial and error could be avoided.

The conceptualization presented here can be used in describing any therapeutic exercise procedure regardless of the approach selected for treatment.

A progressive resistive exercise (PRE) procedure might be described in the following manner:

A. Sitting, knee extension

T. Concentric and eccentric contractions

E. Resistance of gravity and PRE boot

To establish scapular control, the Bobaths, for example, might begin with:

A. Sidelying, scapular protraction

T. Active assistive concentric contraction

E. Manual contacts on key points, scapula and hand

To facilitate synergistic patterns, Brunnstrom might advocate:

A. Sitting, rowing

T. Concentric contractions

E. Manual resistance with manual contacts on wrists/hands

Identifying the component parts of each procedure at first may appear to be tedious and even unnecessary. Consistent thinking in this manner, however, will enable the therapist to readily identify existing similarities and differences among treatment philosophies. Once this step is accomplished, a logical and integrated approach to the treatment planning process can begin.

Glossary of Terms

DEVELOPMENT

Tonic Neck Reflexes Mediated by proprioceptors in the proximal cervical area.

Asymmetrical Tonic Neck Reflex (ATNR) A change in muscle tone of the extremities as a result of head rotation. When the head is turned to one side, extensor tone increases in the extremities on the chin side and flexor tone increases on the skull side.

Symmetrical Tonic Neck Reflex (STNR) When the head is flexed, the motor response is an increase in flexor tone in the upper extremities and in extensor tone in the lower extremities. When the head extends, the motor response is a tendency toward increase in extensor tone in the upper extremities and in flexor tone in the lower extremities.

Symmetrical Tonic Labyrinthine Reflex (STLR) Mediated by the vestibular system. When the head is maintained in extension in a supine position, there is an increase in extensor tone in the extremities. When the head is maintained in flexion in the prone position, there is a decrease in extensor tone or an increase in flexor tone.

Asymmetrical Tonic Labyrinthine Reflex (ATLR) In sidelying there is an increase in flexor tone of the uppermost extremities and an increase in extensor tone of the lowermost extremities which are in contact with the supporting surface.

Righting Reactions Orienting movements of the head, neck, and body to maintain the eyes horizontal, head vertical, and the body in proper relationship to the head. Stimulus may be optical, labyrinthine, or tactile.

Balance Reactions Movements that attempt to maintain the center of gravity (C of G) within the base of support (B of S). Equilibrium reactions are in response to changes in the labyrinthine system and proprioceptive reactions are mediated through the more peripheral proprioceptive receptors.

Protective Extension An extremity movement that changes the B of S if the C of G is moved out of the original B of S.

NEUROPHYSIOLOGY

Autonomic Nervous System (ANS) A motor system that innervates smooth muscle and gland throughout the body. Either through neuronal and/or glandular effects the ANS can influence somatic, cognitive, physiological or psychological behaviors.

Sympathetic Division That portion of the ANS that gives rise to generalized responses, which include acceleration of heart rate and force of heartbeat, increased production by sweat glands, vasoconstriction of cutaneous and visceral blood vessels, and stimulation of adrenal glands. Sympathetic responses are greatest during stress situations. Increased sympathetic stimulation results in a high level of anxiety and a low threshold to pain.

Parasympathetic Division That portion of the ANS that gives rise to localized responses assigned to conserve and restore energy sources of the body. Parasympathetic stimulation results in a low level of anxiety and a high threshold to pain. The interaction of the sympathetic and parasympathetic divisions results in the regulation of the body in such a way that homeostasis results.

Muscle Classification Muscles can be classified according to anatomical, physiological, and metabolic characteristics. On the basis of these characteristics, few muscles can be categorized as pure flexors or extensors. In this text flexor and extensor muscles are defined as follows:

Flexor—Phasic, Type II

- Located superficially, crosses two joints, has long tendinous attachments.
- Composed primarily of large, fast-twitch, motor units that fatigue easily.
- Has a high glycogen content and few oxidative enzymes.

Extensor—Tonic, Type I

- Located proximally, crosses one joint, has broad attachments.

- Composed primarily of small, slow-twitch, motor units that are resistant to fatigue.
- Has low glycogen content and many oxidative enzymes.

Phasic Response A brief muscle contraction. (See Note below.)

Tonic Response A sustained muscle contraction. (See Note below.)

NOTE: Both phasic and tonic responses can be elicited in both flexors and extensors. These responses may be referred to in the following terms: metabolic (high energy, low energy), neurophysiological (sympathetic, parasympathetic), behavioral (away from, toward).

Encapsulated Exteroceptors Cutaneous receptors that are located in the dermis, subcutaneous, and intramuscular connective tissue, periosteum, ligaments, and tendon surfaces. Included in this category are Pacinian corpuscles, Meissner's corpuscles, and Krause end bulbs. These receptors rapidly adapt to touch, pressure, cold, and vibration stimuli and display a short after-discharge pattern.

Free Nerve Endings Cutaneous receptors primarily located in the dermis and around the base of the hair follicles. These receptors slowly adapt to diffuse touch, pain, and temperature stimuli and display a prolonged after-discharge pattern.

A Fibers Fast-conducting myelinated somatic nerve fibers that transmit impulses from excited cutaneous capsulated receptors. These fibers may be associated with the production of phasic or mobilizing responses.

C Fibers Slow conducting, predominantly unmyelinated somatic nerve fibers that transmit impulses from excited free nerve endings. These fibers may be associated with the production of tonic or stabilizing responses.

Proprioceptor A receptor that is located deep within the tissues of the body (for example, muscles, tendons, joints, inner ear) and that responds to changes in position, movement, or deep pressure.

Muscle Spindle A proprioceptor located in skeletal muscle parallel to

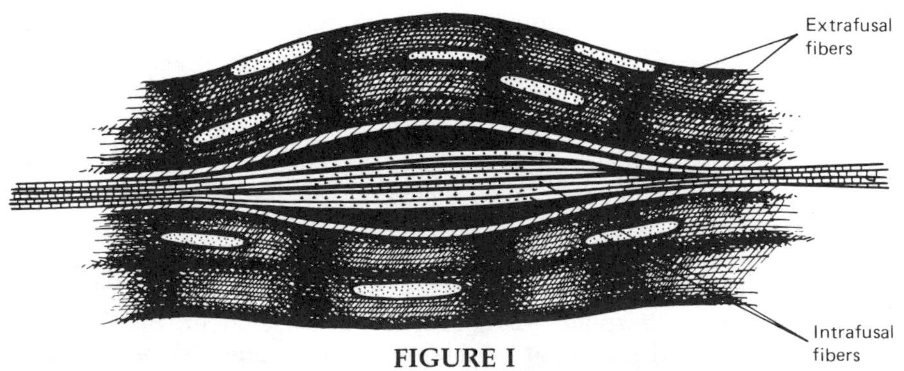

FIGURE I

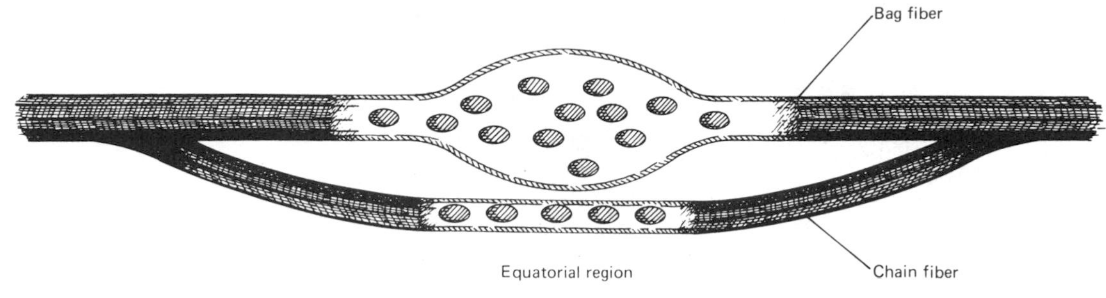

FIGURE II

the extrafusal fibers (Figure I). The main purpose of the muscle spindle is to provide information regarding muscle length back to the CNS.

Intrafusal Fibers Muscle fibers located within the muscle spindle. Two types exist: bag and chain (Figure II).

Ia or Primary Afferent Fiber A large nerve fiber that forms part of the afferent nerve supply from the muscle spindle. The fiber receptor is located in the equatorial or middle regions of both the bag and chain fibers (Figure III). Excitation of the Ia receptors results in autogenetic facilitation (that is,

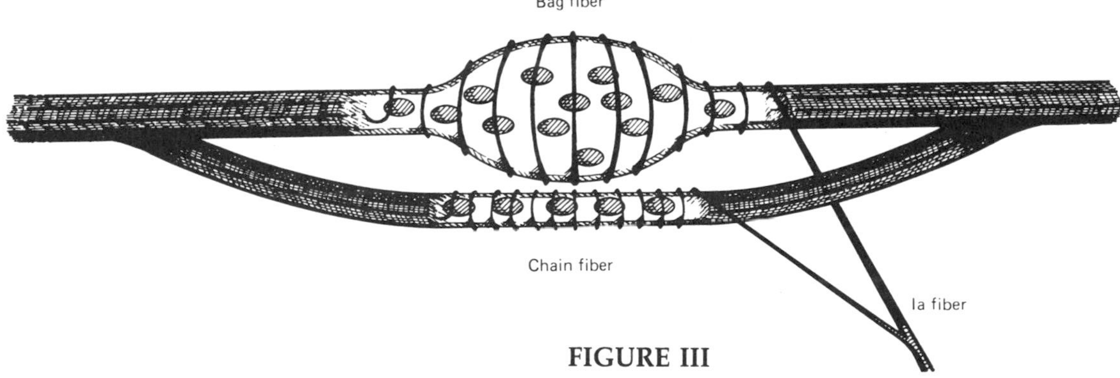

FIGURE III

facilitation to homonym and synergists) and reciprocal inhibition to antagonistic muscle groups (Figure IV). Small changes in movement as well as rates of change or movement are monitored by the Ia receptors.

II or Secondary Afferent Fiber A nerve fiber which, in conjunction with the Ia fiber, makes up the afferent nerve supply from the muscle spindle. The fiber receptor, which is primarily on the chain intrafusal fibers, is located at either end of the equatorial region but is more laterally situated than the Ia receptor (Figure V). Controversy surrounds the function of the II afferent; one theory is that excitation of this receptor in a flexor muscle yields a response similar to that of the Ia fiber, that is, autogenetic facilitation and reciprocal inhibition. In an extensor, however, the result appears

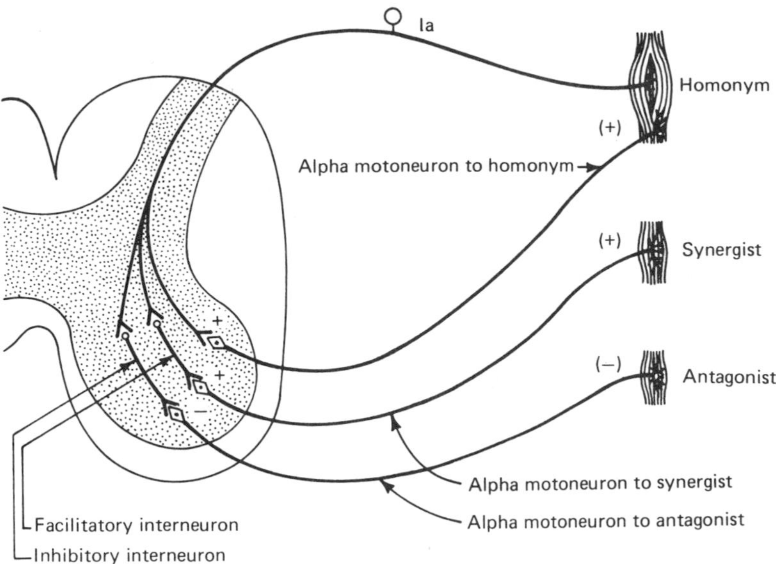

FIGURE IV

to be inhibition to the homonym and facilitation to the antagonist. The II fiber receptor is highly sensitive to slow, maintained stretches in lengthened muscle ranges.

Fusimotor Fibers or Gamma Motoneurons Nerve fibers that form the efferent or motor supply to the muscle spindle. The cell bodies of the gamma motoneurons are located in the ventral horn of the spinal cord, in close proximity with the cell bodies of the alpha motoneurons, and are under the influence of higher centers (Figure VI).

Dynamic Gamma Motoneurons Motoneurons that innervate primarily the polar or contractile regions, primarily of the dynamic intrafusal fibers

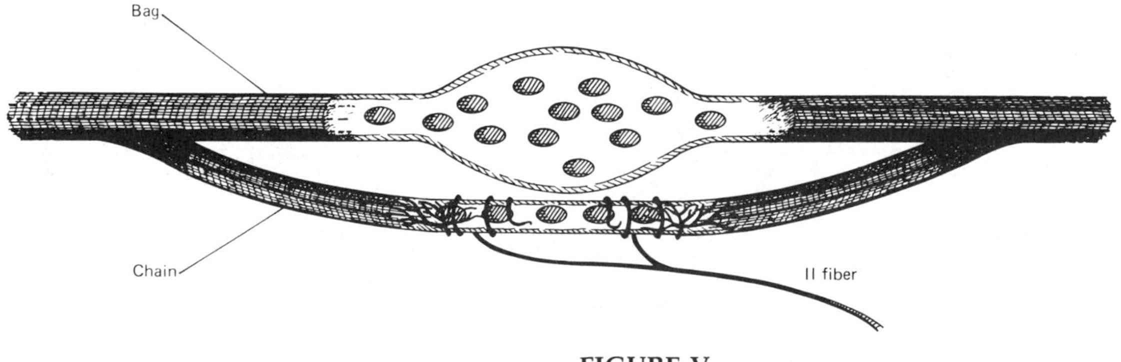

FIGURE V

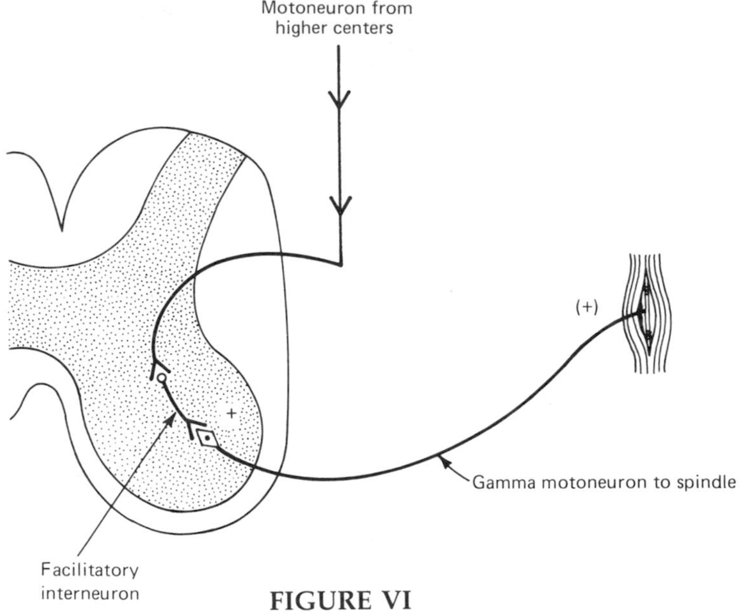

FIGURE VI

(Figure VII). They are associated with increases of the dynamic response of the Ia fiber.

Static Gamma Motoneurons Motoneurons that innervate the juxta- or quasiequatorial regions of both the bag and the chain intrafusal fibers in close proximity to the receptors of the II fibers (Figure VIII). They are associated with biasing or internally stretching the bag and the chain fibers and with maintaining muscle tone.

Internal Stretch or Gamma Bias The active contraction (stretch) of the intrafusal muscle fibers by the static gamma system. Excitation of the static gamma system keeps the spindle fibers taut or "loaded" and thereby responsive to externally applied muscle stretch.

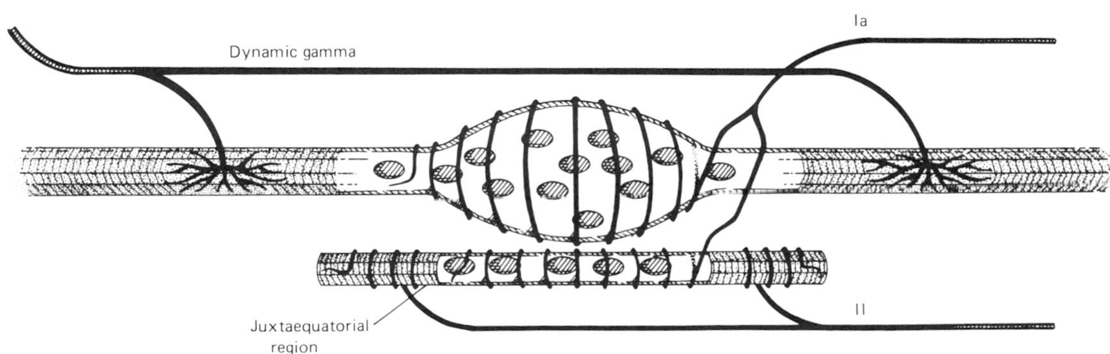

FIGURE VII

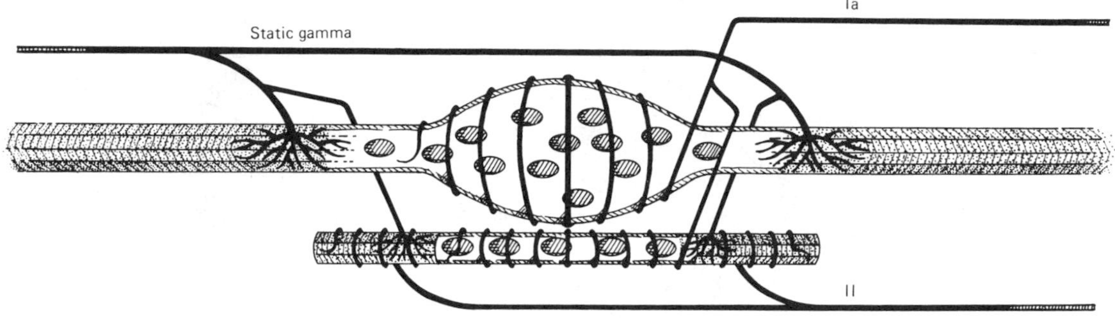

FIGURE VIII

Slack or "Unloaded" Muscle Spindle The passive shortening of the muscle spindle as a result of either extrafusal contraction or of positioning a muscle in shortened ranges. Because of the shortening, the tension on the spindle receptors decreases and consequently the spindle afferent excitation diminishes.

External Stretch Stretch of both the extrafusal and intrafusal fibers by an outside force, for example, quick stretch applied in the lengthened range of a muscle or a pattern of movement. The application of external stretch may help to initiate a muscle contraction, but this contraction cannot be sustained unless internal stretch or maintained gamma efferent activity is present.

Golgi Tendon Organs (GTO) Proprioceptors that are located primarily at musculotendinous junctions in series with the muscle fibers (Figure IX).

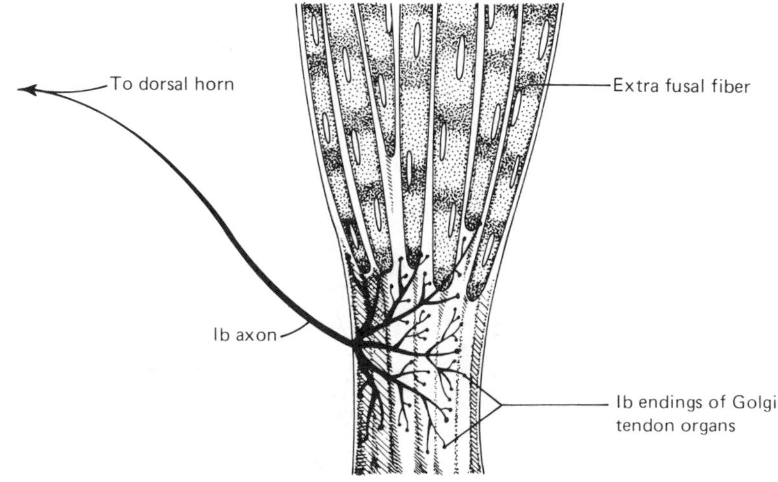

FIGURE IX

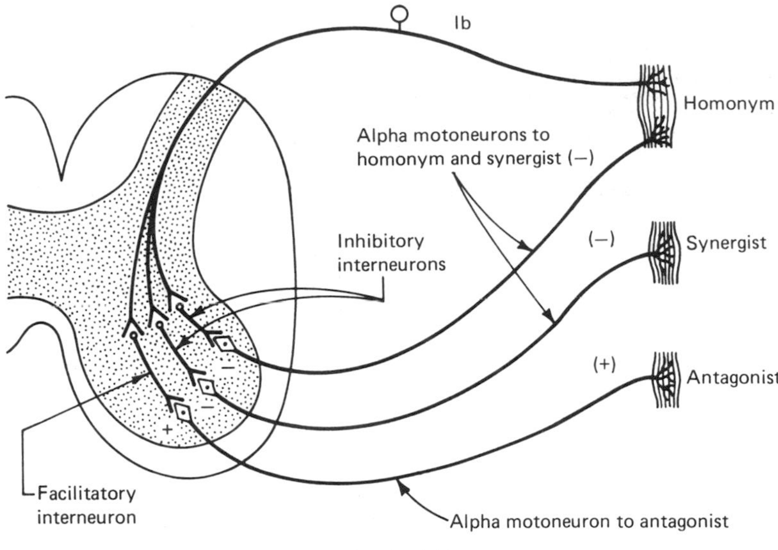

FIGURE X

These receptors are extremely sensitive to muscle tension, particularly when the tension is produced by an active muscle contraction. The response produced by GTO excitation is autogenetic inhibition to the homonym and synergists and reciprocal facilitation to antagonistic muscle groups (Figure X).

Ib Fiber The nerve fiber that forms the afferent nerve supply from the GTO. Unlike the muscle spindles, GTOs do not have efferent innervation.

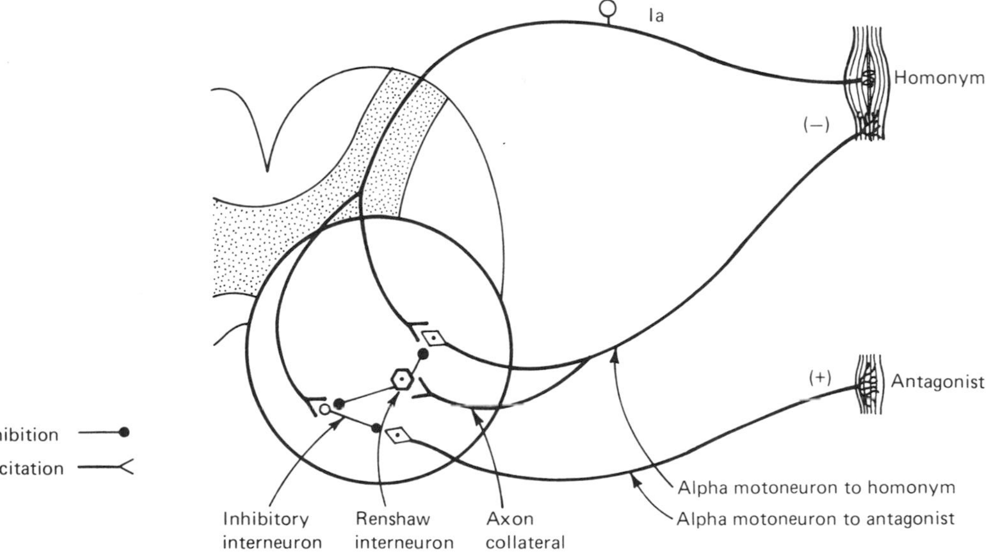

FIGURE XI

Renshaw Interneuron An interneuron that forms part of an inhibitory feedback circuit between the motoneurons to the homonym (usually tonic) and their cell bodies in the anterior horn of the spinal cord. Renshaw cells also exert an inhibitory influence on the inhibitory interneuron that forms part of the final common pathway to the antagonistic musculature—the result of this disinhibition may be equivalent to facilitation of the antagonistic muscle groups (usually phasic) (Figure XI). Renshaw cells can be affected by impulses from higher centers.

Coactivation The simultaneous activation of alpha and gamma motoneurons from higher centers for purposes of initiating or perpetuating muscle contractions.

Cocontraction Simultaneous muscle contractions on both sides of a joint.

Facilitation Lowering the thresholds at synapses of motoneuron pools. Facilitation is not synonymous with activation or the actual firing of motor units.

Adaptation A decline in the discharge frequency of a sensory receptor after the onset of stimulation. The mechanism of adaptation is not known and may differ for various sensory organs. Receptors such as Pacinian corpuscles are said to adapt rapidly, whereas others—such as muscle spindle receptors—adapt slowly.

Tracking The tendency of a part to move in the direction of the sensory stimulus provided by a manual contact.

PROPRIOCEPTIVE NEUROMUSCULAR FACILITATION (PNF)

Direct Approach The application of exercise techniques and elements to an affected area.

Indirect Approach The application of exercise techniques and elements to an uninvolved area to gain overflow excitation or relaxation effects to an affected part. An indirect approach is appropriately used when the patient's involved limbs are either immobilized, weak, or painful.

Procedure A comprehensive term that includes all components of a specific exercise, that is, the activity, the technique, and the sensory input.

Activity Any developmental posture and the movements occurring within that posture.

Technique Type of muscle contraction used in treatment—isometric, isotonic (concentric-eccentric), or a combination of these.

Element Types of sensory input used in treatment to facilitate or inhibit a response.

Mass Pattern The proximal, intermediate, and distal joints of the lower extremity are simultaneously flexed or extended.

Advanced Pattern The proximal and distal joints of the lower extremity are flexed or extended while the intermediate joint simultaneously performs the opposite movement.

Diagonal 1 Flexion Upper Extremity (D_1F UE) Scapula elevation, abduction, upward rotation; combining movements of flexion, adduction, and external rotation occurring at the shoulder; elbow may move in flexion or extension, or may remain extended throughout the movement pattern; wrist and fingers flex and deviate to the radial side and the thumb adducts.

Diagonal 1 Extension Upper Extremity (D_1E UE) Scapula depression, adduction, and downward rotation; combining movements of extension, abduction, and internal rotation occurring at the shoulder; elbow may move in flexion or extension, or may remain extended throughout the movement pattern; wrist and fingers extend and deviate to the ulnar side and the thumb abducts.

Diagonal 2 Flexion Upper Extremity (D_2F UE) Scapula elevation, adduction, and upward rotation; combining movements of flexion, abduction, and external rotation occurring at the shoulder; elbow may move into flexion or extension, or may remain extended throughout the movement pattern; wrist and fingers extend and deviate to the radial side and the thumb extends.

Diagonal 2 Extension Upper Extremity (D_2E UE) Scapula depression, abduction, and downward rotation; combining movements of extension, adduction, and internal rotation occurring at the shoulder; elbow may move in flexion or extension, or may remain extended throughout the movement pattern; wrist and fingers flex and deviate to the ulnar side and the thumb opposes the fingers.

Diagonal 1 Flexion Lower Extremity (D_1F LE) Pelvic protraction; combining movements of flexion, adduction, and external rotation occurring at the hip; knee may move in flexion or extension, or may remain extended throughout the movement pattern; ankles and toes dorsi flex and invert.

Diagonal 1 Extension Lower Extremity (D_1E LE) Pelvic retraction; combining movements of extension, abduction, and internal rotation occurring at the hip; knee may move into flexion or extension, or may remain extended throughout the movement pattern; ankle and toes plantar flex and evert.

Diagonal 2 Flexion Lower Extremity (D_2F LE) Pelvic elevation; combining movements of flexion, abduction, and internal rotation occurring at the hip; knee may move into flexion or extension, or may remain extended throughout the movement pattern; ankle and toes dorsi flex and evert.

Diagonal 2 Extension Lower Extremity (D_2E LE) Pelvic depression; combining movements of extension, adduction, and external rotation occurring at the hip; knee may move into flexion or extension, or may remain extended throughout the movement pattern; ankle and toes plantar flex and invert.

Bilateral Symmetrical Patterns (BS) The bilateral performance of one diagonal pattern (D_1 *or* D_2) by either both upper or both lower extremities. Movement of both extremities occurs simultaneously in the same direction—that is, both limbs flex or extend together.

Reciprocal Symmetrical Patterns or Bilateral Reciprocal (BR) The reciprocal performance of one diagonal pattern (D_1 *or* D_2) by either both upper or both lower extremities. Movement of both extremities occurs in different directions—that is, one limb flexes while the other extends in the same diagonal pattern.

Bilateral Asymmetrical Patterns (BA) The bilateral performance of the two diagonal patterns (D_1 *and* D_2) by either both upper or both lower extremities. Movement of both extremities occurs simultaneously in the same direction—that is, both limbs flex or extend together.

Reciprocal Asymmetrical or Crossed Diagonal Patterns (RA, CD) The reciprocal performance of the two diagonal patterns (D_1 *and* D_2) by either both upper or both lower extremities. Movement of both extremities occurs simultaneously in different directions—that is, one limb flexes in D_1 while the other extends in D_2.

Chop An upper trunk flexion pattern that combines bilateral asymmetrical extensor patterns of the upper extremities—for example, chopping to the right combines D_1 extension of the right upper extremity and D_2 extension of the left upper extremity. Chopping may be easier for a patient to perform than bilateral asymmetrical patterns because the body-on-body contact results in a closed kinematic chain.

Lift An upper trunk extension pattern that combines bilateral asymmetrical flexor patterns of the upper extremities—for example, lifting to the right combines D_2 flexion of the right upper extremity and D_1 flexion of the left upper extremity. Lifting may be easier for a patient to perform than bilateral asymmetrical patterns because the body-on-body contact results in a closed kinematic chain.

Lower Trunk Flexion (LTF) A lower trunk flexor pattern that combines bilateral asymmetrical flexor patterns of the lower extremities—for example, lower trunk flexion to the right combines D_2 flexion of the right lower extremity and D_1 flexion of the left lower extremity.

Lower Trunk Extension (LTE) A lower trunk extensor pattern that combines bilateral asymetrical extensor patterns of the lower extremities—for example, lower trunk extension to the right combines D_1 extension of the right lower extremity and D_2 extension of the left lower extremity. As with the upper trunk patterns, there is a closed kinematic chain in both lower trunk patterns resulting from the body-on-body contact of the two legs in approximation with each other.

Lower Trunk Rotation (LTR) A rotary pattern of movement of the lower trunk performed in hooklying that combines bilateral asymmetrical flexor patterns of the lower extremities from zero degrees to 90 degrees of the movement pattern and bilateral asymmetrical extensor patterns from 90 degrees to 180 degrees of the movement pattern.

ORTHOPEDIC

Contractile Tissue Tissues contributing to joint movement, including the muscle, its nerve, tendon, and bony insertion.

Noncontractile—Inert Tissues involved in maintaining joint stability, including capsule, ligament, meniscus, and the articular cartilage.

Osteokinematic Movement The bone motion occurring in a plane of movement, for example, shoulder flexion.

Arthrokinematic Movement The specific joint movements that occur during an osteokinematic movement. Depending on the joint and the degrees of freedom, a roll, glide, or spin may occur.

End Feel At the end of a normal passive movement the therapist moves the joint slightly beyond the end range and assesses the "feeling" of this movement. Each joint has a characteristic end feel that is physiologically normal for that movement and that depends on the anatomy of the joint. With abnormalities the end feel may vary.

Abbreviations of Terms

The following terms are listed in alphabetical order for your convenience.

AI alternating isometrics
ANS autonomic nervous system
AR agonistic reversals
ATNR asymmetrical tonic neck reflex
BA bilateral asymmetrical
BR bilateral reciprocal
BS bilateral symmetrical
B of S base of support
CD cross diagonal
C of G center of gravity
CNS central nervous system
CR contract-relax
CVA cerebral vascular accident

D_1E diagonal 1 extension
D_1F diagonal 1 flexion
D_2E diagonal 2 extension
D_2F diagonal 2 flexion
GTOs golgi tendon organs
HR hold-relax
HRAM hold relax active movement
LE lower extremity
LE—LI lengthened range of emphasis—initiation
LTE lower trunk extension
LTR lower trunk rotation
MC manual contacts
MMT manual muscle test
NT normal timing
RC repeated contractions
RI rhythmic initiation
ROM range of motion
RP resisted progression
RR rhythmical rotation
RS rhythmic stabilization
SCI spinal cord injury
SE—SI shortened range of emphasis—initiation
SHRC shortened held resisted contraction
SLR straight leg raise
SR slow reversal
SRH slow reversal hold
SRH↗↘RANGE slow reversal hold through increments or decrements of range
STLR symmetrical tonic labyrinthine reflex
STNR symmetrical tonic neck reflex
TE timing for emphasis
UE upper extremity
UTE upper trunk extension
UTR upper trunk rotation

chapter 1

The Treatment Planning Process

INTRODUCTION

Treatment planning is the orderly process of developing the most appropriate treatment for each patient. Each therapist possesses a unique body of knowledge achieved through formal and informal education and clinical experience. By systematically implementing the steps of the treatment planning process, the therapist provides the patient with the best care possible, even though the treatment procedures selected for a given patient may vary from therapist to therapist.

Although the design presented here is applicable to all treatment planning, the discussion will be directed primarily to therapeutic exercise. The main steps of the treatment planning process are illustrated in the flow chart in Figure 1–1.

Four major steps constitute the treatment planning process: evaluate, analyze data, develop treatment plan, and treat patient. Each step is a process in itself. Each has component parts that contribute to the overall effec-

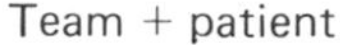

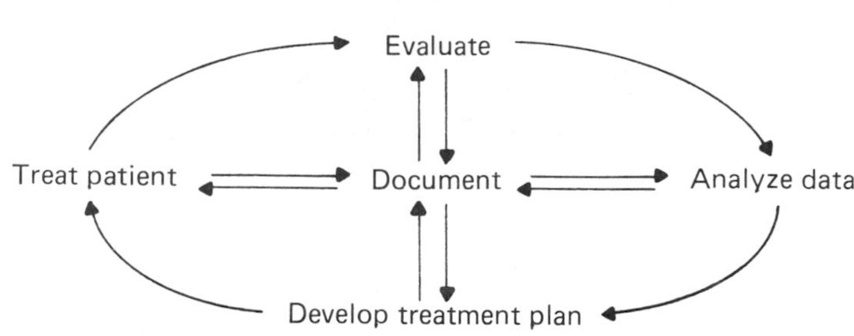

FIGURE 1–1
Treatment planning process.

tiveness of the treatment and that must be completed to successfully conclude the entire treatment planning process.

EVALUATION

The initial stage of evaluation consists of a gross assessment of all systems followed by definitive testing of areas of impairment. Definitive testing of the involved areas might include specific measurements of strength, range of motion, functional ability, sensation, and muscle tone. An evaluation should include assessment of the patient's knowledge of his disorder, mental awareness, emotional reactions, and *personal* goals. All pertinent areas must be thoroughly examined and initial values recorded. Knowledge of the patient's abilities is as important as knowledge of the disabilities.

ANALYZE DATA

Analyzing the data collected during the evaluation is the second major step. Compiling a list of the patient's assets and problems is a way of organizing the evaluation results into a meaningful form. The list is analyzed to discern which problems are primary, that is, to determine which problems influence or cause secondary signs. Problems that require immediate attention and that will respond most favorably to therapeutic exercise are identified. A left hemiplegic patient's problem list, for example, might include decreased sensation of the left side of the body, minimal voluntary control of the involved extremities, edema of the left hand, painful left shoulder, and inability to perform functional tasks such as dressing and transfers. In the therapist's judgment the lack of sensation and voluntary motor control may be the primary problems causing or contributing to the edema, pain, and inability to dress or transfer. Although the emphasis of therapeutic exercise treatment may be on increasing voluntary motor control and sensation, the presence of pain and edema in the upper extremity cannot be ignored when the exercise procedures are being selected. Treatment procedures in addition to exercise may become necessary to overcome the pain and edema of the left extremity. Thus, even though the primary problems may be the chief concern, the secondary problems can also receive immediate attention.

Examples of the patient's assets are good family support, rapid recovery of lost function, and a positive attitude. Once the assets are identified, the therapist can capitalize on them to motivate the patient. The asset list is used in establishing the ultimate functional capacity. The long-range goals for a hemiplegic patient who has a good prognosis, who is motivated, and has employment to which he can return may differ from those of a hemiplegic patient who has a poor prognosis, is depressed, and has no family support.

Establishing goals is the logical conclusion of the analysis of the data. Long-range goals help to delineate the functional abilities that the patient will be expected to perform at the conclusion of treatment. Short-range goals are concerned with the component skills needed to advance the patient from the present level of performance to the desired level.

The goals are sequenced to ensure a proper ordering of component skills. The therapist must therefore know all the factors that make up the hierarchy of motor ability. In order to transfer independently, for example, the patient must have sitting balance, which must be preceded by the ability to roll. In addition to sequencing the functional activities, the therapist must be cognizant of the components of motor control that affect the performance of these activities. Before the goal of rolling can be achieved, for example, tonic reflexes must be integrated, and tone must be balanced so that a reversal of antagonists can be accomplished.

Proper wording of goals is a vital element of good documentation and is critical for the success of the treatment planning process. Goals must describe observable, measurable, and precisely defined expected patient behavior. When expressed in this way, the patient and the team will know exactly what is expected and how perfomance will be measured. A long range goal such as "independent in ambulation" would have to be modified before a common understanding of the patient's ambulatory ability could be reached by the patient, therapist, and all team members. More precisely expressed, this goal might be: "The patient will independently ambulate with a small base quad cane and left-ankle foot orthosis on hard level surfaces for a distance of 300 feet in 3 minutes". Reassessment to determine progress and the effectiveness of an exercise program is possible only when all initial values are accurately recorded and the goals are expressed in terms of observable and measurable behaviors.

DEVELOP TREATMENT PLAN

The third major step of the treatment planning process is to develop the plan of treatment. First, an outline of the course of treatment is prepared. This overview includes such items as plans for interacting with other health personnel; setting of formal reevaluation times; establishing the frequency, duration, and length of treatment; and determining when equipment should be ordered. Next, the general treatment plans for the accomplishment of the short-range goals are developed. The general treatment plan indicates, when appropriate, the type of physical agents, assistive devices, equipment, and exercise that will be employed to reach the goals. Finally, specific treatment procedures are developed. The therapist should not focus on the specific procedures to the exclusion of the other aspects of treatment planning since this may result in a fractionated, uncoordinated rehabilitative process. For the left hemiplegic patient described earlier, the following treatment plan serves to illustrate the third step of the planning process, the development of the plan of treatment. The goals and plans presented are not meant to be comprehensive.

- **Long Range Goals:**

  1. The patient will be independent in self-care (dressing, feeding, and bathing)—performing the tasks in a reasonable period of time without assistance.
  2. The patient will independently ambulate with a standard cane and left-ankle foot orthosis. He will ambulate on all surfaces and stairs for reasonable distances in appropriate times without assistance.

- **Short Range Goals:**

  The patient will

  have a pain-free left shoulder.

  have an edema free left hand and forearm.

  be able to independently roll supine to prone without the use of bed rails.

  be able to maintain the sitting position.

- **Outline of Treatment**

  1. Conference tomorrow with the occupational therapist.
  2. Treat daily for 30 minutes gradually increasing to 1 hour.
  3. Reevaluate with intent to determine equipment needs in one month.
  4. Begin discharge plans.

- **General Treatment Plan**

  1. Apply ice for the painful shoulder.

2. Place elevated armrest on wheelchair for the edematous upper extremity.
3. Begin exercising with total body patterns and progress through the prone, supine, and upright sequences. (These will be described in subsequent chapters).
4. Instruct staff, family, and patient in proper transfer and ROM techniques.

■ **Specific Treatment Procedures**

1. A. Rolling
   T. Rhythmic initiation
   E. Manual contacts: shoulder and pelvis, verbal commands, resistance
2. A. Prone on elbows
   T. Rhythmic stabilization
   E. Manual contacts: shoulder, verbal commands, resistance, approximation

TREAT PATIENT

Implementing the plan by treating the patient is the fourth step of the treatment planning process. During treatment, the therapist continually evaluates the patient's responses. Some modifications of the specific treatment procedures may be indicated and implemented immediately. If, for instance, the patient stabilizes well in prone on elbows with manual contacts on the shoulder, the manual contacts may be moved to head and shoulder to increase the level of difficulty for the patient. Conversely, if the patient is unable to perform at the desired level, one or more of the units of the procedure—activity, technique, or element—can be altered. If, in the above example, the patient is unable to tolerate prone on elbows because of the painful shoulder, the activity could be altered to sitting with the forearms on a table. This position may be less stressful, especially for older patients who may have respiratory or low back problems. Finally, when the patient's ability is at the desired level, facilitation is withdrawn so as to increase the challenge and help to progress the patient.

Periodic formal reevaluations are necessary to determine the progress of the patient and the effectiveness of the treatment, as well as to provide the patient and the team with an accurate picture of the course of recovery. This brings us back to the first step in the treatment planning process, and the cycle is repeated.

The results of both the informal assessment of the patient's immediate response to treatment and the formal reevaluations are used to analyze the treatment planning process itself. The results of the evaluation are compared with the expected results and with the goals. If the observed results are as predicted, the treatment as outlined continues. New goals requiring a progression of the specific treatment procedures are then established. When the desired results are not the observed results, however, each step in the treatment planning process must be reviewed to determine the cause of the failure. Changes in the patient's general medical condition or misinterpretation of earlier evaluative data may be factors. Overestimating a patient's potential might result in the establishment of inappropriate goals, and thereby set into action an inappropriate plan. The initial aspects of treatment planning may be carried out properly but the patient may not respond to specific procedures as predicted. If this occurs, alternative plans and procedures must be chosen. Thus the cycle continues until the predicted results are achieved.

DOCUMENTATION

The hub of the circular treatment planning process is documentation. Documentation must be initiated at the start of the evaluation and must be maintained through each step. Communication, treatment planning, peer review, and research are a few of the processes that depend on adequate documentation of all the patient's responses. Charts and forms, accurately completed, allow the data to be recorded and compared quickly and easily and thus facilitate the treatment planning process.

SUMMARY

Treatment planning is a circular process that depends on proper documentation. The process has four principal steps—evaluation, analysis of data, development of treatment plans, and treatment of the patient. Each major step consists of several phases. The steps are outlined below.

Step 1: Evaluate the Patient

- **A.** Gross evaluation
- **B.** Definitive evaluation

Step 2: Analyze thc Data

- **A.** Problem and asset lists
    - **i.** Organize for interrelationships
    - **ii.** Estimate therapeutic exercise treatment potential
    - **iii.** Determine immediate needs
- **B.** Establish Goals

i. Determine the functional abilities—long-range goals

ii. Select the component skills—short-range goals

iii. Sequence the goals

Step 3: Develop Treatment Plans

A. Overview of plan

B. General treatment plan

C. Specific treatment procedures

Step 4: Treat the Patient

A. Assess response

B. Modify treatment procedures

Step 5: Reevaluate the Patient

A. Perform a definitive evaluation

B. Review treatment planning process

chapter 2

Normal Motor Development

INTRODUCTION

The developmental sequence is the physical manifestation of neural maturation. As each child progresses through the postural activities within the developmental sequence, normal motor control is acquired (1). At the same time, the child gradually acquires sensory-perceptual, cognitive, and personality skills. A discussion of all these aspects of development is beyond the scope of this text. Therefore, the sensory-perceptual and cognitive skills will be discussed only as they relate to the maturation of motor abilities. Since normal motor control is acquired during the developmental sequence, when motor control is adversely affected, a recapitulation of the sequence may be the most effective means of reestablishing control.

Recapitulation of the sequence in its entirety may not always be necessary during patient treatment. The basic assumption underlying the treatment approach presented in this text, however, is that for most types of dysfunction, the gradual rebuilding of control that occurs when a patient progresses through the activities of the developmental sequence and the stages of motor control will rehabilitate the patient to the maximal level of functioning (2).

The following aspects of motor development will be discussed in this chapter:

1. The cephalocaudal, proximal to distal direction of development
2. Autonomic homeostasis
3. From reflex dominance to reflex integration
4. The stages of motor control
5. Sequencing of postures and activities

Many normal variations occur during the development of motor control that can be attributed to both genetic and environmental influences. The information presented here should not be considered an all-inclusive discussion of normal development, but rather an overview of some major concepts derived from the study of normal development that can be related to this treatment approach. The parameters of normal development are summarized in Table 2-1.

TABLE 2–1
Normal Development
cephalocaudal proximal-distal

Age (months)	*ANS*	*Reflex Integration*	*Development of Tone*	*Develop of Motor Control*	*Progression of Postures*
0–3	sympathetic	spinal-tonic	flexion	mobility	supine
3–5	toward parasympathetic	righting	extension	stability tonic holding	pivot prone supine flexion
4–6				stability cocontraction	prone on elbows rolling
6–8		protective extension proprioceptive equilibrium	interaction of antagonists	controlled mobility skill	hands and knees sitting
8–10					modified plantigrade
10–12					standing
12–					walking
	homeostasis				

Parameters of Normal Development

CEPHALOCAUDAL; PROXIMAL-DISTAL

The development of motor control generally proceeds in a cephalocaudal and proximal to distal direction (3, 4). Motor abilities first occur in the face, head, and neck, and progress to the upper trunk, then to the lower trunk. Upper extremity control develops before control in the more caudal lower extremity. Motor control in the upper extremity begins proximally in the scapula and shoulder and progresses distally to the elbow and hand. In the lower extremity motor control progresses from the pelvis and hip to the knee and ankle. In contrast to motor control, tone and reflex development may procede in a caudal cephalic direction.

DEVELOPMENT OF AUTONOMIC HOMEOSTASIS

At birth, the infant appears to be dominated by the sympathetic division of the autonomic nervous system. When awake, the infant is frequently in constant motion and expends a large amount of energy in erratic, reflex-based movements that seem to lack purpose (3, 5). As the nervous system matures, the child is able to perform movements that are maintained, purposeful, and increasingly parasympathetic in nature. A progressive, although not always steady, increase in parasympathetic control continues until a level of homeostasis is reached later in development (6).

FROM REFLEX DOMINANCE TO REFLEX INTEGRATION

At birth, motor behavior is dominated by reflex activity, resulting in primitive stereotyped movement patterns such as the placing, stepping, grasp and tonic neck reflexes (3). Maturation progresses and a greater variety of movements become available to the child as the primitive reflex movements become integrated. Individualized movement occurs when cortical control is gained (3).

In mature motor behavior, the integrated reflexes provide the underlying postural tone necessary for normal movement (7). Righting reactions that dominate behavior at about four months of age, for example, will, as an integrated reaction, assist an adult in maintaining the upright posture. The integration of reflexes follows in an orderly, fairly predictable manner. The domination of spinal and tonic reflexes is followed by righting reactions, which are then superseded by equilibrium and proprioceptive reactions. Timetables for the dominance and integration of these reflexes have been established by many researchers (8–10). Although these reflexes may dominate behavior in normal development, they are never obligatory. An obligatory response is a maintained stereotyped reflex response to a stimulus that occurs every time the stimulus is provided and is indicative of abnormality (11). The dominance of a reflex response is normal at certain stages of development and is characterized by an increase in tone or a reflex movement, which can always be overcome by other random movements.

THE STAGES OF MOTOR CONTROL

The four major stages of motor control are mobility, stability, controlled mobility, and skill (1). Some of these stages are divided into two levels, with transitional levels interposed.

1. Mobility. The random mobility of infancy usually occurs during the first three months. Movement during this stage seems to lack purpose and is erratic and reflex based (3). The mobility stage when describing adult behavior refers to the availability of ROM to assume a posture and the presence of sufficient motor unit activity to initiate a movement. Deficits in mobility can be due to tissue tightness, hypotonia, or imbalances of tone.

2. Stability. Stability is divided into two levels (1, 12)—tonic holding and cocontraction. Tonic holding is the ability of tonic postural muscles to maintain a contraction in their shortened range against gravitational or manual resistance. Tonic stability is developed in the deep postural extensors when the pivot prone posture is maintained against the resistance of gravity. The stretch sensitivity of these muscles is increased as the static gamma motor neurons are facilitated. The pivot prone or prone extension posture is enhanced by the optical and vestibular righting reactions (13). Developmentally, tonic holding of the postural tonic muscles is most evident when the child maintains the pivot prone posture (Figure 2–1). Stretch sensitivity

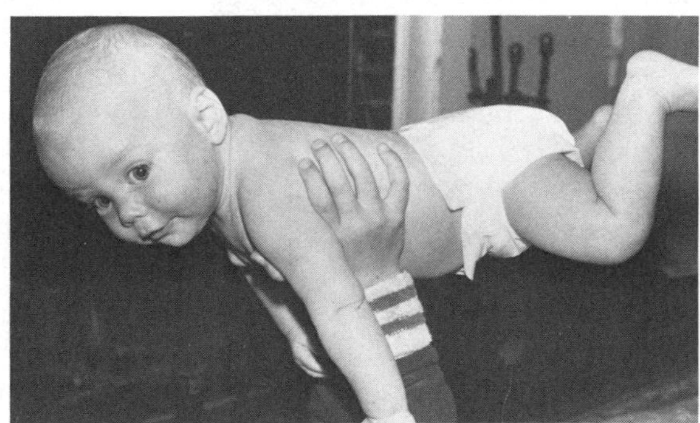

FIGURE 2–1
Pivot prone—prone extension.

of all postural muscles—for example, the abdominals in supine flexion and the soleus as the child stands in plantarflexion—is established as the child progresses through the various postures of the developmental sequence (1).

Tonic holding establishes stretch sensitivity or sets the gamma bias and is preliminary to the second level of stability, cocontraction. Cocontraction is the simultaneous static contraction of antagonistic muscles around a joint to provide stability in a weight-bearing posture or to maintain a midline position. Cocontraction can occur when a stretch-sensitive tonic muscle is positioned in a more lengthened range and the resistance of weight bearing or gravity is superimposed on the contracting muscle (1). The function of the neurophysiological mechanisms involved in cocontraction is not fully understood (14). One explanation states that the maintained lengthened position of the tonic muscle activates the secondary endings of that muscle, that the secondary endings appear to facilitate the antagonistic phasic muscle; the facilitation of the agonist by the Ia endings of its muscle spindle leads to the combined facilitation of muscles on both sides of the joint, that is, cocontraction (1).

Both levels of stability—tonic holding and cocontraction—tend to progress in a cephalocaudal direction. Tonic holding is most commonly observed first in the extensors of the head and neck as the head is maintained in the shortened range of extension in the prone position. The extensors of the upper trunk and proximal upper extremities, then of the lower trunk and lower extremities are also maintained in a shortened position during pivot prone. Once the stretch sensitivity in these muscles is developed, the cocontraction position is attempted. For the head and neck, cocontraction occurs when the head is maintained in the midline, rather than in the shortened position. Cocontraction in the upper trunk and proximal areas of the upper extremity is promoted in prone on elbows, and in the lower trunk and proximal areas of the lower extremity in the quadruped position. The stretch sensitivity of the tonic postural muscles must have been developed in pivot prone to the extent that these midline or weight-bearing positions can be maintained. The child frequently alternates between the positions of tonic holding and cocontraction, especially as higher postures are attempted. Holding the muscles in the shortened range is often repeated seemingly to further enhance stretch sensitivity, since more weight bearing and stretch add stress to the muscle (15).

3. Controlled Mobility. In the third stage of motor control, movement is added to the static posture. For the head, neck, and trunk, controlled mobility refers to the ability to rotate around the long axis. This rotation occurs initially during the rolling and prone on elbows activities. Controlled mobility occurs in the extremities when, in weight-bearing postures, the distal weight-bearing segment is fixed while the proximal component moves over the distal part (1). Rocking in weight-bearing postures, or moving the center of gravity (C of G) over the base of support (B of S), occurs first through small ranges, then through gradually increasing ranges. This expansion of movement is termed rocking through increments of range. Rocking improves the child's ability to independently assume the posture and also develops equilibrium and proprioceptive reactions in the posture. The development of these higher level reactions is necessary before the posture or activity can become functional. During rocking the proximal musculature develops "dynamic stability," which is a prerequisite for the final stage of motor control, skill (1).

Static-dynamic activity is the intermediate stage between controlled mobility and skill. In a weight-bearing activity one of the previously supporting limbs is lifted; the subsequent reduction in the B of S causes the C of G to shift and thus creates a greater demand for stability and balance reactions in the supporting limb(s) (1). Developmentally, the stronger limb generally assumes the static supporting role first because of the increased control needed to support the greater amount of body weight borne through that limb (12).

4. Skill. Skill is the highest level of motor control and includes two functions: the manipulation and exploration of the environment (1). In skilled activities the distal component, the hand or foot, is mobile, while the proximal musculature provides the dynamic stability to guide the limb. The proximal musculature, while providing stability, constantly changes length to allow the limb to move in space. This proximal control, termed dynamic stability, developed during the previous stages of stability-controlled mobility and static-dynamic activities in weight-bearing postures. Dynamic stability control provides the foundation from which distal to proximal timing occurs. Both are integral parts of skilled movements, such as reaching for objects or ambulation.

Manipulating the environment is the major skilled function of the upper extremities. Included in manipulative functions are activities of daily living, as well as other higher level functions. Exploring the environment by means of locomotion is the major skilled function of the lower extremities; however, both the upper and lower extremities participate in lower level exploration such as crawling.

Skill activities require the trunk to have the normal postural reflex mechanisms (11) and the balance reactions to make the necessary small adjustments in tone as the limbs move in space. Although skill is usually discussed in relationship to limb movement, it requires an advanced level of control in the head and neck, trunk, and proximal segments.

SEQUENCING OF POSTURES AND ACTIVITIES

The postures of the developmental sequence are grouped into prone and upright progressions. An overlapping of the stages of control and developmental postures will occur during the acquisition of normal motor skills. Specific activities or entire postural sequences may be omitted by some children (12).

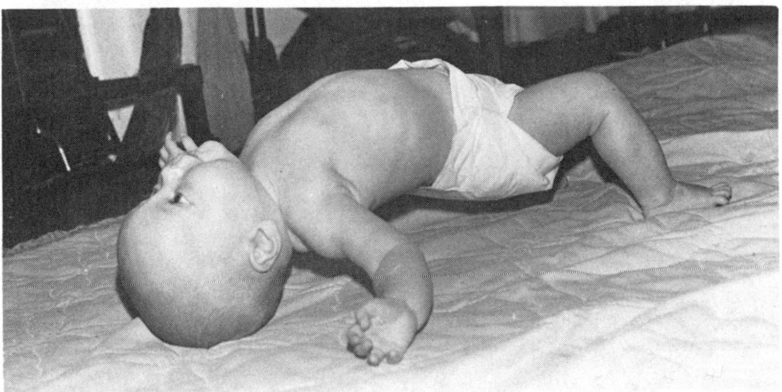

FIGURE 2–2
Supine, total body bridging (modified pivot prone).

During the first three months, an infant is generally in the stage of random mobility. Movements are phasic, reflex based, and uncontrolled, and seem to lack purpose. In prone, neck rotation occurs due to the influence of the primitive neck righting reflex. While awake, many children seem to be most comfortable in **supine**.

During the **pivot prone** activity, tone develops in the postural extensors, as already mentioned (see Figure 2–1). The ability to extend the trunk in prone is facilitated by the optical, vestibular, and body on head righting reactions and indicates an integration of the symmetrical tonic reflexes. Extensor tone may also develop in a supine, total-body bridging position (Figure 2–2).

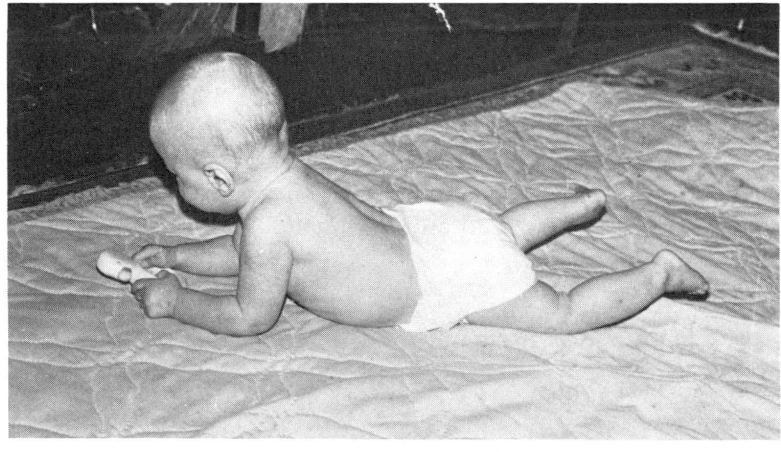

FIGURE 2–3
Prone on elbows.

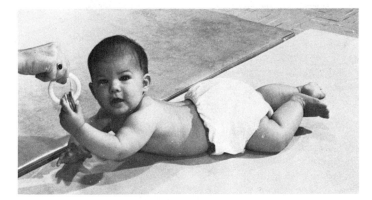

FIGURE 2–4
Prone on elbows—static-dynamic reaching.

Prone on elbows follows pivot prone. The cocontraction level of stability develops in the upper trunk and proximal upper extremities (Figure 2–3). The prone-on-hands posture is a progression of prone on elbows and requires control of elbow extension. In preparation for the increased control needed and the additional body weight supported by the upper extremities, the child may increase the tonic-holding ability of the postural muscles by returning to the pivot prone posture with the elbows extended. In the prone-on-elbows or prone-on-hands posture, the child begins to reach for objects and also to crawl (Figures 2–4 and 2–5).

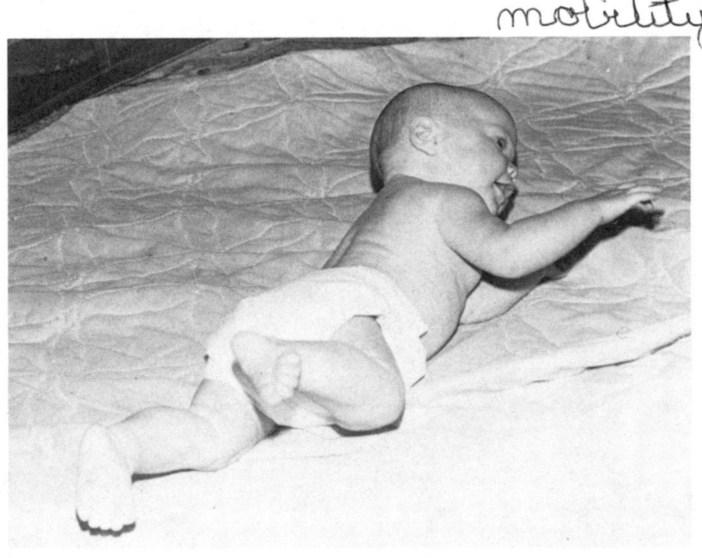

FIGURE 2–5
Crawling.

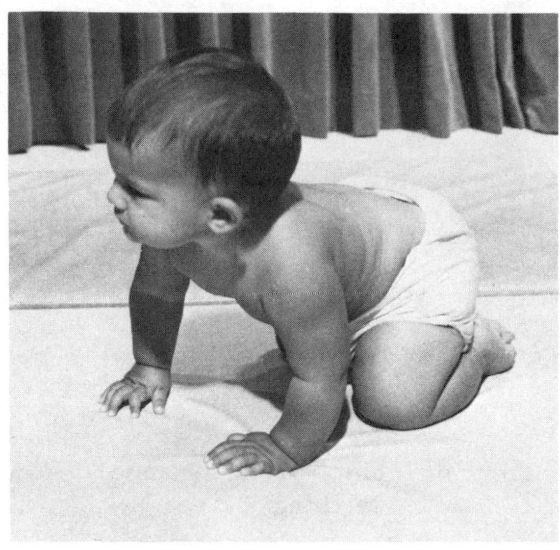

FIGURE 2–6
Quadruped.

Hands and knees or **quadruped** follows prone on hands as control progresses cephalocaudally (Figure 2–6). As previously mentioned, the postural muscles that have been developing stretch sensitivity in their shortened ranges are now able to actively maintain a prolonged stretch position, which facilitates cocontraction around the lower trunk and hips. The weight bearing on the lower extremities is extremely important for the development of the depth of the acetabulum and the growth of the long bones (15), as well as for stimulation of the deep rotators around the hip, which further promotes stability in the posture. In quadruped, due to the elevation of the C of G the amount of weight bearing on all the joints of the upper extremities increases in comparison with prone on hands.

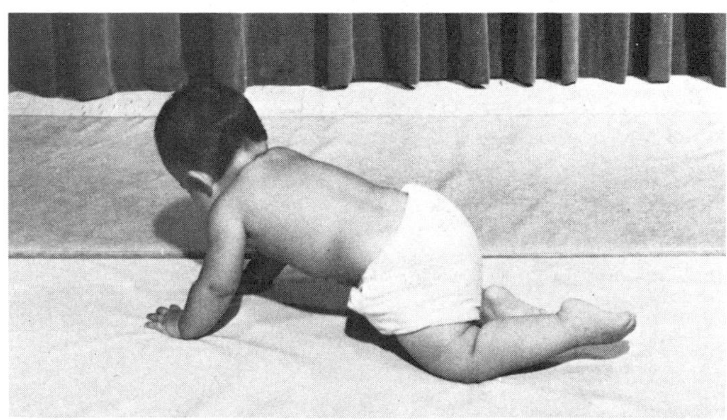

FIGURE 2–7
Creeping.

During these prone weight-bearing postures the child progresses through various stages of motor control: stability is defined as maintaining the posture; controlled mobility is rocking or weight shifting and the independent assumption of the posture; reaching for objects, which is considered the static-dynamic level, occurs when the dynamic limb reaches and the static limb(s) support the posture; and skill is locomotion in any of these activities. Various combinations of movement may be used for either crawling or creeping (Figure 2–7). The most advanced combination is a contralateral pattern requiring reciprocation of the extremities and counterrotation of the trunk.

The child begins to actively interact with the environment by reaching for objects and by exploring the environment during static-dynamic and skill levels of control. The environmental interaction is important for both perceptual and cognitive development (16).

As the child progresses through the prone sequence, parallel activities take place in the upright sequence. The upright postures include supine flexion, rolling, and sitting. **Supine flexion** is similar to pivot prone in that the child is able to control flexion movements in the supine position; this flexion indicates a reduction in the dominance of the symmetrical tonic reflexes. The child uses this posture for a period of time to perform midline upper extremity activities and also to explore its own body, an important aspect of perceptual development (17).

Developmentally, **rolling** first occurs prone to supine through the influence of tonic reflexes and may be accidental (3). The exact sequence of movements may vary. In a prone-on-hands position, head rotation may result in flexion of one extremity and extension of the other. Consequently, the child may fall and roll from prone on hands to supine. Rolling from supine to prone, however, is usually facilitated by righting reactions. The STLR and ATNR must be integrated before the trunk and leading upper extremity can flex across the midline (18). Rotational control of the trunk first occurs during development as the head turns and the body follows to complete the movement. When trunk rotation is produced by head rotation, the result is "log" rolling or rolling of the trunk as a complete unit (Figure 2–8).

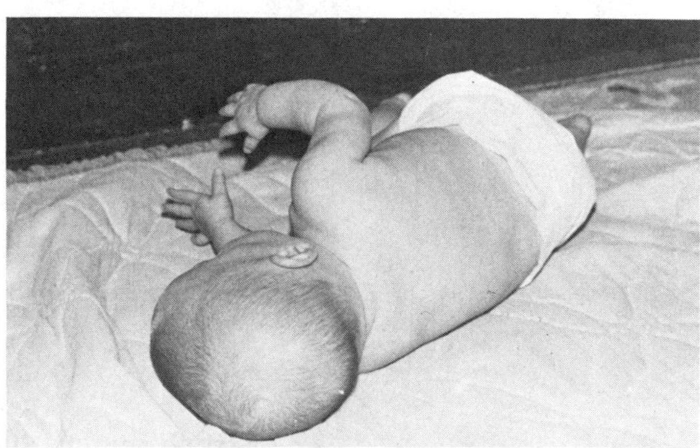

FIGURE 2–8
Log rolling.

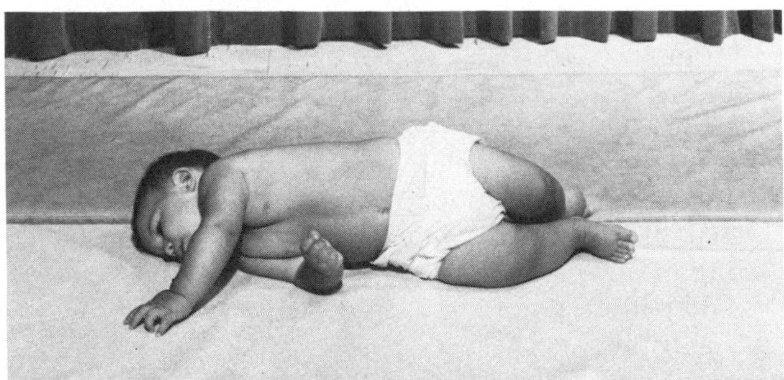

FIGURE 2–9
Segmental rolling.

Segmental rotation develops with the body-on-body reaction (Figure 2–9). When righting reactions have been integrated, head rotation and rolling may not be interdependent—that is, the head may rotate but the body may not follow. At this later stage, independent segmental upper and lower trunk movements occur as rolling progresses from a reflex- or reaction-dominant activity to a purposeful activity. A mature rolling pattern incorporates interaction of the flexor, extensor, and rotational muscles, which precedes control in sitting and locomotion in quadruped.

Sitting follows rolling in the sequence of upright postures. Control in sitting usually occurs at the same time as control in quadruped. Sitting is first assumed and maintained with external assistance (Figure 2–10); later the child can maintain sitting independently but uses both upper and lower

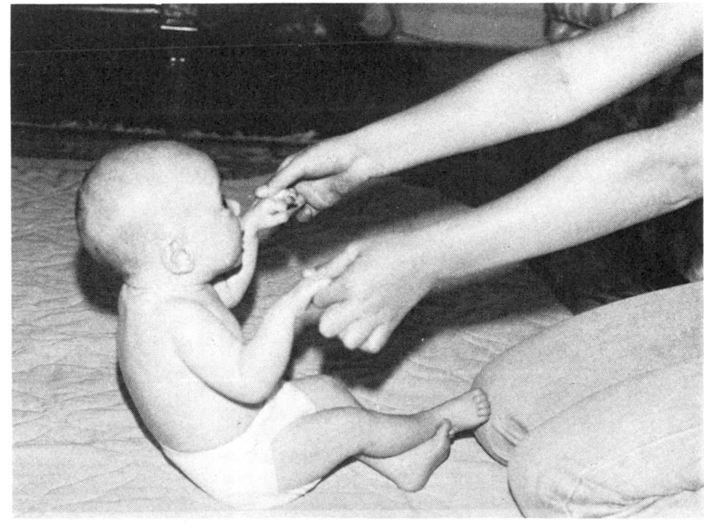

FIGURE 2–10
Assumption of sitting with assistance.

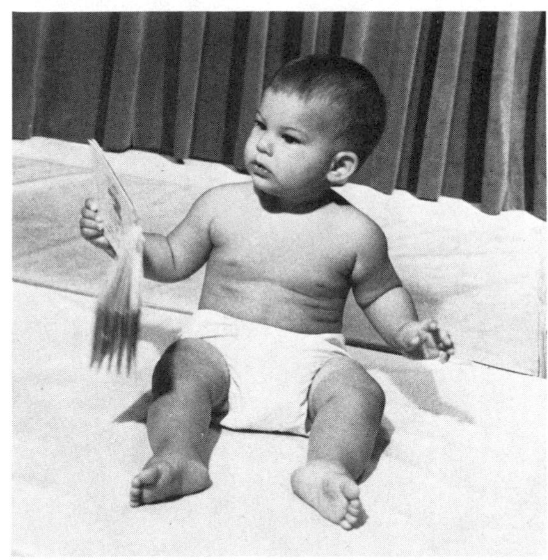

FIGURE 2–11
Sitting—manipulation of objects.

extremities to increase the B of S. As trunk control increases, especially the stability of the lower trunk, the hands are freed from their supporting role and can begin to manipulate objects (Figure 2–11). The activity is then considered to be at the skill level. Trunk control needed for this independent sitting is initially gained both during the sequence of prone postures and during rolling activities. Prior to the freeing of both hands for skilled activities, the child will manipulate objects with one hand while using the other upper extremity for support in a static-dynamic fashion. Such manipulation of objects is initially performed with a primitive hand grasp and progresses to fine dexterity over a period of years (19).

Full or **modified plantigrade** follows the quadruped and sitting postures. Many children use the plantigrade posture for locomotion (Figure 2–12), whereas others use modified plantigrade as the initial supported

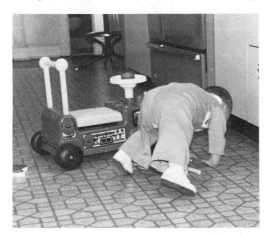

FIGURE 2–12
Full plantigrade.

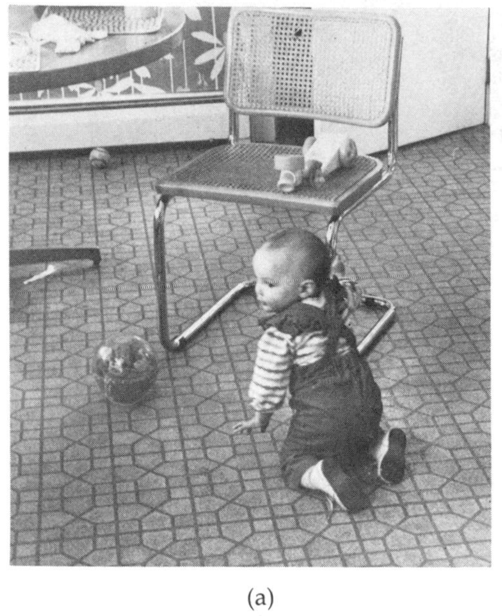

(a)

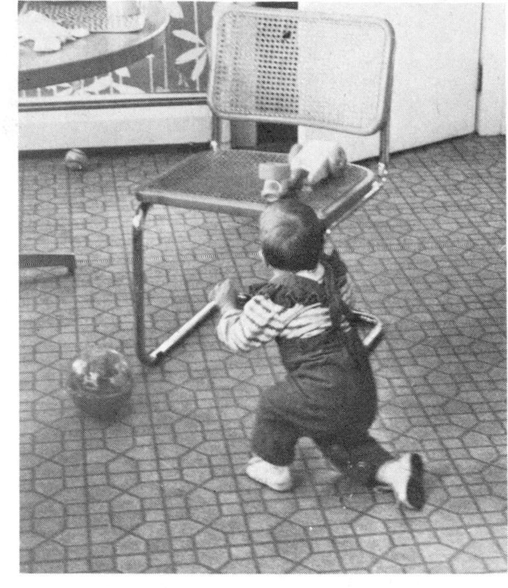

(b)

(c)

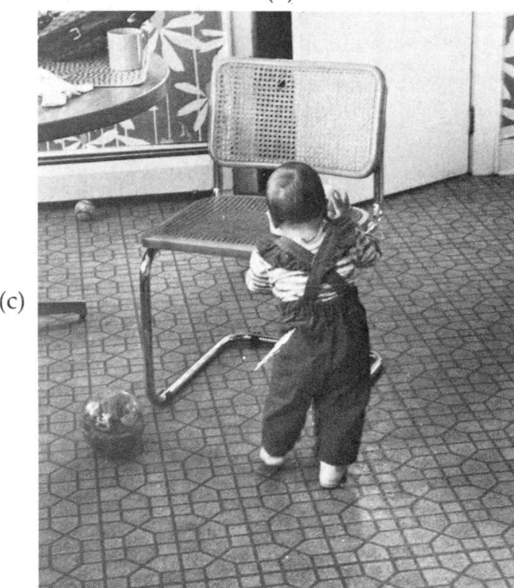

FIGURE 2–13
Assumption of standing.

standing position. Both may be considered intermediate postures between sitting or quadruped and standing (Figure 2–13). During both types of plantigrade activities, weight bearing occurs for the first time through the knee and ankle, and requires cocontraction around those joints. The child commonly stands with the ankles in plantarflexion, a mechanism that may be used to increase the stretch sensitivity in the tonic soleus muscle. As in other activities, development proceeds according to the stages of motor control: stability, which is maintaining the posture; controlled mobility, which is weight shifting or trunk rotation; static dynamic activities, which involve unilateral reaching; and skill, which is locomotion.

As the child develops higher levels of control in **supported standing,** attempts are also made to **stand** unsupported. This combination of activities is an example of the overlapping of postures and levels of motor control. In the less stressful activity of supported standing, the child may be at the static-dynamic level of motor control, while in standing unsupported it may be at the level of stability (Figure 2–13). Walking unsupported begins tenuously after attempts have been made at weight shifting in standing. The child may fall frequently until equilibrium and proprioceptive reactions develop in this high-level posture. The B of S is increased by abduction and external rotation of the legs, and the arms are postured in a retrated and abducted position (Figure 2-14). As control is gained, the B of S narrows, a heel-toe gait is achieved and the arms are held in a more relaxed position, eventually progressing to the mature contralateral reciprocating pattern that requires trunk counterrotation.

The perfection of these basic motor skills proceeds through early childhood, and additional landmarks in motor behavior may include activities such as running, skipping, and jumping. Because these more advanced activities are not routinely part of a therapeutic exercise program, they will not be further described.

The factors affecting progression of the normal motor control are all interdependent. Five basic factors were briefly described in this chapter, but others such as the development of sensory awareness, the ability to maintain contact with the environment, and perceptual and cognitive development are all interrelated and combine to affect the child's growth. Indepth

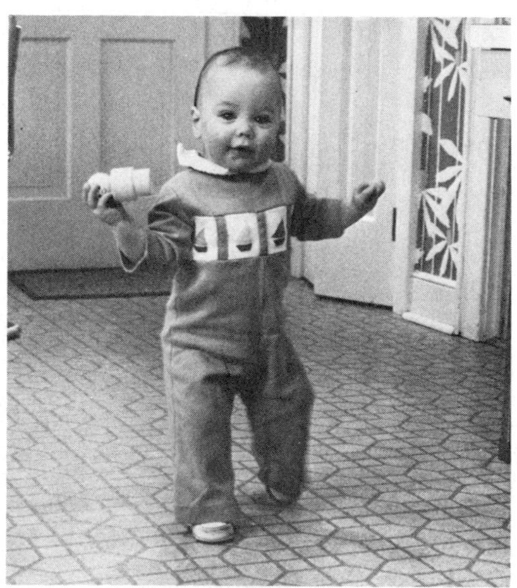

FIGURE 2–14
Walking.

analysis of these factors is beyond the scope of this text. The analysis of normal development is presented in this chapter to provide the reader with a framework for recapitulation of the developmental sequence in treatment when abnormalities of motor control exist. In the subsequent chapters the principles discussed in this chapter will be applied to patient treatment.

REFERENCES

1. Stockmeyer SA: An interpretation of the approach to the treatment of neuromuscular dysfunction. Amer J Phys Med 46:900–956, 1966
2. Voss DE: Proprioceptive neuromuscular facilitation. Amer J Phys Med 46:838–898, 1966
3. McGraw MB: The Neuromuscular Maturation of the Human Infant. New York, Columbia University Press, 1943. Reprinted edition, New York, Hafner Publishing Co., 1963
4. Gesell A, Amatruda CS: The Embryology of Behavior. New York, Harper and Brothers, 1945
5. Hooker, D: Fetal Behavior: The Inter-Relationship of Mind and Body, Baltimore, Williams & Wilkins Co, 1939
6. Stockmeyer SA: Analysis of procedures to improve Motor Control. Unpublished notes from Boston University PT 710, 1979
7. Sherrington C: The Integrative Action of the Nervous System. New Haven, Yale University Press, 1923
8. Hoskins T, Squires J: Development assessment: A test for gross motor and reflex development. Phys Ther 53:117–126, 1973
9. Willson MA: Use of a developmental inventory as a chart of progress. Phys Ther 49:19–32, 1969
10. Bayley N: The California Infant Scale of Motor Development. Berkeley, University of California Press, 1936
11. Bobath B, Bobath K: Cerebral palsy. In Pearson PH, Williams CE (eds): Physical Therapy Services in the Developmental Disabilities. Springfield, IL, Charles C Thomas, 1976
12. Horowitz L: Personal communication September 1978
13. Peiper A: Cerebral Function in Infancy and Childhood. New York, Consultants Bureau, 1963
14. Urbscheit N: Reflexes evoked by group 11 afferent fibers from muscle spindles. Phys Ther 59: 1083–1087, 1979
15. Wolff J: Liber die innere architektur des knochens. Virehows Arch Path Anat 50:389, 1870
16. Stockmeyer SA: A sensorimotor approach to treatment. In Pearson PH, Williams CE(eds): Physical Therapy Services in the Developmental Disabilities. Springfield, IL, Charles C Thomas, 1976

17. Gesell A: The First Five Years of Life, Part 1. New York, Harper and Brothers, 1940

18. Gilfoyle E, Grady A: A developmental theory of somatosensory perception. In Henderson A, Coryell J(eds): The Body Senses and Perceptual Deficit. Proceedings of the Occupational Therapy Symposium on Somatosensory Aspects of Perceptual Deficit. Boston University, Boston, 1972

19. Twitchell TE: Reflex mechanism and the development of prehension. In Connally KH(ed): Mechanisms of Motor Skill Development. New York, Academic Press, 1970

PART I

UNITS OF A PROCEDURE

chapter 3

Activities

FACTORS INFLUENCING THE CHOICE AND PROGRESSION

Activities refer to the postures of the developmental sequence and the movements that occur in those postures. Included in the procedural unit are the activities of trunk and of bilateral and unilateral extremity patterns. The parameters that influence the performance of activities can be divided into three major categories: (1) biomechanical, (2) tonal, and (3) neurophysiological.

■ Biomechanical

An understanding of biomechanical principles is an integral part of the therapist's knowledge of therapeutic exercise, and these fundamental principles should always be incorporated into the planning of a treatment program. They include:

- The size of the base of support (B of S).
- The distance between the center of gravity (C of G) and the supporting surface.

- The number of joints involved in either weight bearing or in a movement pattern.
- The length of the lever arm.

Tonal

Tonal effects refer to the changes in muscle tone caused by both the low-level reflexes and the higher level, more functional reactions. In a normal individual these reflexes and reactions provide the foundation for normal postural tone (1).

Spinal Reflexes. Many reflexes, including crossed extension and positive supporting reactions, are integrated at the spinal level (2). Inter- and intra-segmental connections existing at the spinal level affect normal movement patterns.

Tonic Reflex Influence. Tonic reflexes have been shown to affect tone in normal subjects (3, 4). When muscular weakness exists the effects of the tonic reflexes may be more pronounced. The motor behavior of many patients who have CNS dysfunction is dominated by tonic reflex. The goal of treatment in such cases is to suppress the influence of these reflexes, or to integrate the reflexes by facilitating higher level reactions and more normal movement patterns. Often, however, the changes in tone caused by the tonic reactions may be used advantageously to initiate or reinforce a desired movement (5, 6). Tonic influences must be used cautiously to ensure that the patient is not limited to these movement patterns.

Righting Reactions. Righting reactions may dominate motor behavior and can be just as detrimental to normal movement as dominant tonic reflexes. Obligatory righting reactions are not a common occurrence and treatment goals may include the stimulation of these reactions (7).

Righting reactions as integrated responses assist in the maintenance of upright postures and the development of body position awareness in relationship to the environment (1).

Proprioceptive, Equilibrium, and Protective Reactions. Proprioceptive and equilibrium reactions are responses to small changes in body position and are necessary to maintain the C of G within the B of S (8). Proprioceptive reactions are those postural responses caused by muscle spindle stretch, muscle tension, or changes in joint compression. Equilibrium reactions are responses to changes in the vestibular mechanism. When the C of G is disturbed out of the B of S, protective extension reactions provide a change in the B of S to protect the body from falling or to retard the fall. Only when these three reactions are developed, is a posture considered functional.

Neurophysiological

Motor behavior is controlled by the CNS. During treatment the therapist can influence motor control by manipulating external input and feedback to the CNS. Although many types of stimuli are important, the therapist should pay particular attention to the following factors when designing an activity for a patient.

Resistance. Resistance to an activity may be provided manually or mechanically, or by body weight or gravity. Resistance to a muscle contraction augments proprioceptive feedback (9) from the muscle spindles and gamma efferent activity. If the muscle cannot overcome the resistance of gravity, then a gravity-assisted or gravity-eliminated position is selected. Manual resistance, which can be more finely adjusted to variations of muscular responses than either gravitational or mechanical resistance, can then be used to facilitate the contraction. When the strength of the muscle has increased, a combination of gravitational and manual or mechanical resistive forces can be used. (See Chapter 5.)

The Range in Which Muscles Function. The range in which a muscle functions—shortened, mid-, or lengthened range—depends on whether the muscle is primarily tonic or phasic in composition. During normal activity a tonic or postural muscle functions mainly in the mid- to shortened range. Emphasis during treatment should therefore be placed on exercising these muscles in their most functional range. The stretch sensitivity of a weakened tonic muscle is facilitated in the shortened range by a resisted isometric contraction (10–12). Caution must be taken when positioning or applying resistance in the lengthened range as the inhibitory influences of the secondary afferent endings may increase (13). If the spindle stretch sensitivity of the tonic muscle is not sufficient, these inhibitory influences may predominate over the Ia afferent facilitation. Although the literature contains differences of opinion concerning the secondary afferent influences on muscles that are primarily tonic in composition (14), empirical evidence indicates that a prolonged stretch or positioning in the lengthened range reduces the ability of a tonic muscle to contract. During the initial aspects of the treatment, it appears that a weakened tonic muscle should be facilitated in the mid to shortened range to reduce possible inhibitory influences (13, 15).

In general, muscles that are primarily phasic in composition function in the lengthened to mid ranges. The combined spindle afferent influences on these muscles are mainly facilitatory. Unlike the tonic muscles, which appear to be easily inhibited when placed on a prolonged stretch, treatment of phasic muscles in lengthened ranges does not necessarily result in inhibition (15).

Approximation and Traction Forces. The application of joint approximation or compression facilitates isometric activity of the muscles around a joint and thus enhances stability (13, 16, 17). Joint compression is inherent in all weight-bearing postures and can be further enhanced by manual approximation. Traction may be used to increase isotonic movements, especially of flexor musculature (17). The muscular response to traction or approximation can vary and indications for use in treatment depend on musculoskeletal conditions (see Chapter 5).

Body Contact with Supporting Surfaces. Cutaneous stimulation is one of many stimuli that can alter muscular responses. Both the tactile and pressure stimulation that occurs when areas are in contact with a surface may influence motor activity (18–19).

Type of Muscular Contraction. There are three types of contractions—concentric, eccentric, and isometric—and all can be incorporated into activities. A description of how the different types of muscular contractions can be used in treatment appears in Chapter 4.

Movement Combinations. The extremity movements can be performed in three ways as follows: with the intermediate joint maintained straight, with the intermediate joint flexing, or with the intermediate joint extending. A mass pattern in the lower extremity occurs when all three joints—the hip, knee, and ankle—flex or extend (9, 20). An advanced combination is achieved by simultaneous movement of hip flexion with knee extension or hip extension with knee flexion (17). During the advanced combinations, the two joint muscles shorten over both joints at the same time.

In the upper extremity and trunk the combinations of movement are not as easily defined. The two joint muscles of the upper extremity, the biceps and triceps brachii, shorten over both joints when the shoulder and elbow flex simultaneously or extend respectively. Because of the complex functioning of the upper extremity and the many combinations of movement that are needed for normal activity, mass or advanced patterns will not be analyzed here.

In the lower extremity mass patterns are used to:

- **Initiate movement when generalized or isolated weakness exists.** These patterns may maximize intersegmental overflow and thus enhance muscular contraction. Resistance to mass flexion has been shown to increase the activity of both proximal and distal muscles (21).
- **Balance tone.** For patients having a dominance of mass extensor tone, mass flexor activity may balance tone prior to progressing to a more functional advanced combination.

Advanced combinations are usually the goal of treatment and are the functional combinations needed for higher level activities, especially ambulation.

Although some of the factors described in this section may under certain conditions be more influential than others, all three parameters—biomechanical, tonal, and neurophysiological—affect treatment procedures.

The importance of these parameters varies with the cognitive and motor abilities and deficits of the patient.

Activities are evaluated and chosen so that during the initial treatment sessions as many factors as possible support or enhance the desired posture or movement. When the patient is ready to progress, the parameters can be altered to make the activity more difficult. To initiate hip flexion, for example, the therapist may select the sidelying posture as the starting position because the B of S is large, the C of G low, and the number of joints involved in the activity can be limited. Attention can then be directed to the desired movement and not to the maintenance of the posture. The influence of the asymmetrical tonic labyrinthine reflex (ATLR) will be to facilitate hip flexion (Figure 3–1). Gravitational resistance is eliminated or assists the movement so that fine control can be gained with graded manual resistance. In sidelying, the hip flexors can be exercised in any part of the range—shortened, mid, or lengthened [Figure 3–2(a)]. Mass flexion can be used to help initiate the flexor activity, to strengthen a weakened flexor pattern, or to balance tone if mass extension is present [Figure 3–2(b)]. All three types of muscular contractions can be incorporated during treatment depending on the responses and needs of the patient. The activity would be more difficult in the supine posture, where the biomechanical factors of the B of S, C of G, and number of joints involved are similar but the gravitational and reflex effects are altered. In supine, the hip flexors must contract against the tonal influence of the symmetrical tonic labyrinthine reflex (STLR), and gravity resists the movement. The use of lower trunk or bilateral patterns will increase the number of joints involved and thus could possibly increase the difficulty of the movement (Figure 3–3). At the same time, however, the desired hip flexor activity may be enhanced by overflow from the trunk or contralateral limb. Advanced combinations of movement are a progression from a mass pattern.

Varying the posture, movement combinations, and ranges and types of contractions improves motor control and allows the patient to perform the greatest possible variety of movement combinations.

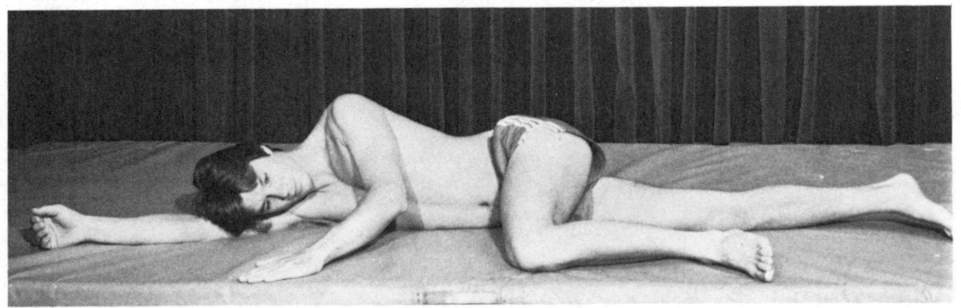

A. Sidelying.

FIGURE 3–1

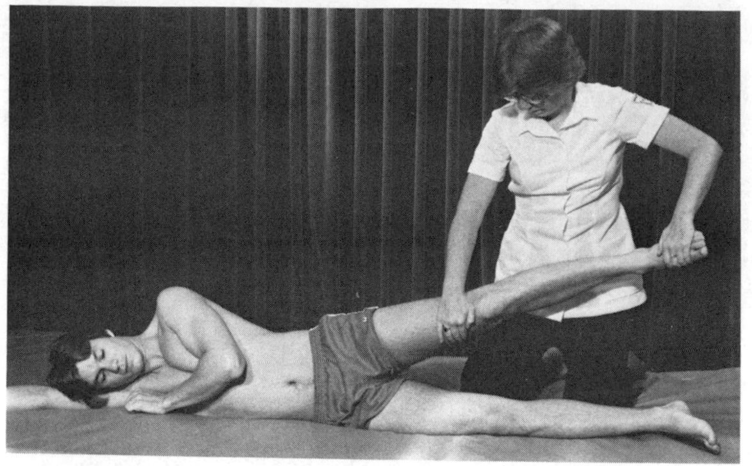

(a)

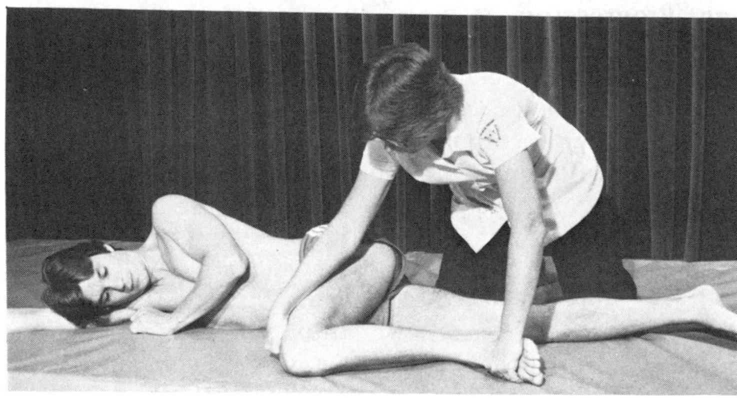

(b)

A. Sidelying: mass flexion lower extremity.
E. MC thigh and foot.

FIGURE 3–2

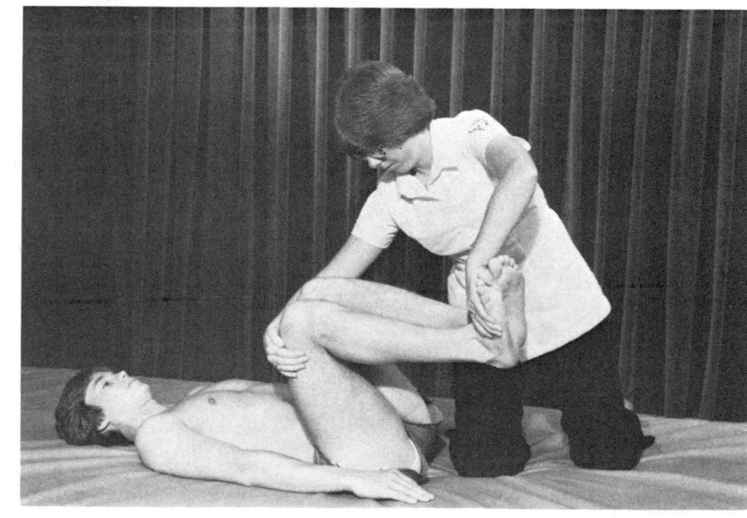

A. Supine: lower trunk flexion, knee flexion.
E. MC thighs and feet.

FIGURE 3–3

ACTIVITIES OF THE DEVELOPMENTAL SEQUENCE

Many of the postures discussed in the preceding chapter will be repeated in this section. The emphasis here, however, will be on the biomechanical, tonal, and neurophysiological influences on the postures and treatment implications for patients with various disabilities. The progression within each posture will follow the sequence of motor control (13). A more extensive discussion of the treatment of patients with specific diagnoses will be presented in subsequent chapters.

Initial Upright Progression

The initial upright progression consists of three postures: sidelying, rolling, and sitting.

1. Sidelying and Rolling. Sidelying and rolling are incorporated into the initial phases of treatment for many patients. The B of S is large, the C of G is low, and no weight bearing occurs through any joints. Any segment of the body, however, can be held or moved within the posture. Sidelying is an appropriate activity when stability or initial control of the trunk or proximal areas is desired. Stability can be enhanced if the B of S is even further enlarged by positioning the uppermost limbs in flexion. Positioning of the upper extremity in contact with the supporting surface also promotes minimal weight bearing through the limb (Figure 3–4). The scapula is pro-

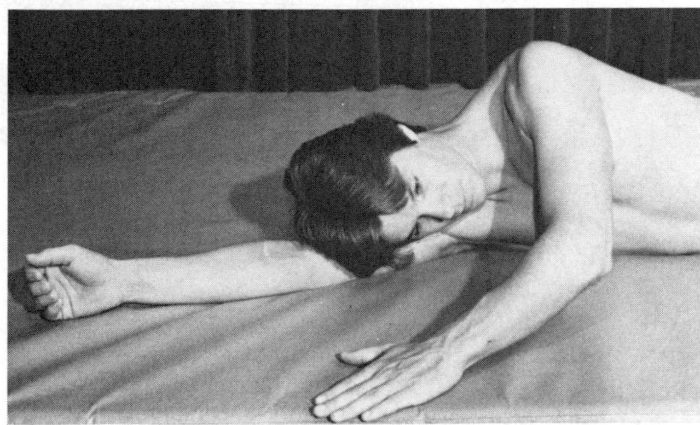

A. Sidelying: upper extremity positioned in flexion.

FIGURE 3–4

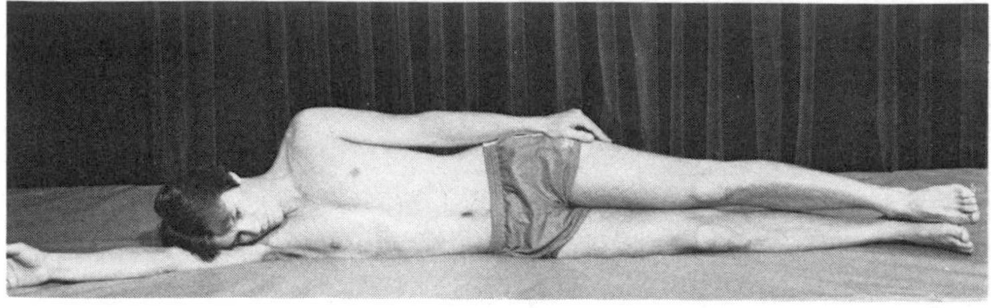

A. Sidelying: without extremity support.

FIGURE 3–5

tracted, the shoulder flexed and adducted, the elbow and wrist are extended, and the volar surface of the hand is maintained in contact with the mat. This combination of joint positions is important for many patients, especially for those with hemiplegia or quadriplegia. As control increases and the trunk is able to cope with a greater challenge, the B of S can be reduced by eliminating the assistance afforded by the extremities (Figure 3–5).

Tonal factors influence the sidelying and rolling activities. In sidelying, the limbs are influenced by the ATLR, which increases flexor tone, or decreases extensor tone in the uppermost extremities. The lowermost limbs or those in contact with the supporting surface exhibit an increase in extensor

(a)

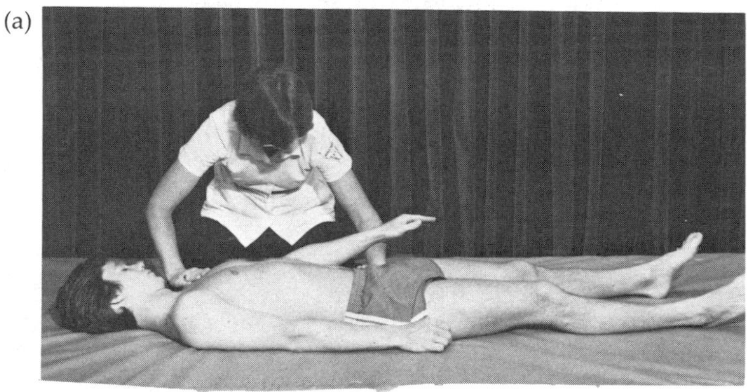

(b)

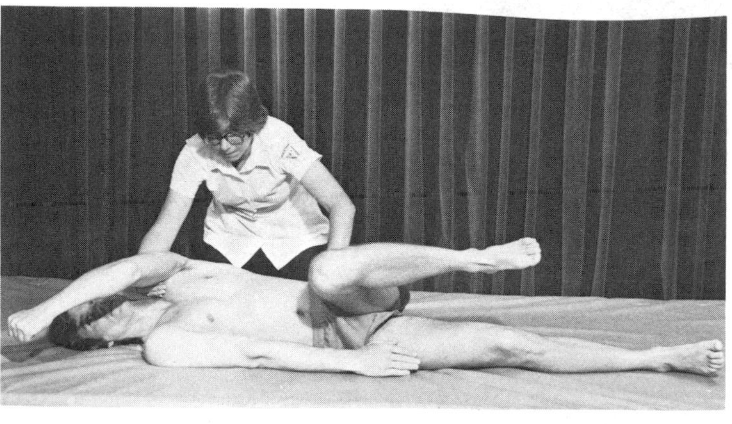

A. Rolling supine toward prone: ipsilateral D_1.
E. MC scapula and pelvis. pelvis.

FIGURE 3–6

tone. Before normal rolling can occur, the tonal influences of both the ATNR and the STLR must be integrated (22). When rolling takes place from supine to prone, the extensor influence of the STLR in the supine position must be overcome so that the flexor muscles can initiate and sustain the movement. The leading limbs must be able to adduct across the midline, indicating a reduction of the influence of the ATNR (Figure 3–6). Rolling toward prone can be used to increase proximal flexor tone and rolling toward supine can be used to increase proximal extensor tone (20). Righting reactions will assist the rolling activity (1). Because of the low C of G and large B of S, very little of the higher level reactions—equilibrium or proprioceptive—are required.

Gravity will resist movements of the trunk from supine or prone to the mid or sidelying position and will assist trunk movements to supine or prone from the sidelying posture. Traction or compression forces are not inherent during rolling.

Stages of Motor Control in Sidelying and Rolling. Trunk movements in sidelying and rolling should progress in a logical sequence according to the stages of motor control: **mobility** is the ability to initiate rolling and implies the availability of ROM through which the patient can move; **stability** is co-contraction of the trunk in sidelying; **controlled mobility** is log rolling through range, that is, movement of the trunk as a whole with rotation around the longitudinal axis of the body (Figure 3–7); **static dynamic activity** is segmental trunk rotation, that is, rotation of either upper or lower portions of the trunk while the other segment is stabilized (Figures 3–8 and 3–9); and **skill** is counter-rotation, which combines simultaneous movements of upper and lower trunk in opposite or adversive directions (Figure 3–10). Certain techniques that can be used to facilitate or reinforce these stages of control will be discussed in Chapter 4.

To enhance rolling activities, the head, neck, and extremities may all be used in combination with the different techniques. Because rolling toward prone is a flexor dominant activity, head and neck flexion with rotation can be used to initiate movement in this direction. The upper extremity must cross the midline when rolling toward prone. Therefore the two adduction

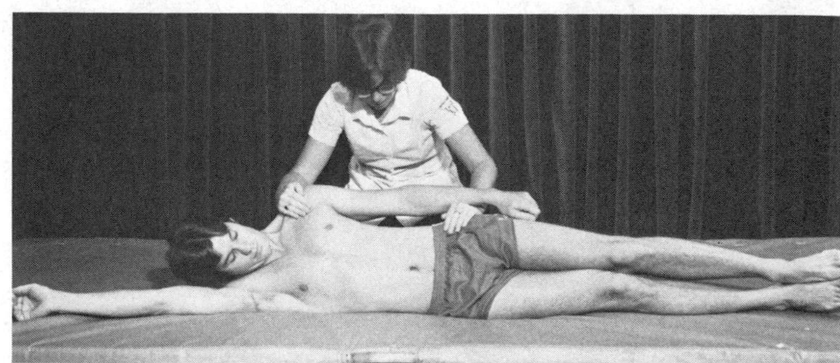

A. Log rolling.
E. MC scapula and pelvis.

FIGURE 3–7

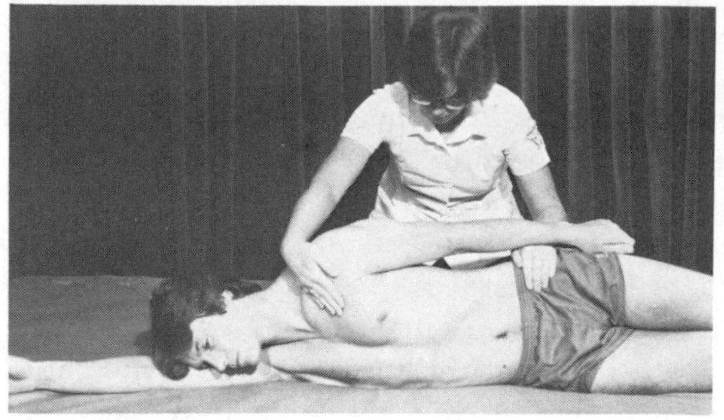

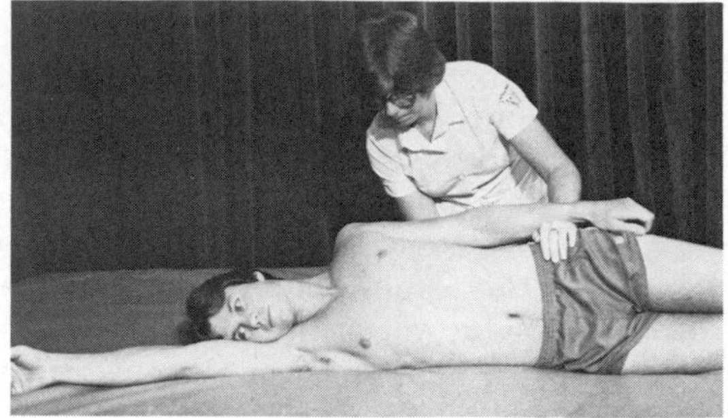

(a) (b)

FIGURE 3–8

A. Sidelying: upper trunk motions.
E. MC scapula and pelvis.

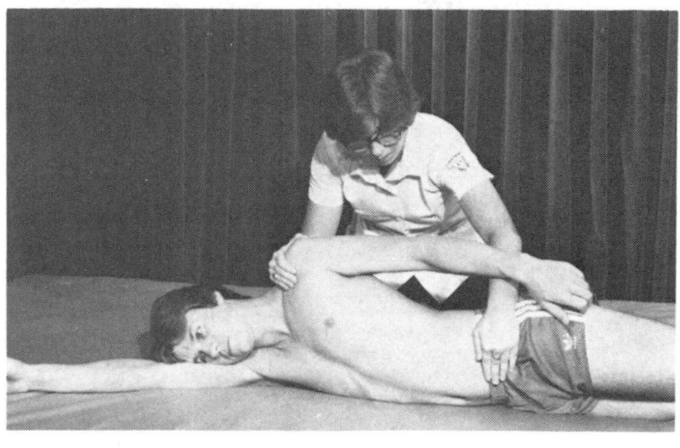

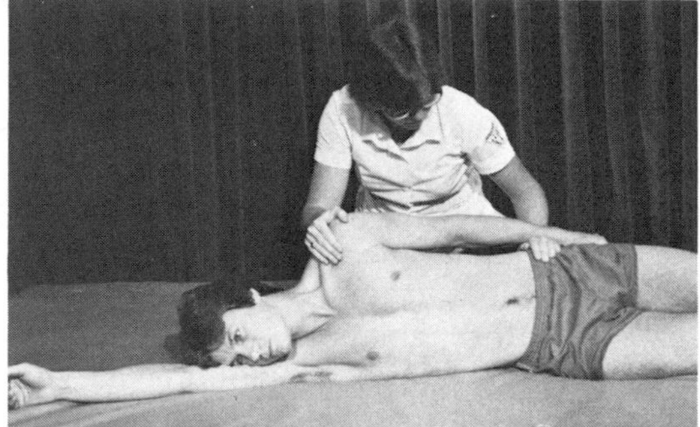

(a) (b)

A. Sidelying: lower trunk motions.
E. MC scapula and pelvis.

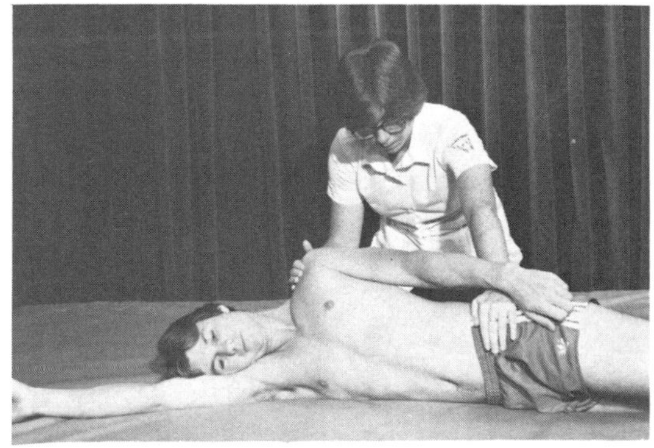

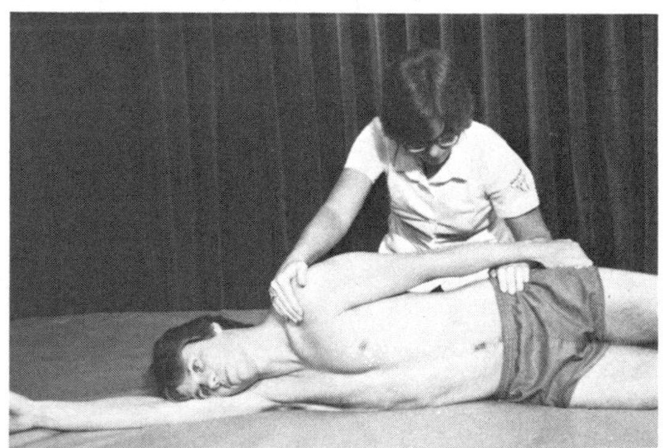

(a) (b)

FIGURE 3–10

A. Sidelying: counter-rotation, adversive movements.
E. MC scapula and pelvis.

patterns of Diagonal 1 Flexion (D_1F) [Figure 3–11] or Diagonal 2 Extension (D_2E) [Figure 3–12] can be used to enhance the movement. The upper trunk patterns of a chop [Figure 3–13] or reverse chop [Figure 3–14] can also be used to facilitate rolling toward prone while a lifting pattern can be incorporated into rolling toward supine [Figure 3–15]. The lower extremity consistently performs a D_1 pattern (20) (see the section "Extremity Patterns").

Clinical Implications. Rolling is an important functional activity that may be needed for dressing, relieving pressure, and improving bed mobility. The control gained in sidelying and rolling is necessary for the assumption of other postures such as sitting (23).

The rotational movement that can be facilitated in sidelying or in rolling has positive clinical effects. Log rolling in a slow rhythmical fashion has been found empirically to promote relaxation in patients experiencing spasticity or rigidity (16). This relaxation has been attributed to the influence of the vestibular system and its effect on the reticular activating system (24). Segmental rolling emphasizes spinal rotation and is appropriate when movement is lacking in the upper or lower trunk. If upper trunk extension with rotation is deficient, as it is for a patient having Parkinsonism, this upper trunk motion can be promoted in sidelying while the lower trunk is being stabilized (25) (See Figure 3–16). The scapula motions that occur during upper trunk rotation are important for various patients, including hemi-

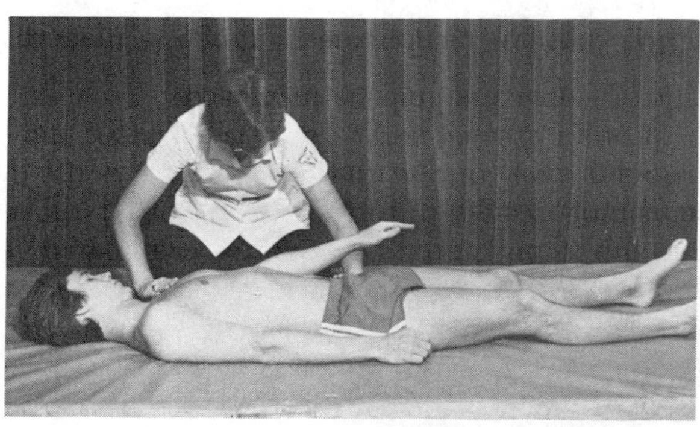

(a)

A. Rolling: supine toward prone, ipsilateral D_1F.
E. MC scapula and pelvis.

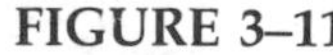

FIGURE 3–11

(b)

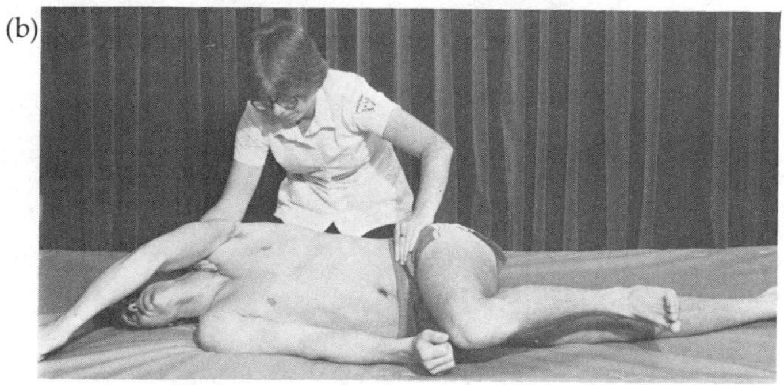

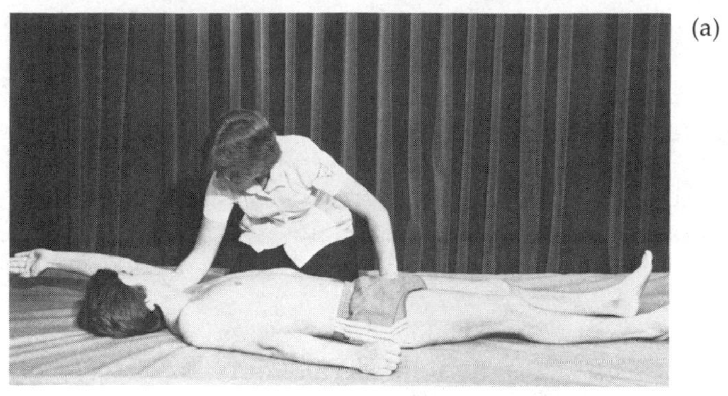

(a)

(b)

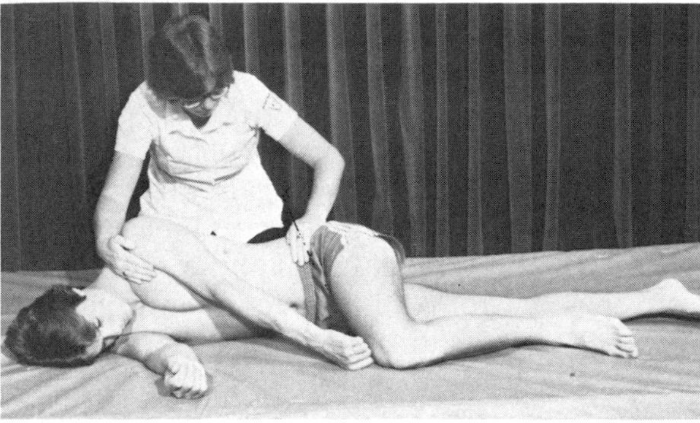

A. Rolling: supine toward prone, D_2E, UE; D_1F, LE.
E. MC scapula and pelvis.

FIGURE 3–12

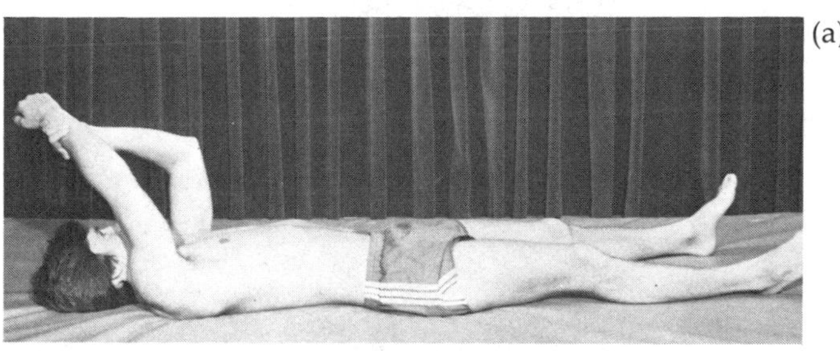

(a)

(b)

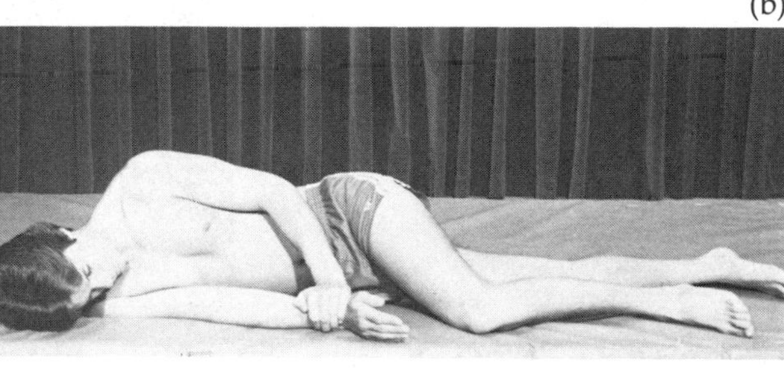

A. Rolling: supine toward prone, chop; D_1F, LE.

FIGURE 3–13

(a)

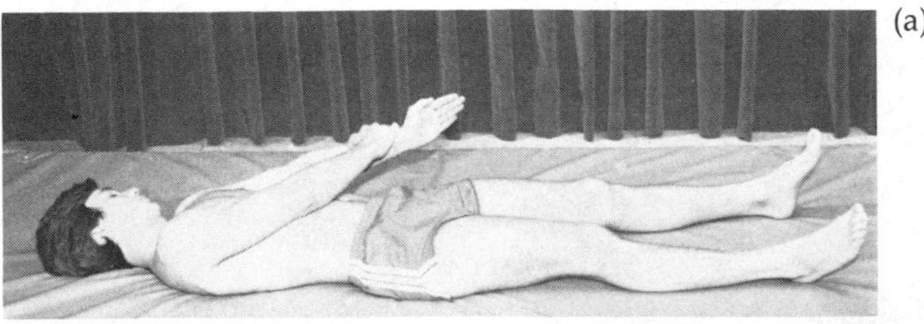

(b)

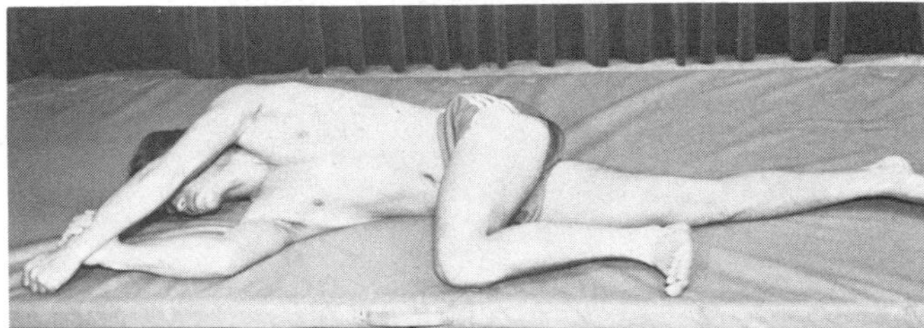

A. Rolling: supine toward prone, reverse chop, D_1F, LE.

FIGURE 3–14

plegics and those having shoulder disabilities (7, 26) (see chapters 8 and 10). Many patients are unable to protract or rotate the lower trunk forward; this deficiency may be most noticeable during gait. Segmental lower trunk rotation with emphasis on protraction in particular can enhance this motion. Once this movement is facilitated, counter-rotation of the trunk and movements combining forward pelvic rotation with hip flexion can be attempted (Figure 3–17). Segmental trunk motions may also assist in integrating tonic reflexes by reducing the mass tonal effects of these reflexes. Counter-rota-

(a)

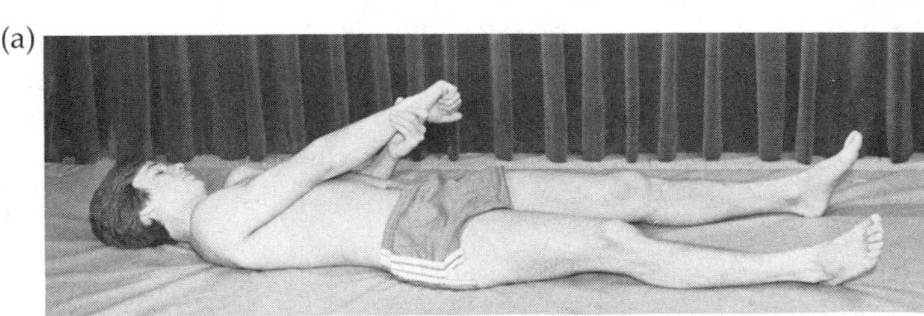

(b)

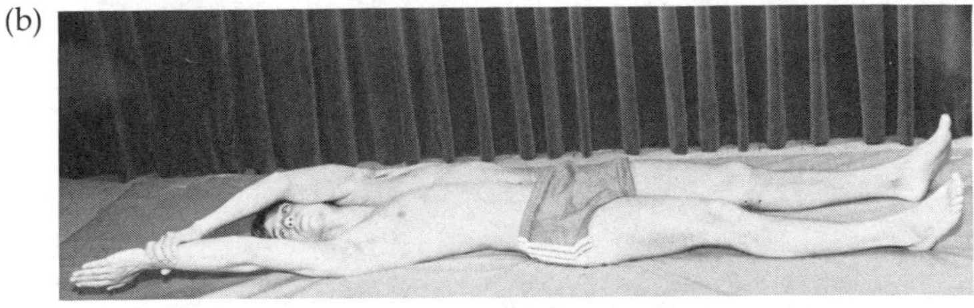

A. Rolling to supine: lift.

FIGURE 3–15

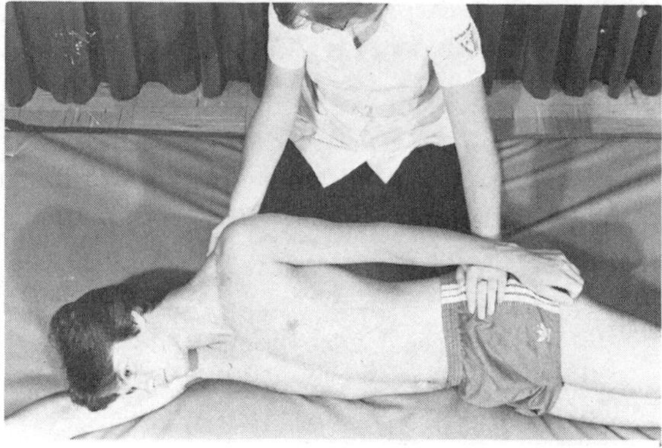

A. Sidelying: UTE.
E. MC scapula and pelvis.

FIGURE 3–16

tion of the trunk is indicated for many patients, especially when improved ambulation is a long-range goal.

As already mentioned, specific extremity and trunk patterns can be used to influence the tone of the activity. Many patients with multiple sclerosis (MS), for example, experience increased extensor tone and thus have difficulty rolling from supine to prone. Any of the previously discussed movement patterns—head flexion with rotation, D_2E or D_1F of the UE, chopping, D_1F LE—can be used to increase proximal flexor tone. Hemiplegic patients, on the other hand, frequently neglect their involved arm when they roll, and a reverse chop, which is an upper trunk pattern, will improve their body awareness and assist in bringing the involved arm across the midline. Patients with hypotonia, such as those with Guillain-Barré, may need to increase extensor tone, and can do so by combining a lifting pattern with rolling toward supine. These few examples illustrate that the pattern of rolling may be adapted to meet the needs of the patient. If the therapist finds that certain movement combinations are efficient and successful, those patterns can be reinforced; otherwise, some of the examples given here might be used to enhance the desired movement. Stability techniques in sidelying

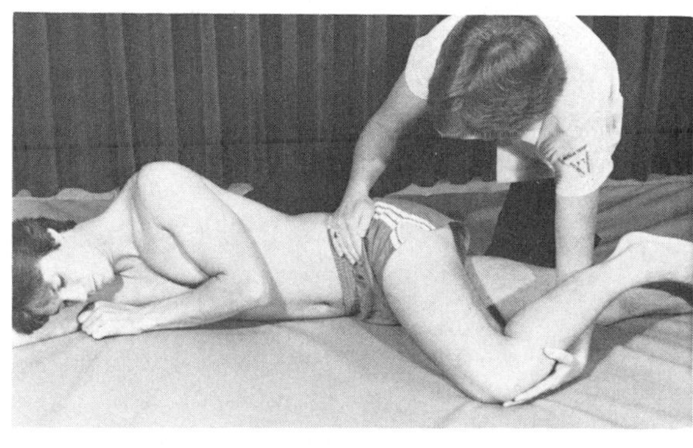

A. Sidelying: LT protraction with hip flexion.
E. MC pelvis and knee.

FIGURE 3–17

can promote cocontraction of the trunk musculature, an important consideration for patients with low back pain (27) (see Chapter 12).

In summary:

- Rolling is an important functional activity for dressing, bed mobility, and the assumption of sitting and other postures.
- The B of S is large, the C of G is low, and no weight bearing occurs through the joints.
- Segmental trunk rotation can enhance specific trunk motions.
- Trunk counter-rotation, which is necessary for normal gait, can be promoted in sidelying.
- Trunk rotation can assist in the integration of tonic reflexes and promote the righting reactions needed for rolling.
- Various trunk and extremity patterns can facilitate specific proximal musculature and enhance the rolling movements.

2. Sitting. The sitting posture follows rolling in the initial upright progression. The size of the B of S is smaller than in sidelying or rolling and may be varied according to the amount of extremity support. Longsitting will increase the B of S anteriorly, and may be specifically useful for patients with spinal cord injury (Figure 3–18) (see Chapter 9). Longsitting may be difficult for other patients because of inflexibility in the lower trunk and extremities. The upper extremities can be used to: 1) assist the trunk in maintaining the posture by increasing the B of S in the posterior (Figure 3–19), lateral (Figure 3–20), and anterior (Figure 3–21) directions either in long or short sitting; and 2) increase upper extremity control (7). When the arms are positioned posteriorly, the extensors of the upper trunk and upper extremities may be facilitated in their shortened range (Figure 3–22). An increase in joint compression that will enhance the holding of these muscles can be achieved either by manual approximation or by weight shifting toward one side. A minimal stretch is placed on the proximal postural mus-

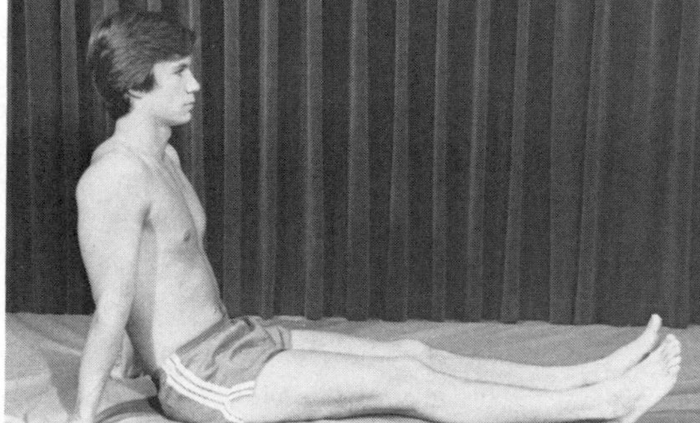

A. Longsitting.

FIGURE 3–18

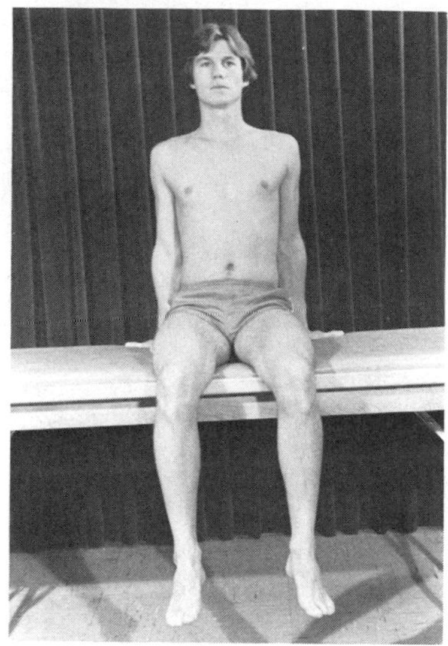

A. Sitting: UE support posterior.

FIGURE 3–19

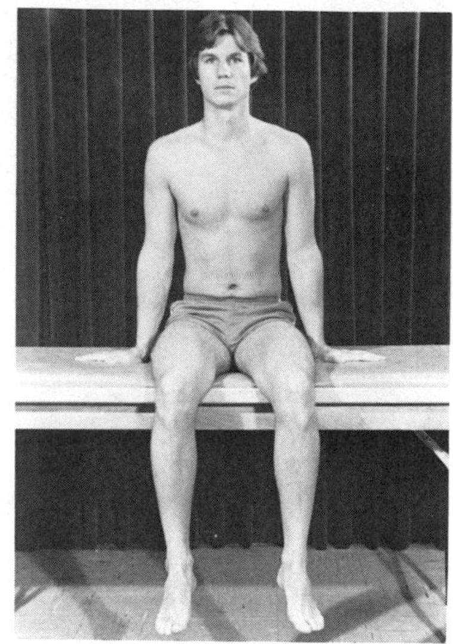

A. Sitting: UE support lateral.

FIGURE 3–20

cles by positioning the arms laterally and then anteriorly to the trunk.

In this posture the C of G is higher than in rolling and sidelying. The number of joints involved in sitting may vary and may include those of the trunk and the upper extremities, depending on the movements performed.

The tonic reflexes are not a major influence in sitting if the head is maintained in the midline position (23). Righting reactions help the patient to maintain this upright posture. Because of the variations in biomechanical factors, such as C of G and B of S, higher level equilibrium, proprioceptive and protective extension reactions are prerequisites to functioning in the posture (8).

In the sitting posture the effects of gravity tend to be balanced. For this reason, sitting is appropriately used to promote control of weakened head and neck musculature before progressing to postures such as prone on elbows, in which the resistance provided by gravity is increased (Figure 3–23). The vital functions of chewing, swallowing, and feeding can also be promoted in sitting or semisitting postures (see Chapter 8).

The tactile input from the supporting surfaces, the buttocks, and thighs is very important in helping the patient to maintain a vertical position. When tactile input that is normally used to orient to the position is not equal, as in the case of hemiplegic patients, it becomes difficult to maintain balance (7). Manual approximation through the trunk may improve both the tactile and proprioceptive input.

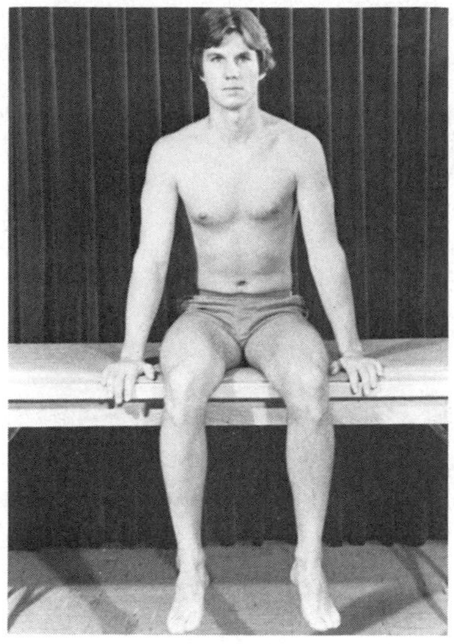

A. Sitting: UE support anterior.

FIGURE 3–21

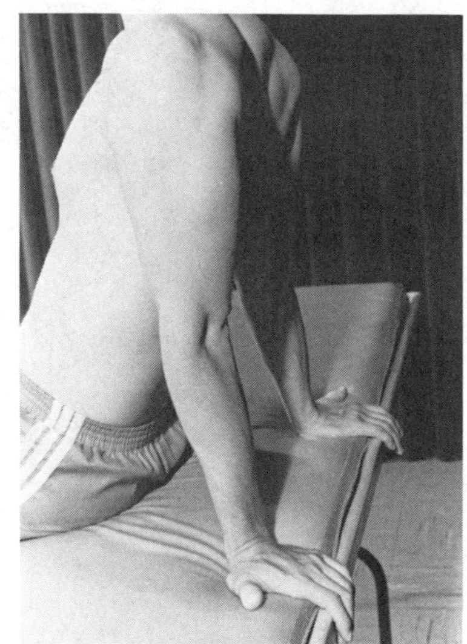

A. Sitting: upper extremities posterior.

FIGURE 3–22

Stages of Motor Control. The various sitting activities can be related to the levels of motor control. Stability in sitting is the maintenance of the posture with or without upper extremity assistance. Without upper extremity assistance, obviously more trunk control is needed. The tonic phase of stability can be gained in the upper trunk when the trunk extensors are positioned in their shortened range. Cocontraction occurs when the upper extremities are weight bearing or when the manually resistive force facilitates

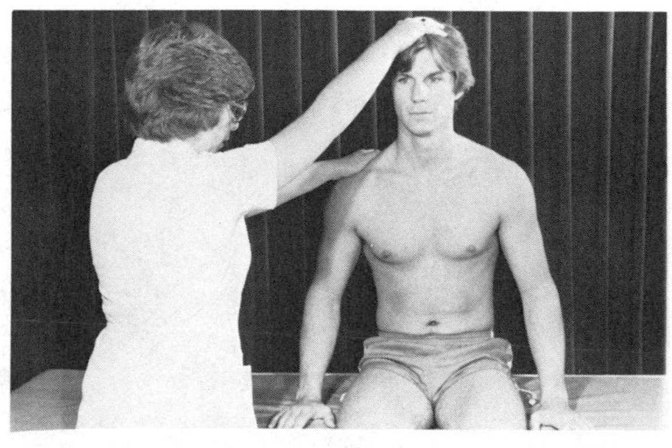

A. Sitting: with arm support.
E. MC head and scapula: approximation.

FIGURE 3–23

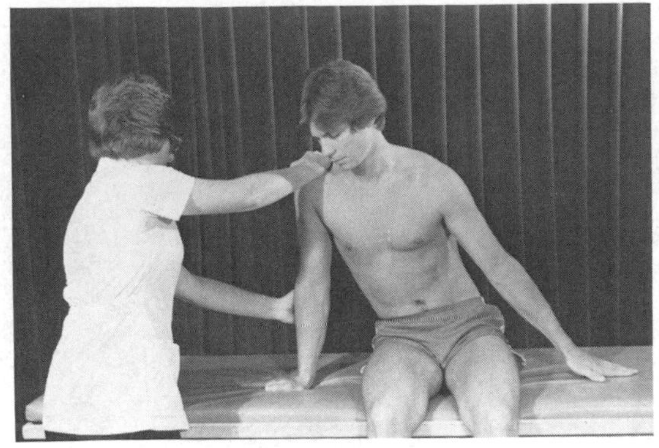

A. Sitting: with arm support, lateral weight shifting.

FIGURE 3–24

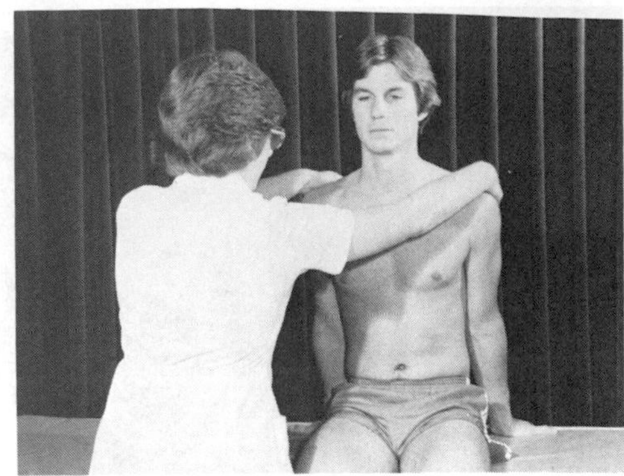

A. Sitting: with arm support.
T. AI resistance to trunk extension.
E. MC scapula.

FIGURE 3–25

cocontraction (13). Controlled mobility is achieved by movement within the posture, either by rocking over the supporting upper extremities (Figure 3–24) or by moving the trunk without extremity assistance. The level of control reaches the point of skill when the upper extremities can be freed to perform functional activities (13). The trunk control that is needed at this skilled stage is termed dynamic stability, providing a stable yet constantly changing base in response to extremity motions. Proximal dynamic stability is promoted during the controlled mobility procedures when the equilibrium and proprioceptive reactions are facilitated in preparation for the skilled functional level of control.

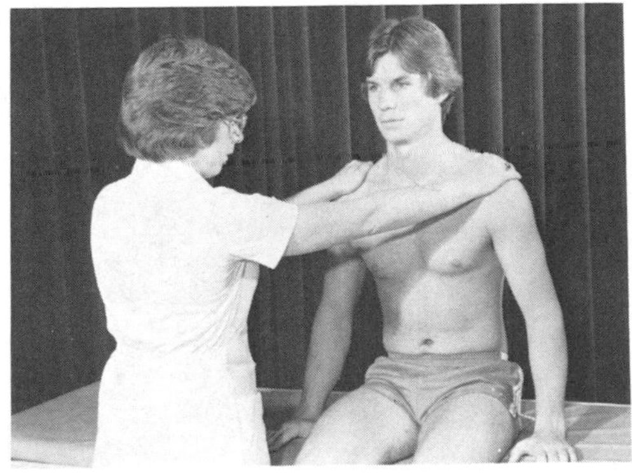

A. Sitting: with arm support.
T. RS.
E. MC scapula.

FIGURE 3–26

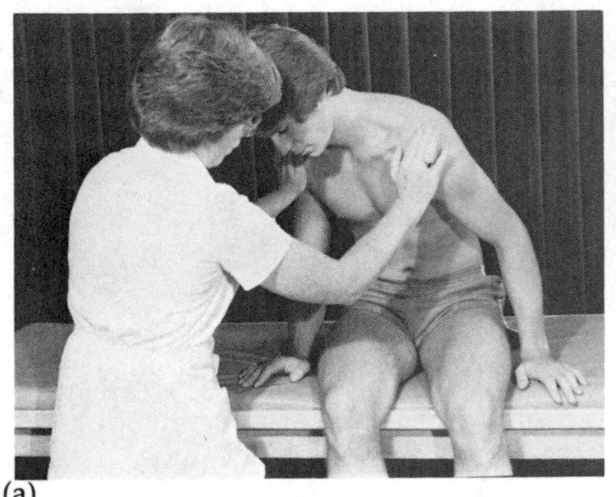
(a)

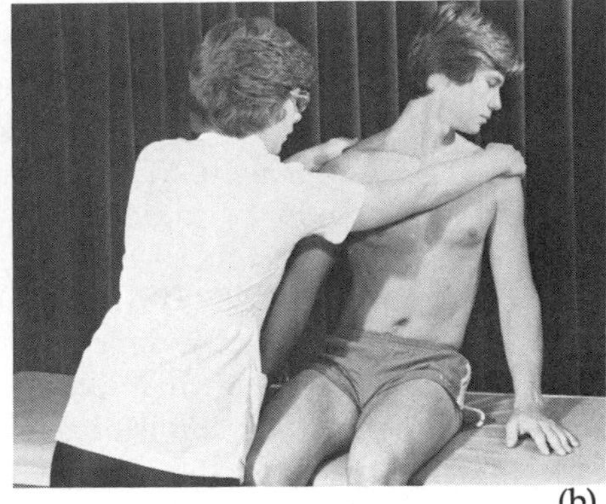
(b)

A. Sitting: with arm support, upper trunk flexion, and extension with rotation.
E. MC scapula.

FIGURE 3–27

Clinical Implications. Clinically, sitting can help many patients reach a number of goals. As previously stated, head and neck control, vital functions, and facial muscle facilitation can be promoted through sitting. The use of a mirror may improve feedback if other sensory mechanisms are deficient (17). During stability (Figures 3–25 and 3–26) and controlled mobility procedures, trunk flexion, extension, lateral shifting, rotation, or a diagonal combination of these motions can be emphasized (Figures 3–27 and 3–28). Improved trunk control is a goal of a great number of patients, including most patients with CNS dysfunction and many with orthopedic problems. In the case of patients with CNS dysfunction, reduced trunk control com-

A. Sitting: with arm support, upper trunk rotation.
E. MC scapula.

FIGURE 3–28

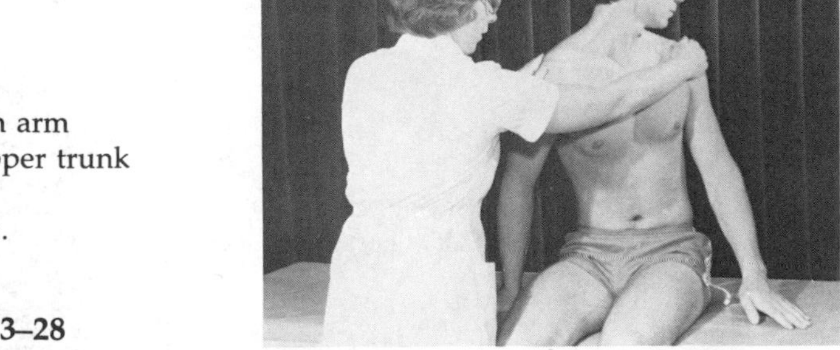

monly occurs as a result of an imbalance of tone. As already noted, the treatment of patients with Parkinsonism usually involves extension with rotation (25). In addition to resisting a rolling pattern toward supine, the therapist can emphasize extension with rotation in sitting. Conversely, for patients with MS who demonstrate increased extensor tone, flexor motions would be indicated. Patients with orthopedic back problems may initially need isometric strengthening of the trunk musculature, which can be accomplished during stability procedures in sitting (27).

When independent sitting balance is a goal—as is common with patients with hemiplegia, Guillain Barré, brain injury, or spinal cord injury—a very gradual progression of procedures may be needed. Procedures that promote stability are followed by controlled mobility movements through increments of range to improve body awareness, muscular tone, and to promote righting and balance reactions that are needed for functional independence in sitting.

Sitting with upper extremity support also may be appropriate for patients with reduced upper extremity control. When the upper extremity is positioned posteriorly, the scapula retractors, the shoulder, elbow, wrist, and finger extensors are positioned in the shortened range. Isometric holding of these primarily tonic muscles can be facilitated both by manual re-

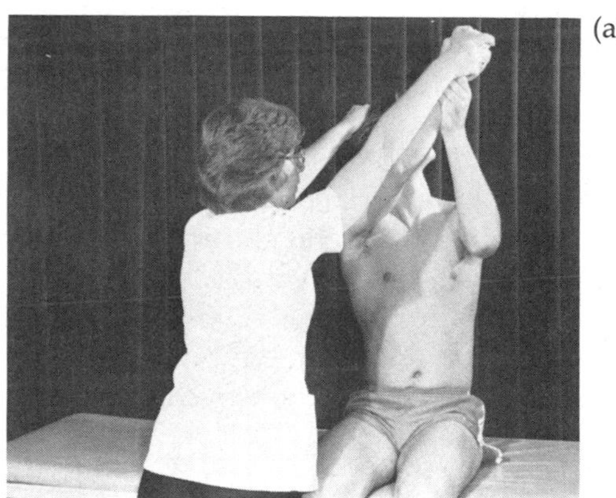

(a)

(b)

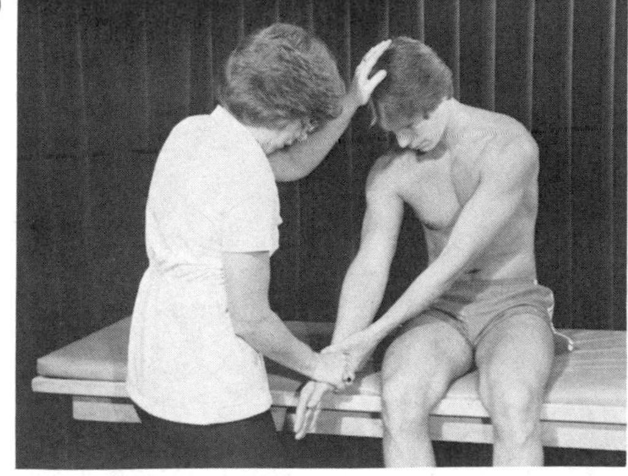

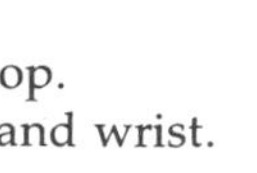

A. Sitting: chop.
E. MC head and wrist.

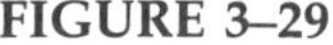

FIGURE 3–29

sistance or by increasing weight bearing. If hypertonia is present in the elbow, wrist, and finger flexors, a balance of tone may be facilitated by increasing the activity of the extensor muscles in this weight-bearing position. As activity of the extensor muscles gradually increases, the arms may be positioned more anteriorly to increase the stretch on the proximal extensor muscles and the amount of weight-bearing resistance can be increased (see Chapter 8). Patients with shoulder dysfunction from orthopedic conditions who have a deficit in proximal stability and controlled mobility functions could also benefit from this progression (see Chapter 10).

As in rolling, many upper trunk or extremity patterns can be added to the sitting activity to emphasize specific trunk or proximal musculature. The difficulty of performing these patterns varies between rolling and sitting because of the gravitational changes, the tonal variations, and the altered B of S and C of G. A patient with weak trunk musculature, for example, must overcome the resistance of gravity when rolling with a chop from supine to prone. With the assistance of gravity, the same chopping motion may be performed more easily in sitting (Figure 3–29), but because the B of S is smaller and the C of G higher, balance in the sitting position may be more difficult. When trunk balance is inadequate the feet should be supported to help the patient maintain balance.

Lower extremity patterns, either bilateral or unilateral, can be performed in sitting (see the section "Extremity Patterns"). Various combinations of patterns can be used specifically to emphasize knee or ankle control (see the section on "Extremity Patterns") or indirectly to challenge the patient's sitting balance.

In summary:

- The sitting posture can be used to promote vital functions as well as to improve activities of daily living.
- The B of S can be increased by the placement of the limbs on the supporting surface either to assist trunk stability or to specifically emphasize extremity control.
- The number of joints involved in sitting depends on whether the extremities participate in weight bearing or in controlled movement patterns.
- The tonic reflex influence in sitting is minimal. Righting reactions assist maintenance of the posture.
- The higher level balance reactions—equilibrium and proprioceptive—are required to move within the posture and to perform skilled activities.
- The progression through the stages of motor control promotes the functional use of the posture.
- Various combinations of head, neck, trunk, and extremity patterns can be performed to reach a number of goals.

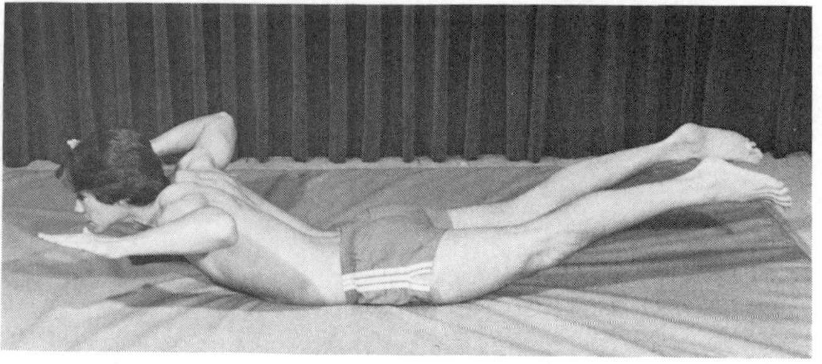

A. Pivot prone.

FIGURE 3–30

The Prone Progression

The prone progression consists of the pivot prone, prone on elbows, and quadruped postures.

1. Pivot Prone. Developmentally, the prone progression begins with the pivot prone position (Figure 3–30) (28). During pivot prone all the tonic postural extensors isometrically contract against the resistance of gravity in their shortened ranges and theoretically increase the stretch sensitivity of their muscle spindles (13), therefore developing the first stage of stability-tonic holding (see Chapter 2). Pivot prone may not be possible for many patients who have decreased ROM in the trunk and hips. Severe hypotonia may also prevent patients from overcoming the effects of gravity. When these conditions exist, a modified pivot prone posture in supine (Figure 3–31), sidelying (Figure 3–32), or supported sitting (Figure 3–33) may be substituted to promote a shortened, held, resisted contraction of the tonic extensor muscles (15). Before weight-bearing postures can be successful, the postural muscles must be able to maintain the body weight against manual resistance or the resistance of gravity (see Chapter 4).

2. Prone on Elbows. The prone-on-elbows posture (Figure 3–34) is a progression from pivot prone. The extensors that were made stretch sensitive in pivot prone are now on prolonged stretch, which may cause excitation of the spindle Ia and II afferents. Such excitation seems to result in cocontraction of the muscles of the head and neck, scapula, and shoulder. Weight bearing may also enhance the contraction of the deep tonic postural muscles (13, 29, 30).

The large B of S and low C of G of prone on elbows minimize the need for balance reactions. The scapula and shoulder joints are the only weight-bearing joints. Head control and neck control are required, however, to

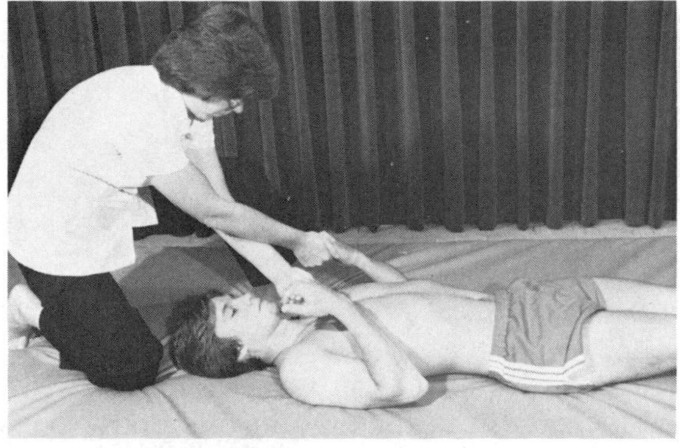

A. Supine: BS D_1 withdrawal.
T. SHRC.
E. MC hands.

FIGURE 3–31

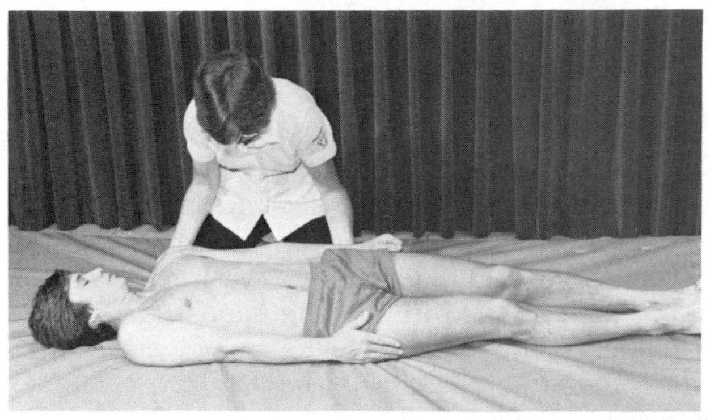

A. Sidelying trunk extension.
T. SHRC.
E. MC scapula and pelvis.

FIGURE 3–32

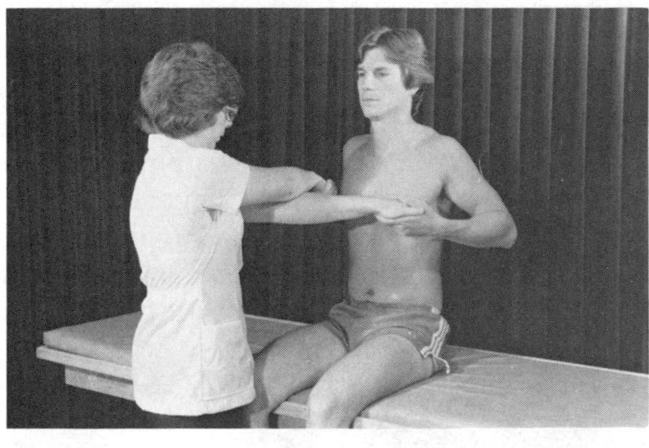

A. Sitting: BS D_1 withdrawal.
T. SHRC.
E. MC hands.

FIGURE 3–33

maintain the midline position against the resistance of gravity. Maintenance of the head in the vertical position may be resisted by gravity but assisted by righting reactions. The support afforded by the biomechanical factors in prone on elbows makes this posture appropriate for patients with reduced motor control. Many of these patients, especially those who have CNS dysfunction, may experience an increase in the dominance of lower level re-

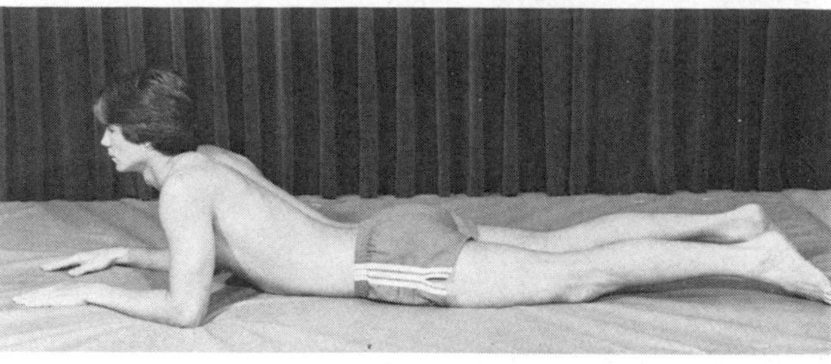

A. Prone on elbows.

FIGURE 3–34

flexes. A generalized increase in flexor tone in this prone posture may be due to the effects of the STLR. The tonic neck reflexes may also be dominant. Neck extension may cause an increase in upper extremity extensor tone, which will be most evident in the elbow extensors (Figure 3–35). Neck rotation may also alter upper extremity tone by means of the ATNR (Figure 3–36). Varying head position, without allowing a change in the posturing of the arms, will help the patient to integrate the tonic reflexes in this posture.

Some neurophysiological mechanisms affecting the prone-on-elbows posture have already been discussed. Gravity adds resistance to the head, neck, and upper trunk extensors. Manual approximation added to the scapula and shoulder appears to increase the holding of the postural muscles around those joints. The triceps is positioned in the lengthened range with weight bearing on the triceps tendon. Both of these factors may increase the inhibitory influences to the elbow extensors (13) (see Chapter 5).

In the prone-on-elbows position, the lower extremities are in a mass extensor position, which is frequently desirable for patients having hypotonic or lower extremity flexor spasticity. Patients who demonstrate an increase in extensor tone may need to have the lower extremity position altered. This can be accomplished by flexing the knees with a support under the lower leg (7). The leg is thus positioned out of mass extension and into an advanced combination of hip extension and knee flexion.

In this prone posture, lower extremity patterns are performed with the hip remaining in extension (7, 17) (See Figure 3–37). The effects of gravity, reflexes, and muscle length differ from the supine and sitting positions, in

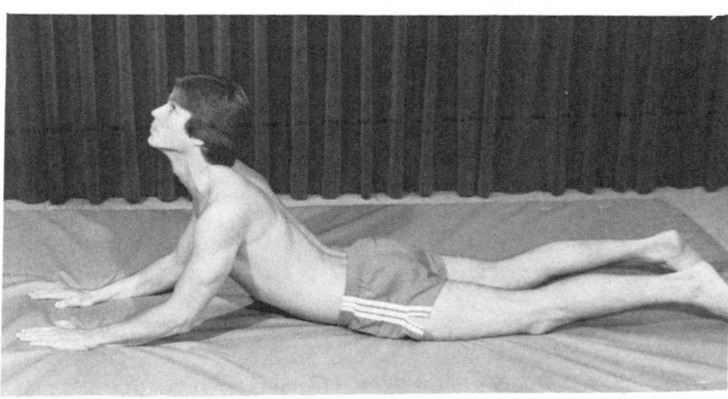

A. Prone on elbows: neck extension with increased elbow extension (STNR).

FIGURE 3–35

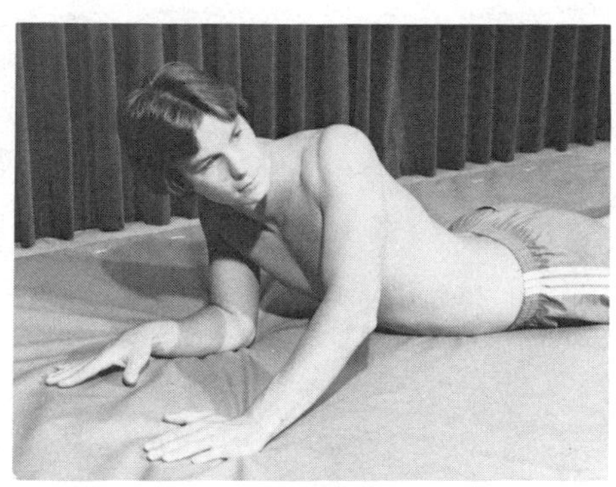

A. Prone on elbows: neck rotation, increase in extension one UE (ATNR).

FIGURE 3–36

which leg patterns are also frequently performed. When the quadriceps are below a fair range, they can be easily exercised in prone against manual resistance with the assistance of gravity. As the hamstrings shorten over both joints and flex the knee against gravity, active insufficiency can occur (31). Therefore resistance in the shortened range should be avoided to prevent cramping. The passive insufficiency of the rectus femoris can reduce the amount of knee flexion. A unilateral D_2 mass flexion pattern of the lower extremity can also be performed in this posture to facilitate a creeping movement (20).

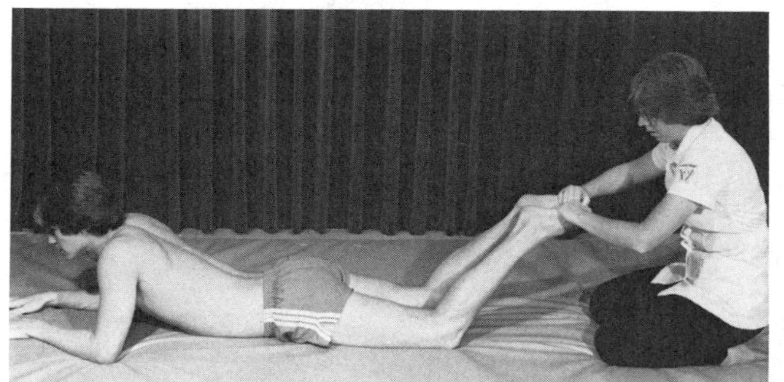

(a)

(b)

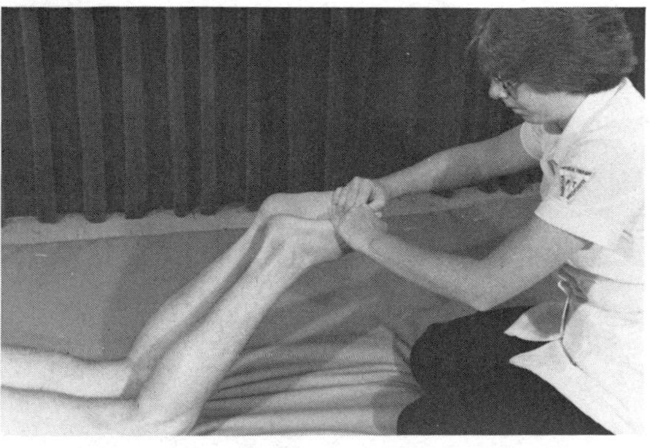

A. Prone on elbows: bilateral leg patterns.
E. MC feet.

FIGURE 3–37

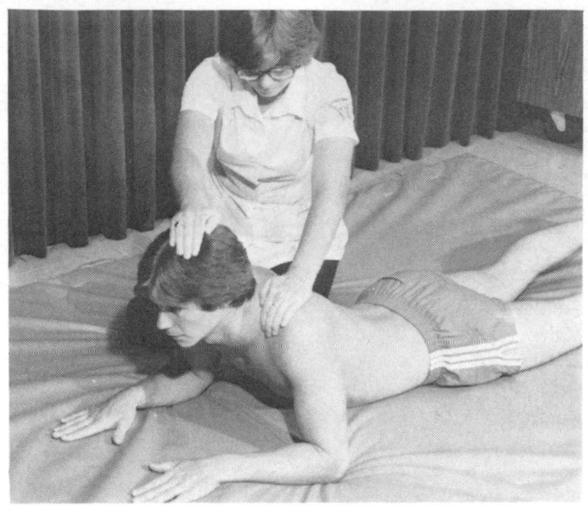

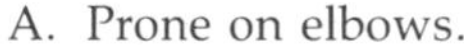

A. Prone on elbows.
T. RS.
E. MC head and scapula.

FIGURE 3–38

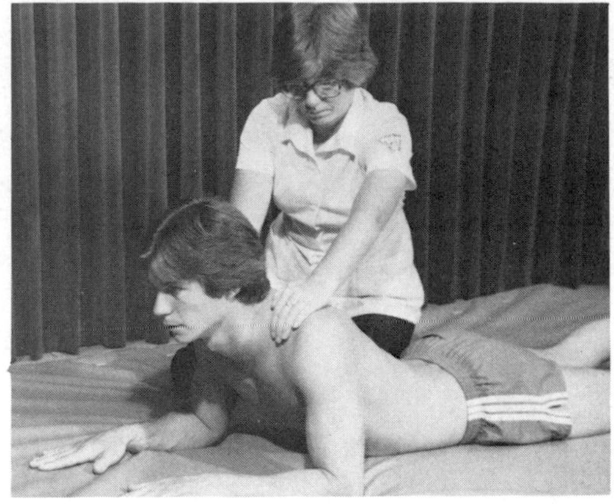

A. Prone on elbows.
T. RS.
E. MC scapula.

FIGURE 3–39

Stages of Motor Control. Clinically, a gradual progression of the stages of motor control in prone on elbows may be most useful for patients with spinal cord injury, brain damage, or any disability resulting in a lack of proximal stability, such as multiple sclerosis or cerebral palsy. Patients with shoulder disability will also need the proximal stability and controlled mobility that can be developed in this posture. By altering manual contacts, techniques that enhance isometric holding and cocontraction—such as alternating isometrics (AI) and rhythmic stabilization (RS) (see Chapter 4)—can be applied to increase stability at the head, neck, and scapula (Figures 3–38 and 3–39). The head has reached controlled mobility or skill level of control when it can rotate independently in a midline position (13, 15). Controlled rotation of the head can be promoted by combining neck patterns with facilitative techniques. Controlled mobility or weight-shifting activities will facilitate scapulohumeral rhythm (Figure 3–40). The increased weight bearing on one upper extremity should enhance activity of the deep rotators, an important consideration for patients with shoulder pathology. Weight shifting may be enhanced by head rotation in the direction of the weight shift (33). Although weight shifting in a lateral direction is most easily accomplished, other directions may be indicated for some patients. Static-dynamic activities will promote unilateral weight bearing as well as dynamic stability that is necessary for skilled activities (5, 26) (see Figure 3–41). Quadriplegic patients may also use this static-dynamic position to initiate rolling from prone to supine. Crawling or walking on elbows is the skill level of control and may be functional for patients with spinal cord injury (see Chapter 9). Crawling in this posture is not a particularly functional activity for other patients, however, and may be omitted.

Clinical Implications. As stated, the prone-on-elbows posture can help some patients develop head, neck, upper trunk, scapula, and shoulder control. Cocontraction around these joints may be promoted by the stretch on the postural muscles or the resistance of body weight (13, 32). The gravitational resistance provided in this prone posture is greater than that in sitting, in which initial head and neck control was developed. The 45-degree angle of shoulder flexion also makes prone on elbows a progression from the sitting position, where weight bearing at the shoulders occurs at around 0 degrees of flexion, which is usually less stressful. Because the elbow is flexed in prone on elbows, however, the length of the lever arm of the upper extremity is reduced, making it easier for some patients to exert control in this posture than in sitting.

Like pivot prone, prone on elbows may not be appropriate for some patients. The lordotic curve created in the low back cannot always be tolerated. Hemiplegic patients may experience an increase in spasticity or pain in the shoulder; these reactions indicate that the posture is too stressful. Patients with respiratory deficiency or hip flexion contractures may find this position difficult to attain or maintain. Positioning a pillow under the abdomen may alleviate some of these problems. When necessary, the scapula and shoulder control provided by this posture can be promoted either in modified prone-on-elbows activities (13), such as sitting with arm support, or, if lower extremity control is present, in modified plantigrade on elbows.

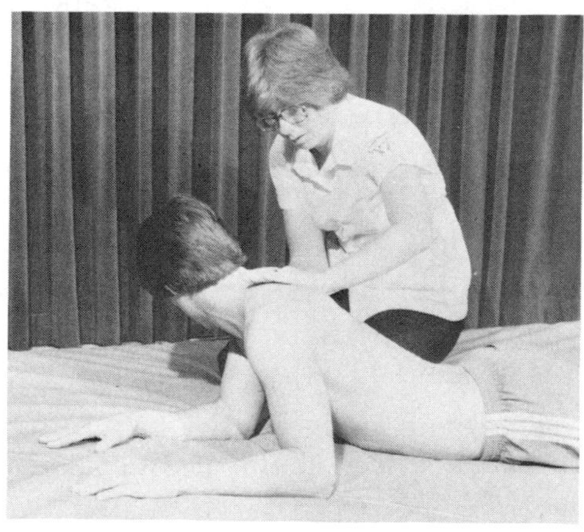

(a)

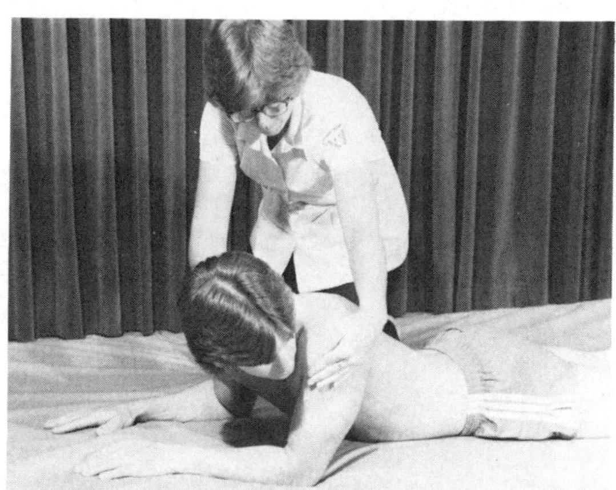

(b)

A. Prone on elbows: head rotation, lateral shifting.
T. SR, SRH.
E. MC scapula.

FIGURE 3–40

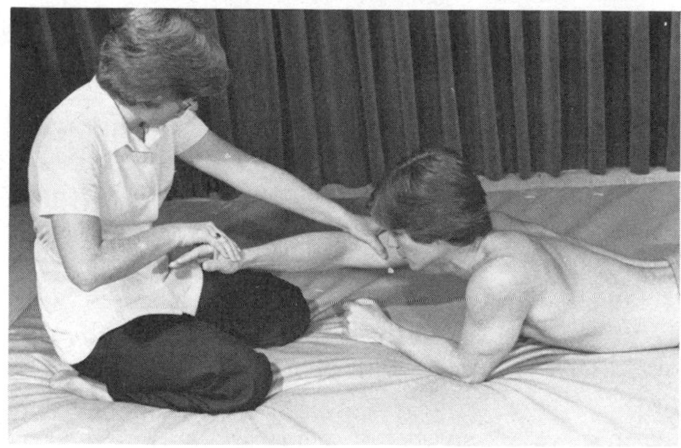

A. Prone on elbows: D_1 thrust.
E. MC hand and arm of dynamic limb (or hand of dynamic limb and scapula of static limb).

FIGURE 3–41

In summary:

- The prone-on-elbows posture has a large B of S and low C of G. The head, neck, scapula, and shoulder joints are directly affected by gravitational resistance in this posture.
- Tonic reflex influence may be evident in some patients. Varying head position while maintaining a constant UE posture may help to integrate tonic reflexes. Righting reactions will help to maintain the head position. Higher level reflexes are not essential to maintaining this posture.
- The scapula and shoulder muscles previously shortened in pivot prone are positioned on stretch and thus may facilitate cocontraction.
- The approximation force through the elbows may increase activity of the tonic muscles and deep rotators and can be further enhanced by manual approximation to the shoulders.
- Stability, controlled mobility, and static-dynamic control can be developed when the shoulder is in about 45 degrees of flexion.
- The lower extremities are positioned in mass extension, which may be appropriate for some patients; for others, the position may be modified by flexing the knee.
- Lower extremity patterns of movement can be used specifically to emphasize knee control.
- If prone on elbows is too difficult to attain, a modified position in sitting or modified plantigrade may be substituted to improve proximal control.

Prone on hands is a posture observed in the course of normal development, but it is not commonly used for adult patients because it creates increased hyperextension of the low back.

3. **Quadruped.** Developmentally, the quadruped posture follows the prone-on-elbows position (28) (see Figure 3–42). Compared with prone on elbows, quadruped has a smaller B of S, higher C of G, and involves more joints, specifically the elbow, wrist, hand, lower trunk, hip, and knee joints.

As in prone on elbows, flexor tone may be increased in quadruped owing to the influence of the STLR. The increased stress of the posture may cause the effects of any tonic reflexes to be more pronounced. Because the B of S is decreased and the C of G is raised, equilibrium, proprioceptive, and protective extensor reactions are necessary for the patient to maintain and move within the quadruped posture.

Maintenance of the posture is resisted by the effects of gravity. The extensors of the upper trunk are stretched more than in prone on elbows, and because the upper extremities support more body weight, there is more resistance to the postural muscles. The elbow and wrist extensors, holding in the shortened range, support more weight than in sitting, where they hold in a similar range. The extensors of the lower trunk, hip, and knee are now on a prolonged stretch and weight bearing occurs through the hip, which should promote cocontraction (13, 32). Activity in the abdominals, important in maintaining the posture, may be facilitated by the stretch on the extensors.

The hand and finger flexors are maintained in contact with the supporting surface. Prolonged pressure on the long flexor tendons can decrease flexor tone, an important consideration for patients with spasticity in those muscle groups (13). Weight bearing also occurs on the patella tendon and may increase inhibitory influences to the quadriceps (15) (see Chapter 5). The position of the lower extremity is in mass flexion. Movements of the lower extremity in this posture are most easily performed in either a mass flexor or extensor pattern.

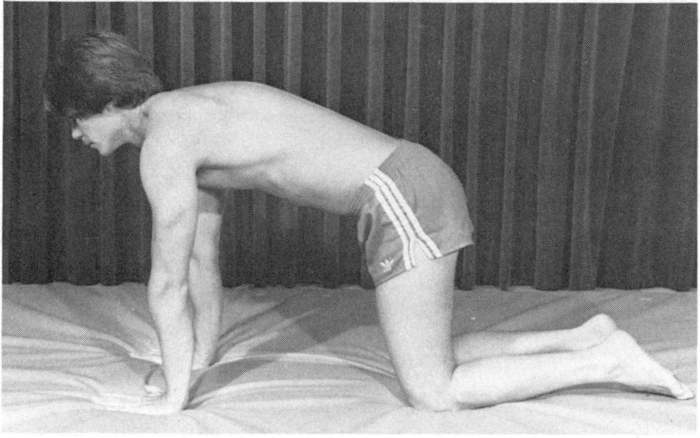

A. Quadruped.

FIGURE 3–42

Stages of Motor Control. Cocontraction can be enhanced at various segments by altering manual contacts from the head to the scapula or pelvis (Figure 3–43). The areas of emphasis will depend on the specific problem.

Controlled mobility—rocking through increments of range—will enhance equilibrium and proprioceptive reactions and will increase range at all the proximal and weight-bearing joints. Rocking also influences proximal muscle tone: rocking backward enhances flexor tone, while rocking forward enhances extensor tone. Rocking performed in lateral and diagonal direc-

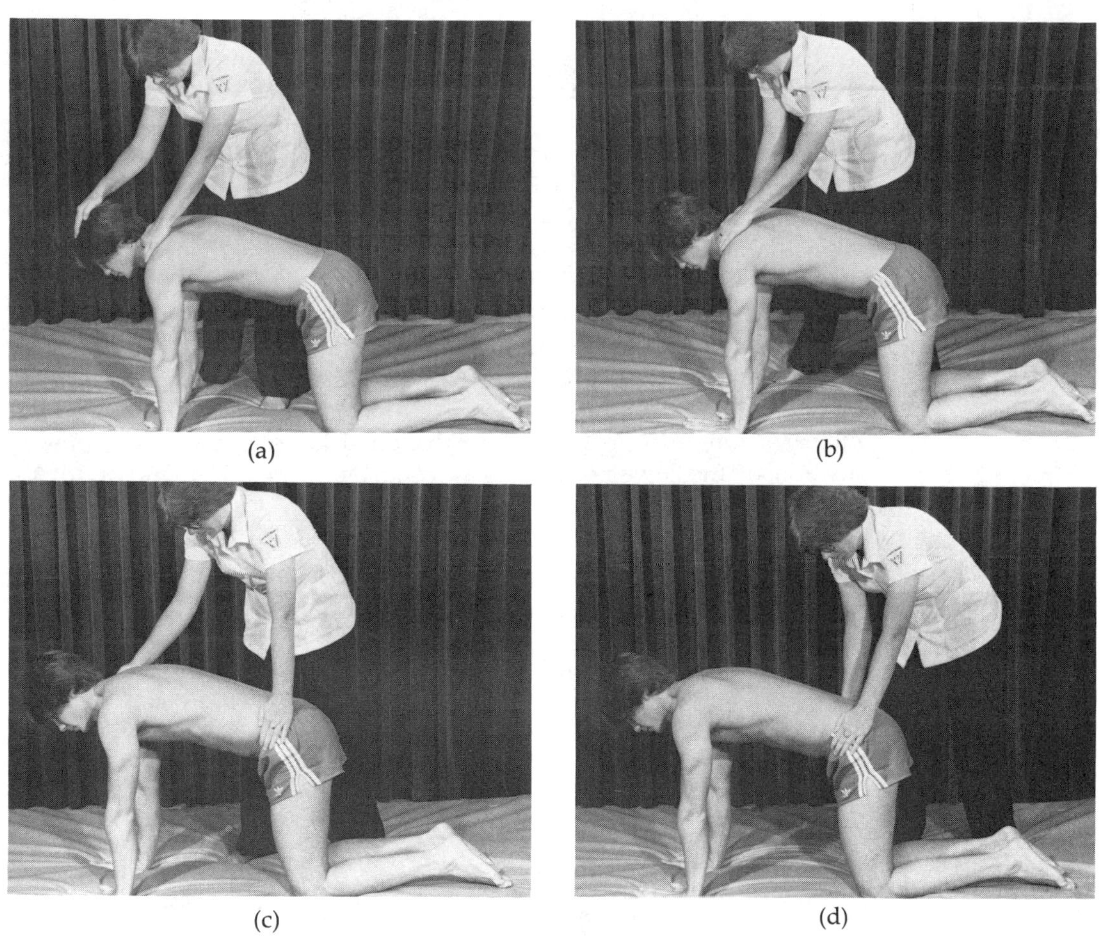

(a) (b) (c) (d)

A. Quadruped.
E. MC head and scapula, scapula, scapula and pelvis, pelvis.

FIGURE 3–43

(a)

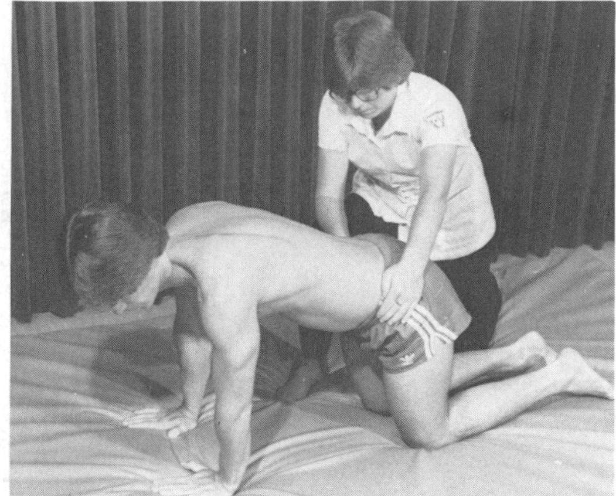

(b)

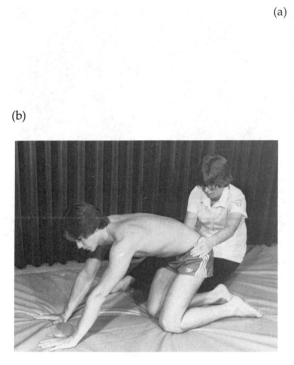

A. Quadruped: diagonal rocking.
T. SR, SRH.
E. MC pelvis.

FIGURE 3–44

tions increases range in specific movements and alters the amount of weight bearing on the extremities (13, 17) (see Figure 3–44). Rocking forward and backward results in alternate weight bearing on the upper and then the lower extremities and simultaneously increases the range of the extension and flexion motions; rocking side to side produces alternate weight bearing on the right and left limbs and promotes abduction and adduction; movement in a diagonal direction incorporates rotation with movements in both the frontal and saggital planes so that diagonal patterns of both upper and lower extremities are elicited. Rocking forward toward the right, for example, results in D_2 extensor patterns of the right upper and lower limbs and D_1 extensor patterns of the left limbs.

Static-dynamic activities of both the upper (Figure 3–45) and lower extremities (Figure 3–46) can increase the dynamic stability of the trunk and supporting extremities as well as strengthen the dynamic limb. While indicated for many patients, these activities can be particularly useful for scoliotic patients who need extension or flexion with rotation or lateral bending. Upper extremity movements can be performed to emphasize upper trunk motions while lower extremity patterns can be used specifically to facilitate lumbar movements.

Creeping is the skill level of control in this posture (Figure 3–47). As in all activities, the quality of the movement should be noted. A contralateral combination of extremity movements that incorporates trunk rotation is the desired sequence of movements.

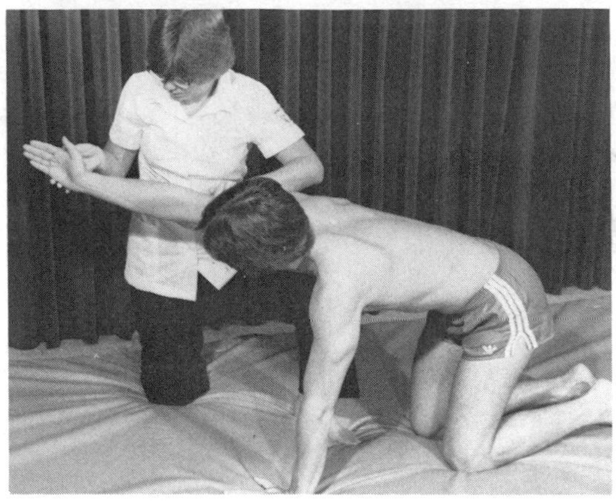

(a)

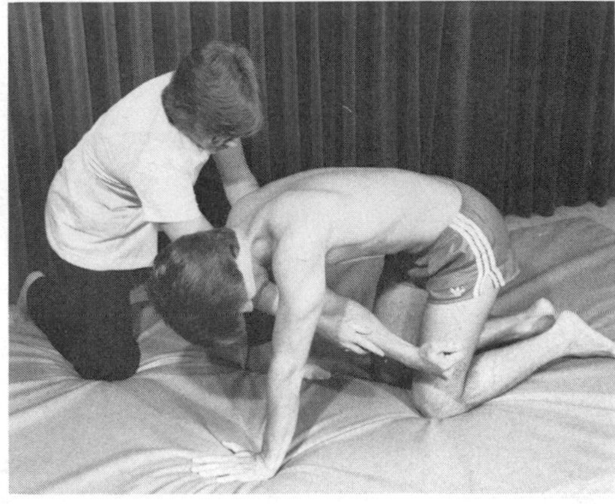

(b)

A. Quadruped: D_2 UE.
T. SR, SRH.
E. MC arm and shoulder.

FIGURE 3–45

Clinical Implications. The clinical implications will be discussed in a cephalocaudal direction. The effects on the head are similar to those in prone on elbows. The scapula retractors are in a more lengthened position compared with prone on elbows and the shoulders are in about 90 degrees of flexion. Patients with shoulder disability frequently have difficulty with muscular control in this 90-degree range. Facilitation of the deep rotators and postural muscles by the compression force of weight bearing can help to promote control in this range. The elbow and wrist extensors, as we have noted, contract isometrically in their shortened range and thus promote stretch sensitivity of the muscle spindles, which is an important consideration if those muscles are weak or if the antagonistic flexors are spastic.

Cocontraction may be developed in the lower trunk and hips by the prolonged stretch placed on the extensor muscles in the posture. The trunk flexors are facilitated not only by the stretch but also by the resistance of gravity as they contract to maintain the trunk alignment. Cocontraction and particularly facilitation of the lower abdominal muscles are often important goals for patients with low back problems. The maintained stretch on the back extensors may also reduce any tightness present in those muscles. If a patient is unable to maintain quadruped because of a lack of proximal stability, the stretch sensitivity of the tonic postural muscles may need to be increased in pivot prone or in modified pivot prone postures.

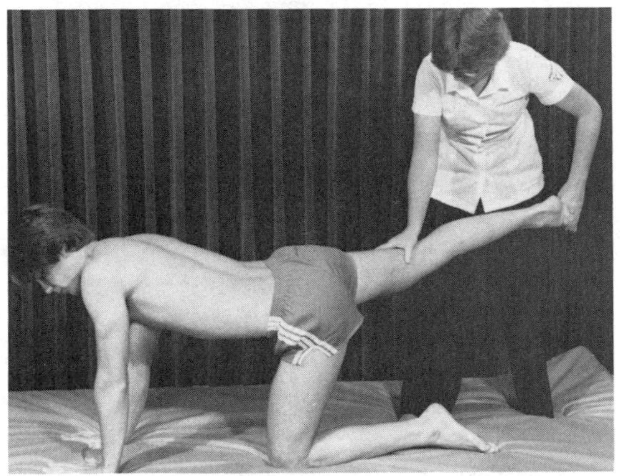

(a)

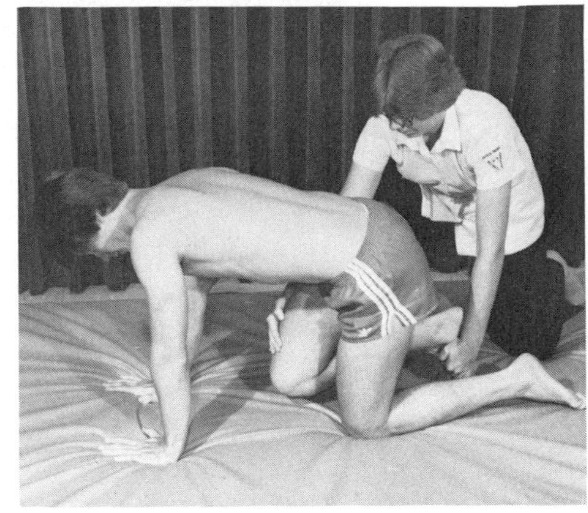

(b)

A. Quadruped: D_1 LE.
T. SR, SRH.
E. MC thigh and foot.

FIGURE 3–46

The inhibitory influences occurring as a result of pressure on the patella tendon and maintained stretch to the quadriceps may be indicated for patients who have a dominance of extensor tone. In contrast, for a patient with quadriceps weakness the inhibitory influence produced by this posture may not be consistent with the goal of increasing quadriceps strength during initial treatment sessions. If one of the goals of treatment is to increase tone of hip, knee, or ankle flexors, a mass flexor pattern performed with gravity assistance and manual resistance might be helpful.

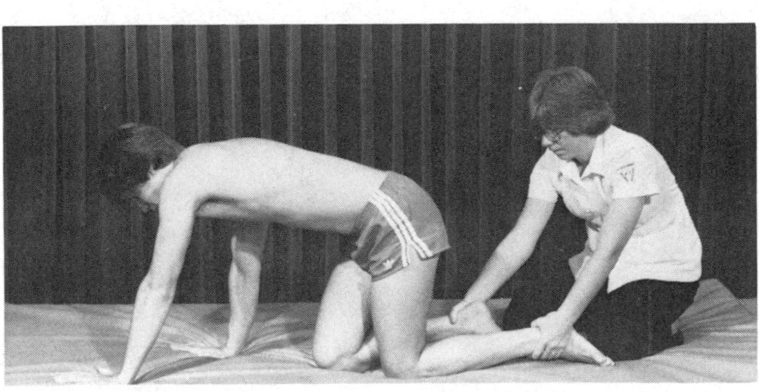

A. Creeping.
T. RP.
E. MC feet.

FIGURE 3–47

In summary, the quadruped position compared with prone on elbows has the following characteristics:

- The B of S is smaller, the C of G higher, and more upper extremity, trunk, and lower extremity joints are involved in quadruped.
- The changes in joint position in quadruped alter the ranges in which the muscles contract.
- The reflex influences are similar in both positions but because the biomechanical factors have been altered in quadruped, higher level reactions are required to maintain this posture.
- Because more joints are involved, quadruped is more useful for a greater variety of patient problems.

Lower Trunk Progression

The postures that constitute lower trunk progression are: lower trunk rotation, bridging, kneeling, and half-kneeling. A tonic holding procedure should precede any of these lower trunk activities.

1. Lower Trunk Rotation. This supine activity (Figure 3–48) has a large B of S and a low C of G. The lower extremities are directly involved, whereas the upper trunk and upper extremities are only indirectly involved as stabilizers.

Extensor tone in the supine posture may be increased because of the influence of the STLR. Because the entire foot is in contact with the support-

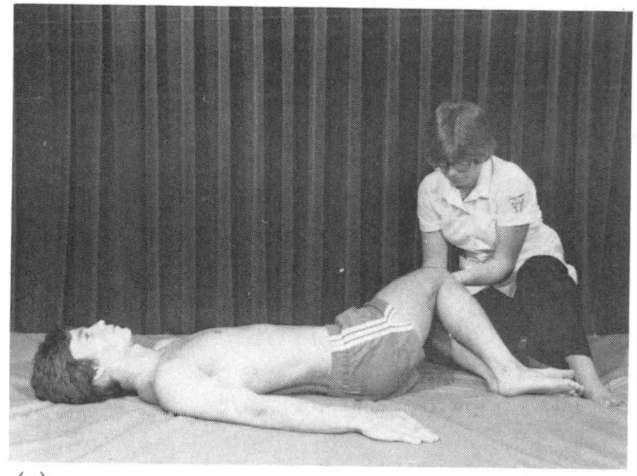

(a)

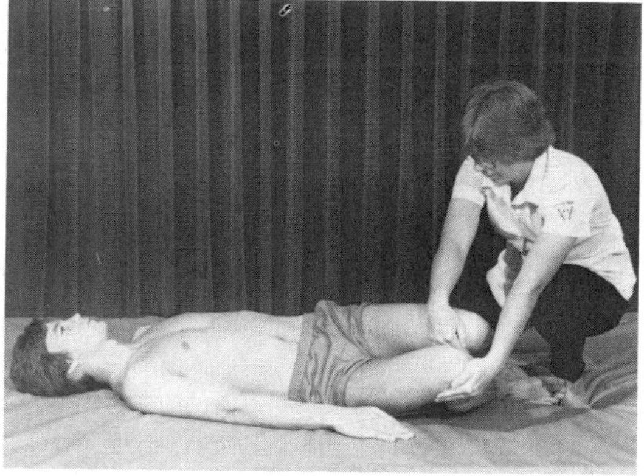

(b)

A. LTR.
E. MC knees.

FIGURE 3–48

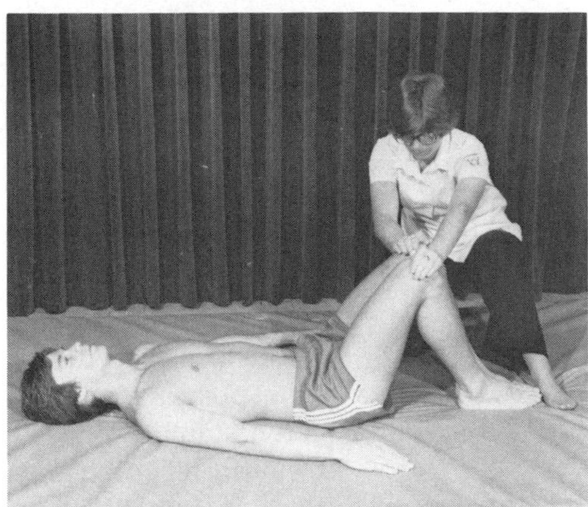

A. LTR: midline position
E. MC knees.

FIGURE 3–49

ing surface, the extensor tone in the lower extremities may be further enhanced through the effects of the positive supporting reaction. To reduce this extensor influence, flexion of the hips and knees can be increased and the foot position altered so that weight bearing occurs primarily through the heel. The therapist may need to support the feet if the patient has difficulty maintaining the posture.

The activity of lower trunk rotation (LTR) can be divided into a flexor and extensor phase (17, 34) and in a modified form incorporates the diagonal patterns of the lower extremities. As the knees move against gravity from the lengthened range toward the midline (Figure 3–49), the leading or abducting leg flexes in D_2 and the adducting limb follows in D_1. Once the knees cross the midline, gravity assists the movement. When manual resistance is provided, the abducting leg extends in a D_1 pattern and the adducting limb extends in D_2. Because of the variation in gravitational resistance, the manual resistance provided by the therapist must also be altered during the two phases. During the flexor phase of the activity the lower abdominals—the internal obliques—are highly active, and during the extensor phase the lower back extensors are most active.

Clinical Implications and Stages of Motor Control. Patients with imbalances of tone can benefit from the reversal of antagonists that occurs during the flexor and extensor phases of the movement. In addition, crossing of the midline by the lower extremities facilitates interaction of the two sides of the body, which is specifically indicated for patients experiencing perceptual deficits or unilateral neglect.

The mobility phase of motor control indicates that the patient has the strength to initiate the pattern and full ROM to complete the movement. LTR together with the mobility techniques of rhythmical rotation or rhythmical initiation (see Chapter 4) is an appropriate procedure to increase ROM in the low back and hips when either spasticity or rigidity limit movement.

The posture of the entire body should be constantly monitored, especially in the upper trunk and upper extremities. Associated reactions in the upper extremities may occur if an activity attempted in the lower extremities is too stressful (7). Patients with trunk rigidity may have difficulty isolating movements of the lower trunk and may tend to rotate the trunk as a unit. If total trunk movement occurs, LTR should be applied through small ranges that can be increased gradually as relaxation becomes evident. To initiate movement in patients with hypotonia, the technique of hold-relax-active-movement (HRAM) is appropriate (35) (see Chapter 4).

A stretch is placed on the lower trunk, hip, and knee extensors in the hooklying posture, which may in itself facilitate cocontraction. Cocontraction or the stability phase of control can be further promoted by means of the isometric techniques of AI and RS. AI (Figure 3–50) produces greater amounts of alternating muscular activity, particularly in the lower abdominals and lower back extensors, whereas RS (Figure 3–51) produces less muscular activity but enhances cocontraction of the muscles. Isometric strengthening of these lower trunk muscle groups may be most appropriate for patients with weakness around the low back area. The stability gained in this usually nonstressful posture may be a precursor of the stability needed by some patients in the higher level activities of sitting and quadruped.

The stability procedures in hooklying can be made more difficult by changing the angle of hip and knee flexion and by moving the manual contacts one joint more distally to the ankles. As the lower extremities move further into extension, the challenge to patients with extensor spasticity is

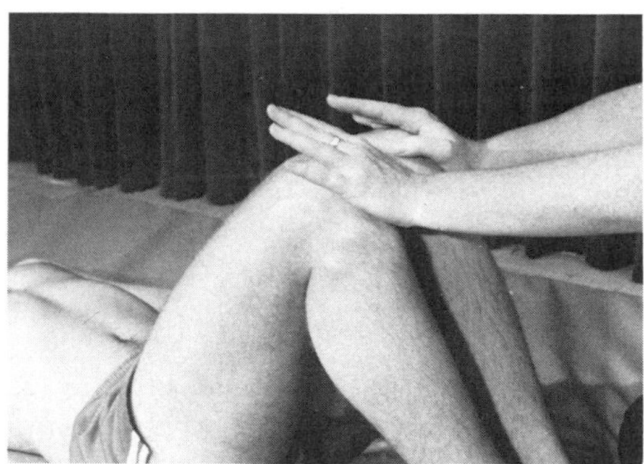

A. Hooklying.
T. AI.
E. MC knees.

FIGURE 3–50

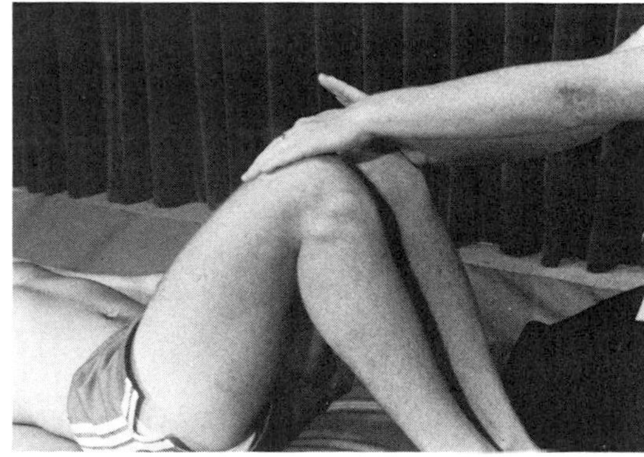

A. Hooklying.
T. RS.
E. MC knees (fingers should remain in contact with the knees).

FIGURE 3–51

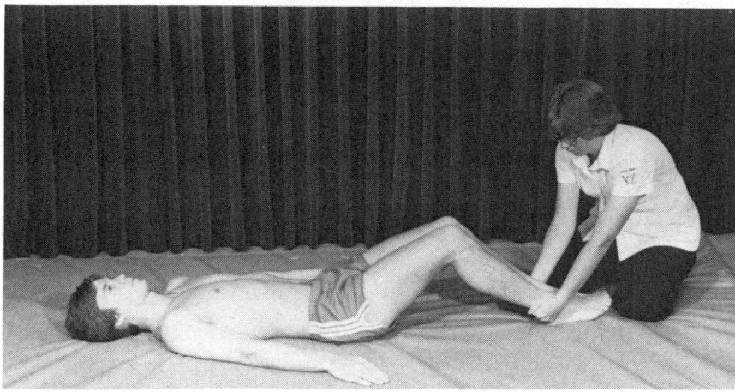

A. Hooklying: knees in further extension.
E. MC ankles.

FIGURE 3–52

increased. As the maintained stretch on the quadriceps is lessened, the inhibitory influences of the secondary endings may also decrease. For a spastic quadriceps such a reduction in angle may increase the tendency for a spastic response when the quadriceps contracts. Conversely, patients having weak quadriceps may find that holding with the knees in a more extended position against resistance is less difficult than in the flexed position. Resistive force applied on the ankles with manual contacts will most directly affect the activity of the knee and ankle musculature (Figure 3–52).

Emphasis in treatment on the controlled mobility level of motor control will promote a smooth reversal of antagonists of lower trunk and extremity musculature and segmental lower trunk rotation. Techniques can be applied during the different phases of the movement to strengthen either the trunk or hip muscles. When the patient can hold the extremities in the shortened range of the extensor phase against manual resistance and simultaneously begin to raise the hip from the supporting surface, then the patient can progress to the next activity—bridging.

In summary:

- LTR can be utilized to increase ROM in the lower trunk when muscle tightness, spasticity, or rigidity limit motion.
- LTR promotes crossing of the midline of the lower extremities and a reversal of antagonists of lower trunk and lower extremity musculature.
- LTR increases both isometric and isotonic activity of the lower trunk and lower extremity muscles.

2. **Bridging.** This posture (Figure 3–53) is a common progression from LTR, and will be compared to that activity in this section. The hips are elevated over the supporting surface and thus create a higher C of G and smaller B of S; the patient needs control of balance reactions to maintain or move within the posture. Because the lower extremities are now in a weight-bearing position, more joints are involved. Extensor tone may be increased in these two supine activities of LTR and bridging owing to the influence of the STLR. In bridging, both the low back and hip extensors isometrically contract in their shortened range against the resistance of gravity and thereby increase the muscle spindle stretch sensitivity of these postural muscles. Extensor tone in the upper trunk and upper extremities may also be enhanced as these muscles continue to perform a stabilizing function. The quadriceps remain on a prolonged stretch at the knee, causing inhibitory influences to increase. The leg is now in an advanced combination of hip extension and knee flexion.

Clinical Implications and Stages of Motor Control. Bridging is a functional activity that can be used to improve bed mobility, bed pan use, and, for some patients, dressing. Although these functional implications are important for many patients, the therapeutic indications of the posture need to be considered. Most importantly, bridging activities can be used to enhance the control needed for the stance phase of gait (33). Many of the determinants of gait (36)—including pelvic forward motion; pelvic lateral shift; pelvic rotation; advanced lower extremity combination of hip extension with knee flexion; and variations in ROM at the knee and ankle—can be either initiated or reinforced in this posture. These components of gait can be emphasized individually or in combination with one another. First they are promoted by means of the isometric techniques of AI and RS for the purpose of stability, and then by means of isotonic techniques such as slow reversal hold (SRH) for controlled mobility. Pelvic forward motion is promoted when the posture is assumed. The forward control can be further enhanced if the technique AI is applied with resistance in a sagittal plane. Rotation is also first promoted isometrically, then with isotonic motions (Figure 3–54). AI applied in a frontal plane is preliminary to lateral weight shifting, which can be promoted with SRH (Figure 3–55). Pelvic shifting should be emphasized and total trunk movements discouraged during this activity. These three pelvic motions—forward control, rotation, and lateral shift—are finally combined with the isometric technique of RS before movement through range is promoted to simulate the pelvic motions occurring during weight acceptance in gait. Eccentric control, which is a necessary component of gait, can be promoted by the technique of agonistic reversals (AR), during which the patient slowly alternates between concentric contractions of hip extensors against manual resistance and eccentric contractions of these same muscles against the slowly applied downward resistance of the therapist. The eccentric control of the extensors promoted in bridging will improve the patient's ability to sit from a standing position.

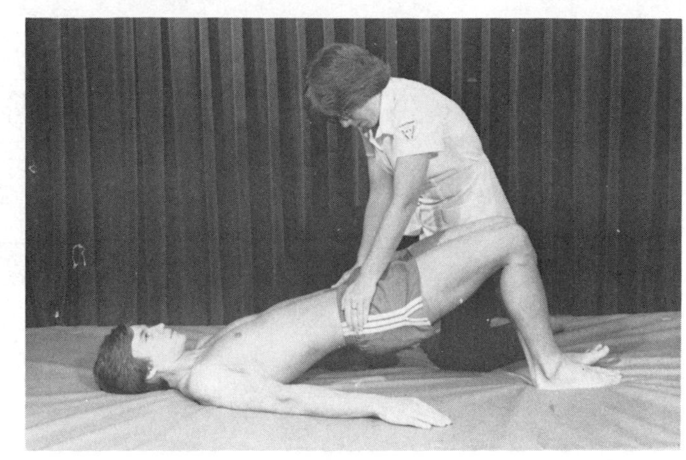

A. Bridging.
E. MC pelvis.

FIGURE 3–53

A. Bridging: pelvic rotation.
T. AI, SRH.
E. MC pelvis.

FIGURE 3–54

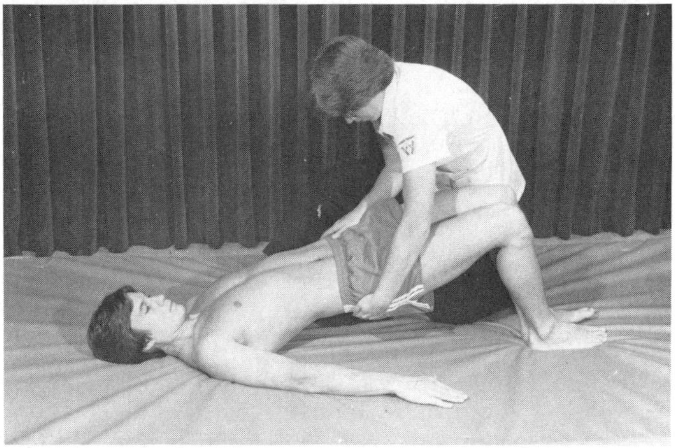

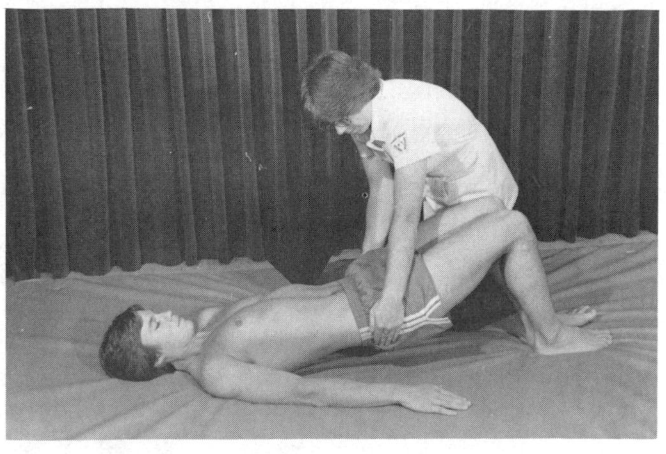

A. Bridging: lateral shifting.
T. AI, SRH.
E. MC pelvis (lateral aspect).

FIGURE 3–55

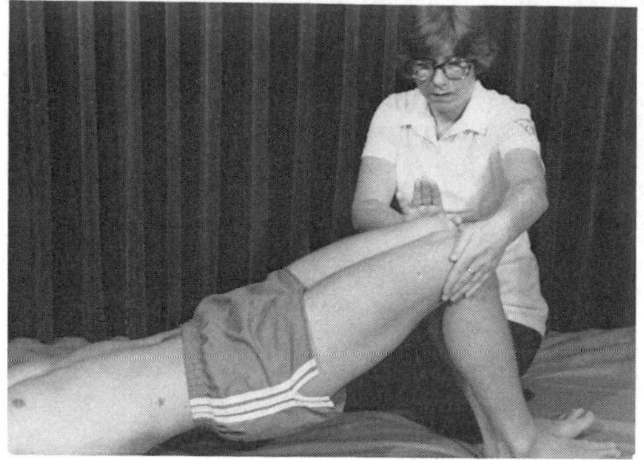

A. Bridging: symmetrical abduction and adduction.
T. AI.
E. MC knees.

FIGURE 3–56

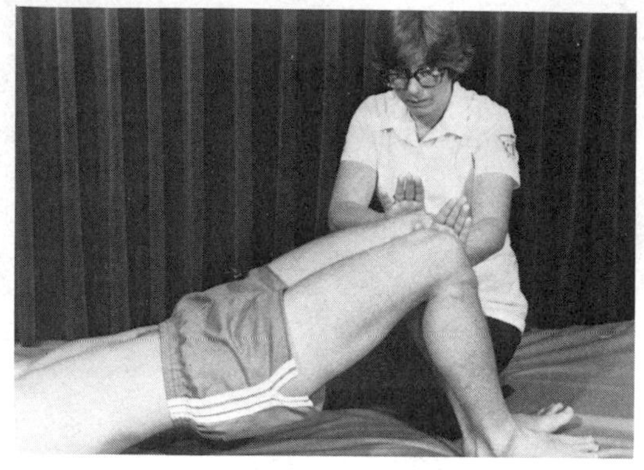

A. Bridging: asymmetrical abduction and adduction.
T. AI.
E. MC knees.

FIGURE 3–57

The demands of the procedure can be varied by altering the manual contacts from the pelvis to the knees and then to the ankles. The resistive force of manual contacts on the knees can facilitate hip abduction and adduction symmetrically (Figure 3–56) or asymmetrically (Figure 3–57). Isometric resistance can also be given in a diagonal direction to enhance quadriceps and hamstring activity. Stability is achieved by means of isometric contractions and controlled mobility is accomplished by means of resisted isotonic movements through range. Lateral weight shifting improves eversion-inversion movements at the ankle. The activity of the knee musculature is further facilitated when resistance is applied in a symmetrical or reciprocal direction with the manual contacts placed at the ankles (Figure 3–58).

As in the case of LTR, the bridging activity can be modified by changing the base of support. This change in the B of S can be accomplished by decreasing the angle of knee flexion, weight bearing on elbows (Figure 3–59) or hands, or by performing static-dynamic activities. These adaptations of the posture provide a more difficult challenge that requires greater upper trunk and upper extremity control. Single-limb lower extremity support will increase the demands on the weight-bearing limb and simulate the control needed during the stance phase of gait. When the activity is made more difficult by decreasing the B of S, the techniques and the placement of manual contacts may have to be modified to ensure that the total procedure will not be too stressful. These changes in the bridging activity are especially useful for younger patients or athletes when increased difficulty during mat exercises is indicated.

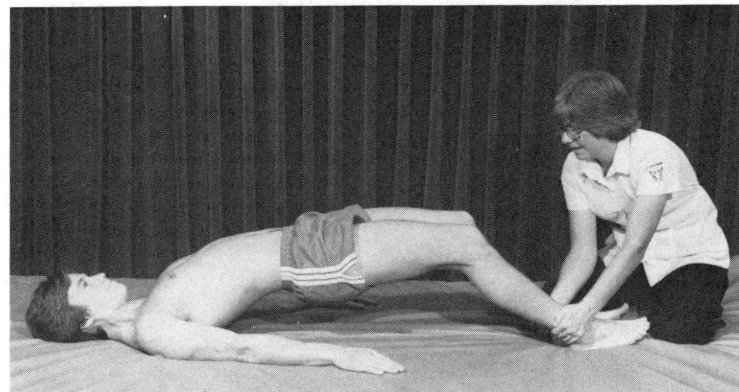

A. Bridging: knees extended.
T. AI.
E. MC ankles.

FIGURE 3–58

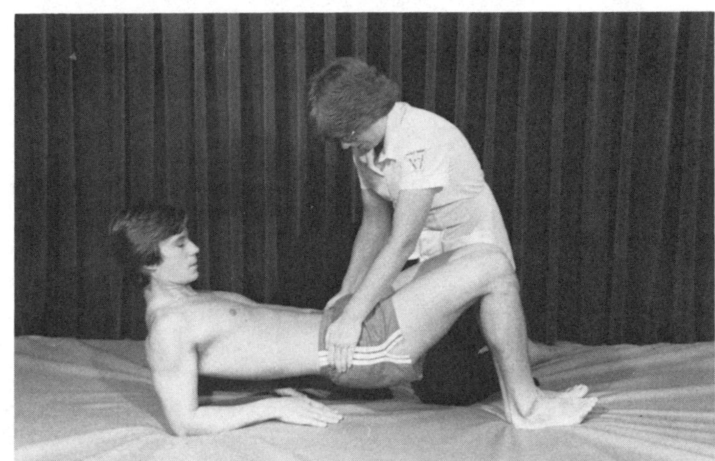

A. Bridging: on elbows.
E. MC pelvis.

FIGURE 3–59

In summary:

- The bridging position may be incorporated into a patient's program whenever improved lower trunk or lower extremity control is needed.
- The B of S is large and C of G low. Both can be altered to increase the level of difficulty of the activity.
- Many of the determinants of gait can be promoted with the lower extremity weight bearing in the advanced combination of hip extension with knee flexion.
- Emphasis can be placed on all of the joints of the lower extremity by altering the placement of manual contacts.

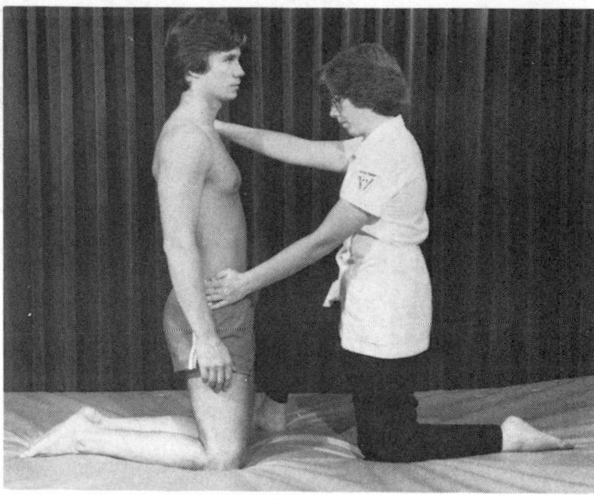

A. Kneeling.
T. RS.
E. MC scapula and pelvis.

FIGURE 3–60

3. **Kneeling.** The kneeling posture (Figure 3–60) has been described as upright bridging (17). In both activities the lower extremity is in an advanced combination of hip extension with knee flexion. In addition, both can enhance lower trunk and pelvic control. The two activities differ, however, in the parameters influencing their performance.

In contrast to bridging, kneeling is characterized by a reduction in the B of S that is beneath and posterior to the C of G. Balance can be easily disturbed anteriorly because of the decreased B of S in that direction, and thus kneeling can be a difficult activity for some patients. The C of G is higher in kneeling than in bridging and more upper trunk control is needed to maintain the posture. Because of the upright position, STLR has little effect on muscle tone in kneeling. The alteration of biomechanical factors necessitates integrity of higher level reactions to maintain and move within the posture. Instead of being on the feet, weight bearing is on the knees. As in bridging, the quadriceps are on a prolonged stretch at the knee and hip. In kneeling, however, the weight bearing that occurs on the quadriceps tendon may further increase the inhibitory influences to that muscle (15). The shortening of the hamstrings at both the hip and knee joints results in active insufficiency. In this shortened position the hamstrings contract in a tonic postural manner to keep the hip in extension and to help prevent the patient from falling forward. Patients with decreased hamstring and hip extensor tone may find this posture difficult, if not impossible, to maintain.

When the kneeling position is assumed from heelsitting, there is an initial flexor phase as the upper trunk moves forward; then an extensor phase of the trunk and hip complete the motion. The flexor phase can be enhanced by the trunk pattern of a chop (Figure 3–61) and the extensor phase by a lift (Figure 3–62). The choice of patterns depends on the patient's deficit and the desired goal.

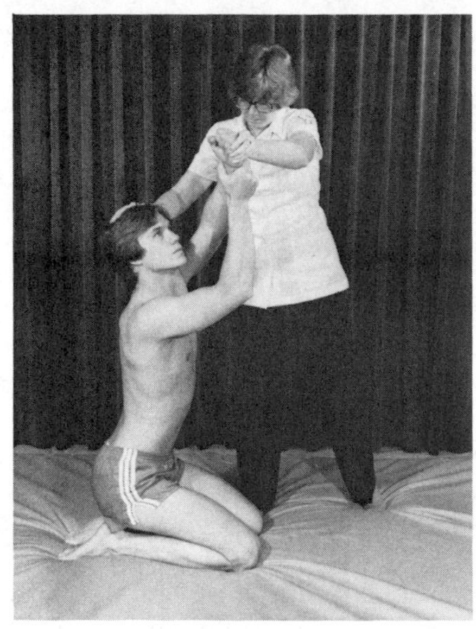

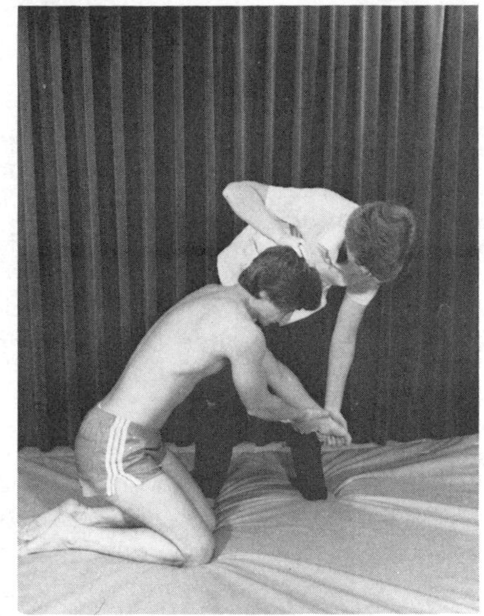

(a) (b)

A. Kneeling with a chop.
T. Assumption of posture.
E. MC head and wrist.

FIGURE 3–61

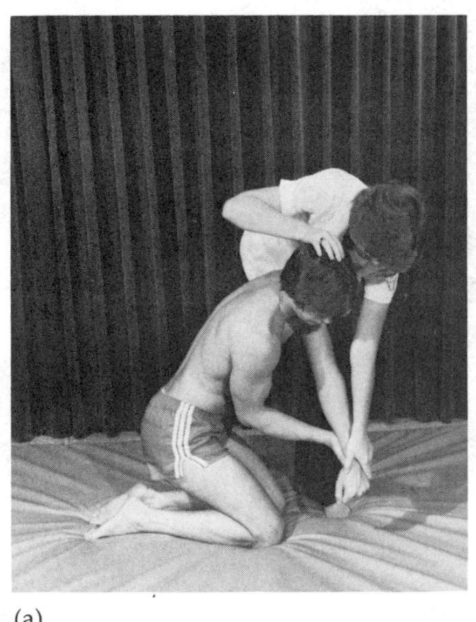

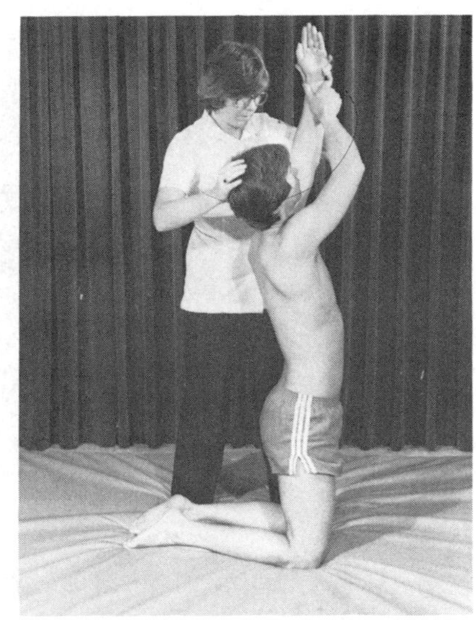

(a) (b)

A. Kneeling with a lift.
T. Assumption of posture.
E. MC head and wrist.

FIGURE 3–62

Clinical Implications and Stages of Motor Control. The increased inhibitory influence to the quadriceps, the lack of pressure on the ball of the foot, and the reduced influence of the STLR may make kneeling a less difficult activity than bridging for a patient with increased extensor tone of the lower extremities. In contrast, if quadriceps weakness is the problem, these influences may conflict with the goal of strengthening. When increased quadriceps activity is the goal, the kneeling activity should be used only during the later phases of rehabilitation. If sufficient quadriceps tone is first achieved, the danger of inhibitory influence predomination may not be as great.

Stability can be enhanced at the pelvis and in the entire trunk by altering the placement of manual contacts. Resistance, especially when applied in the forward direction, must be carefully graded to reduce the possibility of disturbing balance.

As in bridging, controlled mobility activities can emphasize the pelvic motions needed during gait, including pelvic forward motion, lateral shift, and rotation (Figure 3–63). Because the upper trunk is not stabilized in this posture, many patients tend to substitute total trunk movements for individual pelvic motions, particularly if trunk rigidity or spasticity is present. If the goal of the procedure is to isolate lower trunk motion, trunk substitution should be discouraged, especially during the lateral shift and rota-

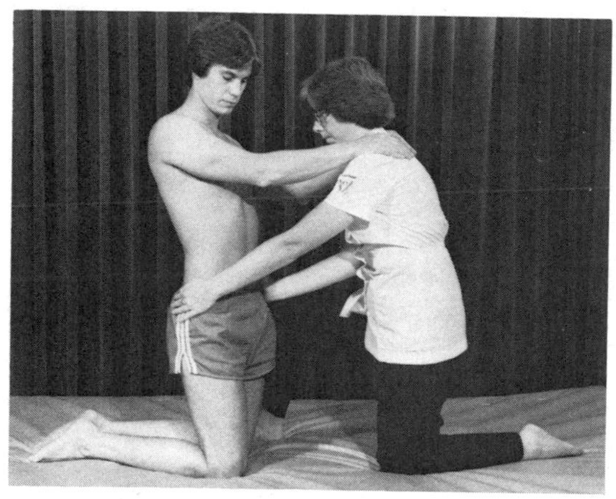

(a)

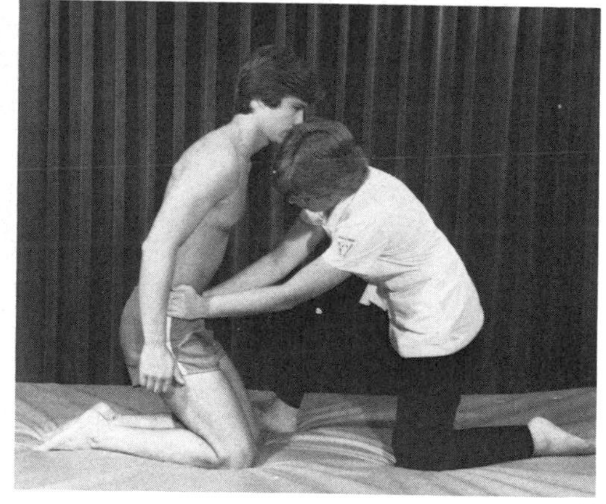

(b)

A. Kneeling: pelvic movements.
T. SRH.
E. MC pelvis.

FIGURE 3–63

tional movements. Positioning the patient's arms on the therapist's shoulders will enhance stabilization of the upper trunk and allow the patient to initiate the appropriate pelvic movements more easily. Independent assumption of the posture—a controlled mobility level of motor control—may be accomplished with the trunk patterns of a chop or a lift, as described earlier. The patient's ability to move from kneeling to heelsitting can be increased by the technique of agonistic reversals, which promotes eccentric and concentric contractions of the lower trunk, hip, and knee extensor muscles. The eccentric control that is promoted in the hip and especially in the knee extensors will improve the patient's ability to perform other activities such as descending stairs or moving from standing to sitting. Like many controlled mobility procedures, the excursion of movement is gradually increased as control is developed.

Unilateral weight bearing is a static-dynamic activity, and kneewalking is the skill level of control.

In summary:

- The activity of kneeling requires control of equilibrium and other high level reactions because the B of S is beneath and posterior to the C of G.
- The quadriceps are on a prolonged stretch and weight bearing occurs on the patella tendon.
- The hamstrings are in a position of active insufficiency while acting tonically to support this posture.
- Lower trunk pelvic and hip control can be achieved by progressing through the stages of motor control.

4. **Half-kneeling.** The posture that is a progression from kneeling is half-kneeling (17) (see Figure 3–64). In this position, the height of the C of G remains the same as in kneeling but the B of S is altered. The base of support is now anterior and posterior, but only in one diagonal direction. The anterior lower extremity is now weight bearing through the foot, while the posterior leg remains weight bearing on the knee.

The reflex influences are almost the same as during kneeling. The altered B of S requires less equilibrium control in the anterior posterior direction but more control laterally.

The factors influencing the posterior lower extremity are the same as those in kneeling; more weight is now borne through the posterior supporting limb, however, so that half-kneeling is more challenging in preparing for the stance phase of gait. The hips are in a reciprocal position, the posterior supporting limb is in an advanced combination of hip extension with knee flexion, and the anterior lower extremity is in mass flexion. The quadriceps in this forward limb are still on a prolonged stretch, but the inhibitory influence of weight bearing on the tendon is eliminated.

Clinical Implications and Stages of Motor Control. Half-kneeling is an important functional activity in the sequence of assuming standing from the prone position. The application of stability techniques will further enhance the control needed at the extended supporting hip. Manual contacts can be placed on the trunk, pelvis, or the forward knee.

Controlled mobility procedures can emphasize range of motion at the hips, knees, and the supporting forward ankle (Figure 3–65). Patients who have pain when bearing weight on the knee may find this activity less stressful when their involved lower extremity is flexed forward so that weight bearing is on the foot. The focus of the weight shifting in this posture can be directed toward the movement of the ankle. Dorsiflexion can be enhanced by forward rocking, which emphasizes flexion of the tibia over the fixed talus. Because the knee is flexed, dorsiflexion will not be limited by any tightness that may be present in the gastrocnemius. When rocking

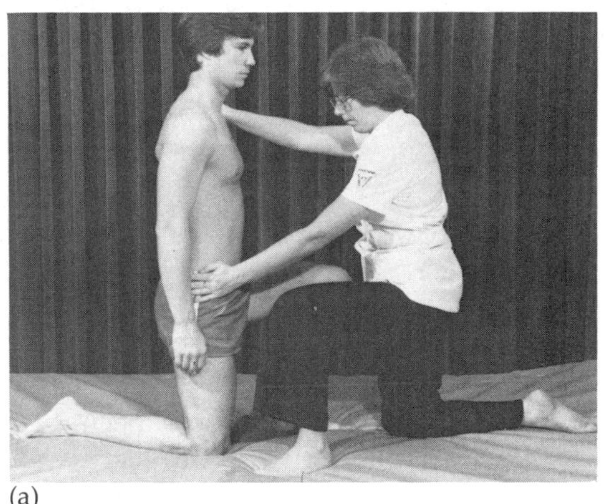
(a)

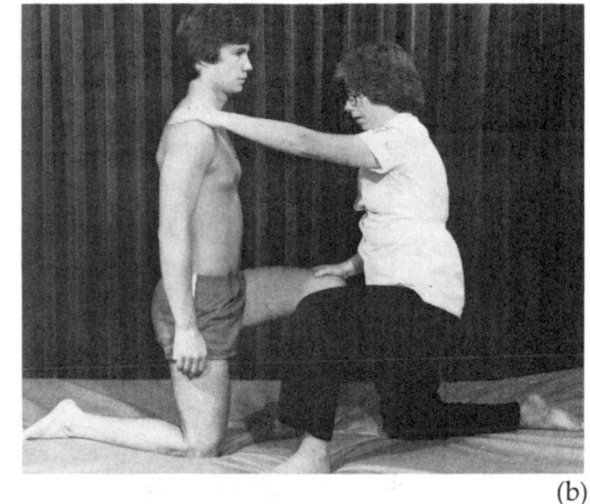
(b)

(c)
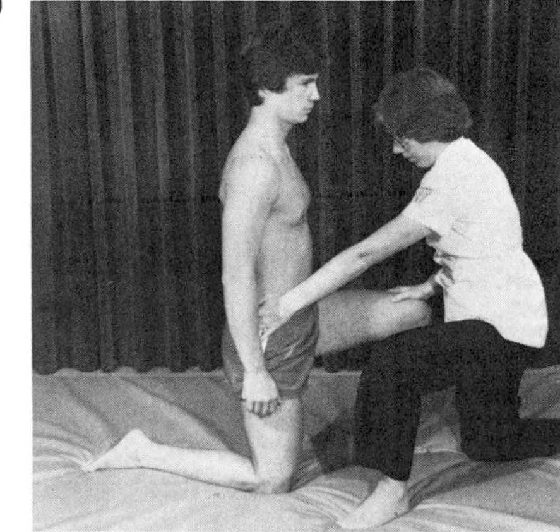

A. Half-kneeling.
T. RS.
E. MC shoulder and pelvis, shoulder and knee, pelvis and knee.

FIGURE 3–64

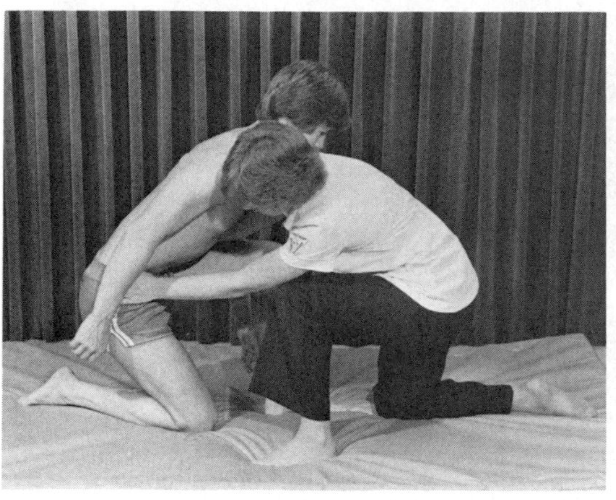

(a)

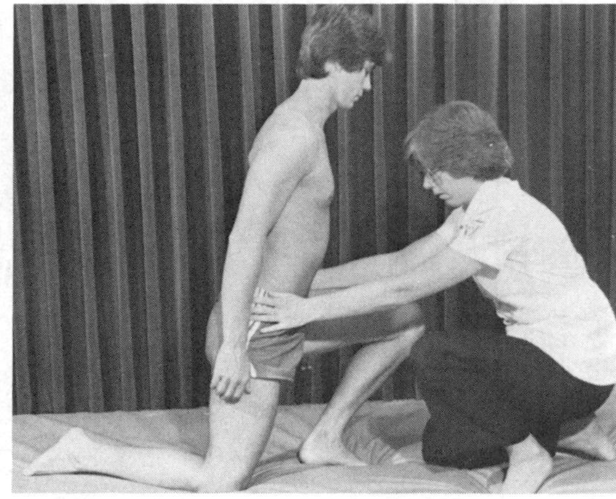

(b)

FIGURE 3–65

A. Half-kneeling: rocking.
T. SR.
E. MC pelvis.

is performed in half-kneeling, the upper trunk should be allowed to flex as the patient rocks backward to maintain the C of G near the B of S. Such trunk movement will reduce the stress of this controlled mobility activity.

■ Advanced Upright Progression

1. Modified Plantigrade. Modified plantigrade (Figure 3–66) frequently precedes standing and walking (33). The lower extremities are weight bearing through all the joints. Because the B of S is small and the C of G high, control over equilibrium and proprioceptive reactions is required. The upper extremities are weight bearing and there is approximately 30–60 degrees of shoulder flexion; this weight bearing increases the B of S and also promotes upper extremity control. The lower extremity is in the advanced position of hip flexion, knee extension, and ankle dorsiflexion; thus the quadriceps are put in the shortened range and the gastrocnemius and soleus on a prolonged stretch.

Stages of Motor Control. As in other postures, stability techniques can be applied in modified plantigrade to emphasize various segments. The placement of manual contacts may be altered and manual approximation applied to the shoulders and pelvis to enhance the stability of both the upper and lower extremity musculature (Figure 3–67).

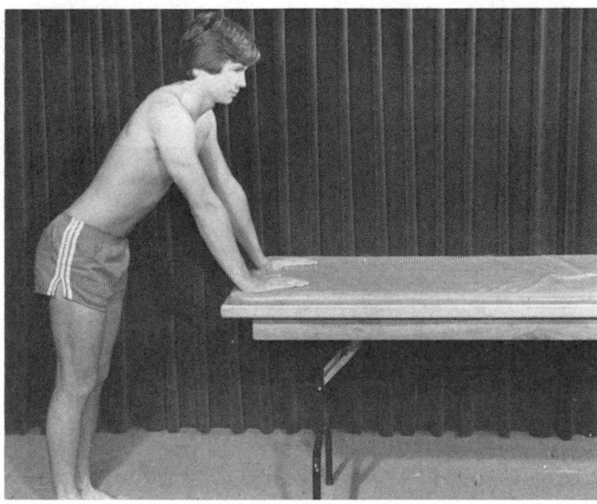

A. Modified plantigrade.

FIGURE 3–66

Controlled mobility techniques may be useful to improve the range of motion at both the distal and proximal joints while maintaining the intermediate joints—the elbow and the knee—in extension. In addition, rocking in various directions specifically increases weight bearing on the limbs while emphasizing specific movements at the distal and proximal joints similar to rocking in quadruped (Figure 3–68).

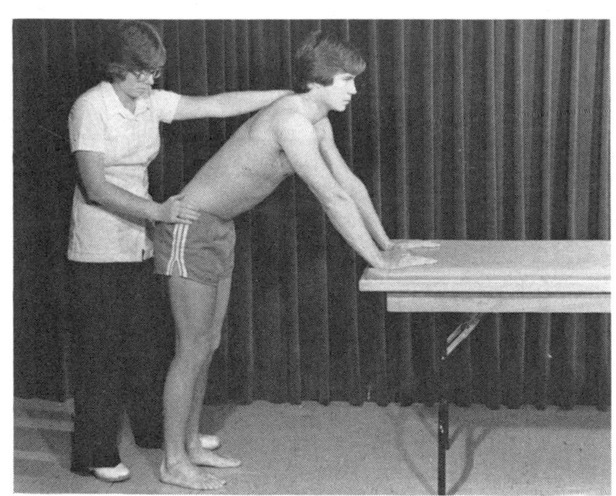

(a)

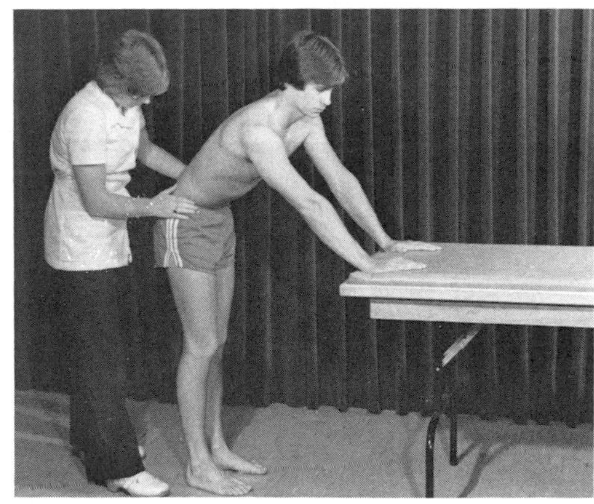

(b)

A. Modified plantigrade.
T. RS.
E. MC scapula and pelvis, pelvis.

FIGURE 3–67

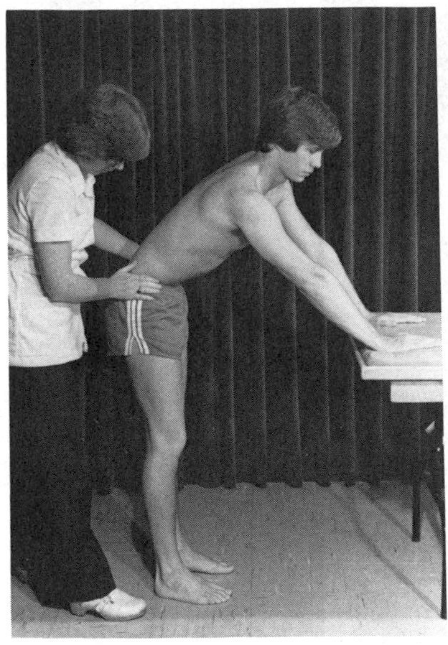

(a)

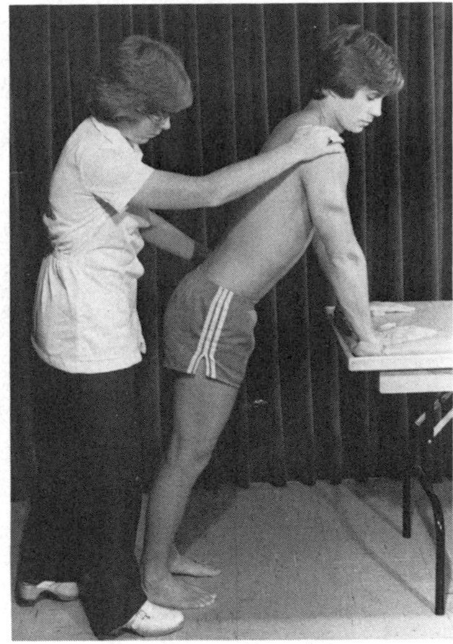

(b)

A. Modified plantigrade: rocking.
T. SR, SRH.
E. MC scapula and pelvis, pelvis.

FIGURE 3–68

In preparation for gait, the lower extremities can be placed in a stride (Figure 3–69) position during controlled mobility movements. Weight shifting in a forward direction will simulate the midstance to heel-off phase of gait in the posterior limb. The tibia flexes over the talus and places the triceps surae on stretch. This important ankle movement is commonly limited by tightness or hypertonia in the posterior muscles, and may result in hyperextension of the knee during gait (33). The eccentric control of the triceps surae, which increases the angle of dorsiflexion, can be promoted in this less stressful posture of modified plantigrade before progressing to full standing. Allowing the posterior knee to flex will increase the angle of dorsiflexion but at the same time will reduce the stretch on the gastrocnemius. On the anterior limb, weight acceptance can be emphasized. Attention is directed proximally so that lateral shifting onto the forward limb and rotation of the contralateral pelvis can be promoted. The knee of the anterior weight-bearing leg must be monitored to discourage excessive flexion or hyperextension.

Static-dynamic activities can be performed to achieve any of the following goals: flexion or extension with rotation of the trunk, movements of the

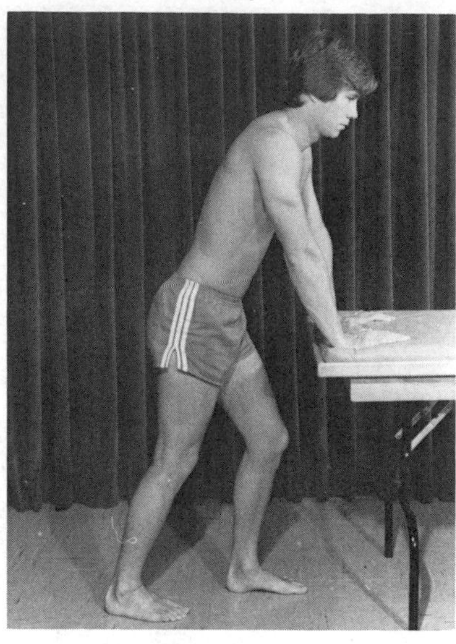

A. Modified plantigrade: feet in stride.

FIGURE 3–69

dynamic limb, or an increased amount of weight bearing on the three static limbs (Figure 3–70).

Clinical Implications. Modified plantigrade is a useful activity for a variety of conditions. The goals of treatment will determine where in the sequence of procedures modified plantigrade is appropriate.

When the goal is the development of upper extremity control, the modified plantigrade posture may be incorporated into treatment between sitting and quadruped. The amount of weight bearing that occurs through the upper extremity and the range in which the scapula and shoulder muscles function are the factors that are varied in this sequence of activities. Sitting with upper extremity support requires the least amount of control. Quadruped, in which both the amount of weight bearing and the proximal ROM are the greatest, is the most demanding developmental posture for the upper extremities. The sequencing of the modified plantigrade and quadruped postures may be similar for a patient with quadriceps weakness. Facilitation of quadriceps activity in the shortened range, which occurs in modified plantigrade, may precede the prolonged stretch position of quadruped (see Chapter 11).

Patients with generalized weakness or impaired balance reactions may find the quadruped posture less stressful than modified plantigrade because of the differences in the B of S and the C of G. The mass flexor position of the lower extremity in quadruped may not be indicated for patients exhibiting a flexor withdrawal response or increased flexor synergy during the swing phase of gait. For those patients, modified plantigrade that promotes an advanced lower extremity combination would be a more appropriate posture (see Chapter 8).

In summary:

- Modified plantigrade has a B of S that is relatively small and a high C of G that requires control of balance reactions to maintain or move within the posture.
- This posture promotes weight bearing and consequently the stability of all joints in the four extremities.
- It improves proximal stability, and when rocking movements are superimposed on the posture, ROM and proximal dynamic control are increased.
- Modified plantigrade prepares the lower extremities for the different phases of gait.

2. Standing and Walking. The standing and walking activities (Figure 3–71) are the culmination of the developmental sequence and are the functional goals for many patients. In comparison with the other postures, here the B of S is smallest, the C of G highest, and many joints and segments are involved. Because of the decreased biomechanical support, higher level balance reactions are vital to maintain and move within these activities.

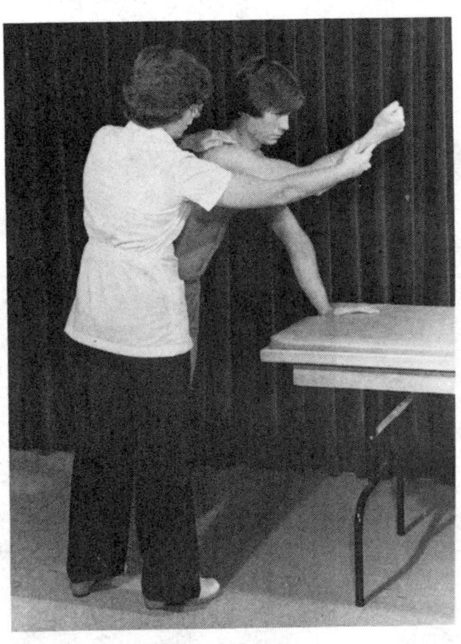

(a)

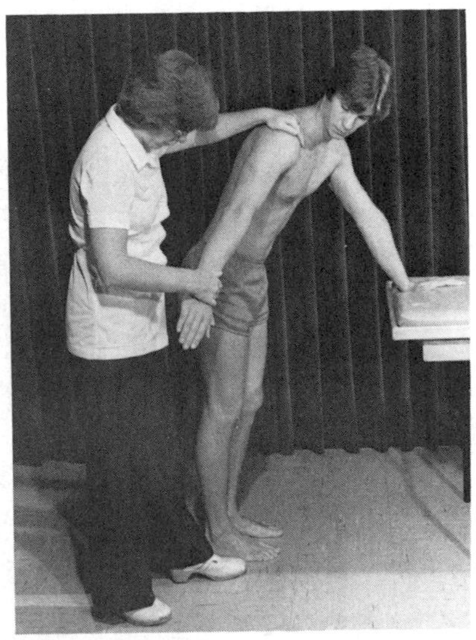

(b)

A. Modified plantigrade: D_1 UE.
T. SR, SRH.
E. MC scapula and forearm.

FIGURE 3–70

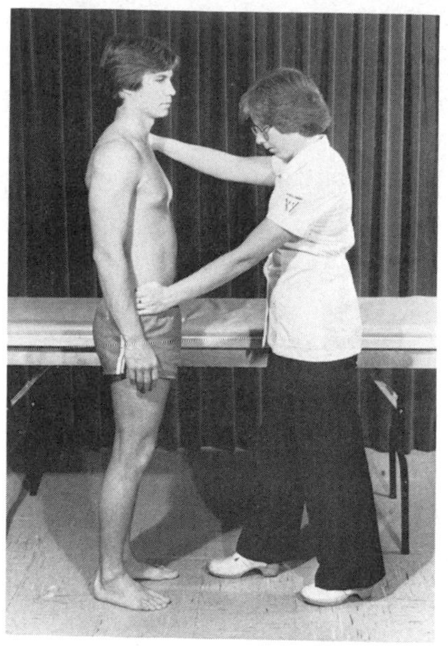

A. Standing.
T. RS.
E. MC scapula and pelvis.

FIGURE 3–71

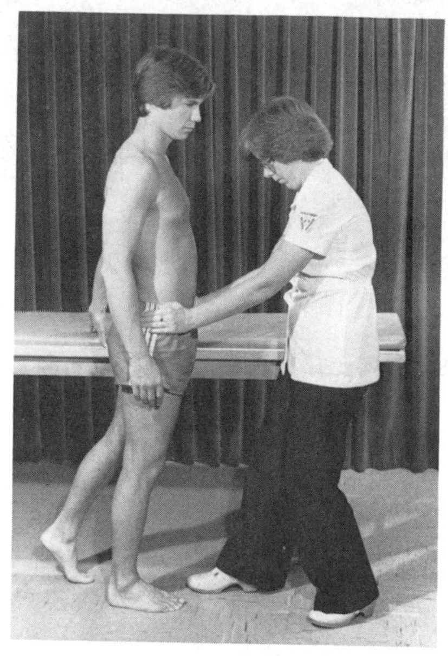

A. Standing in stride: pelvic motions.
T. RP.
E. MC pelvis.

FIGURE 3–72

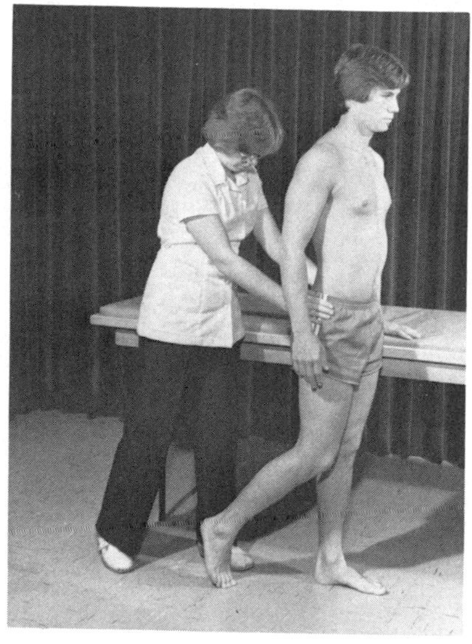

A. Walking backward.
T. RP.
E. MC pelvis.

FIGURE 3–73

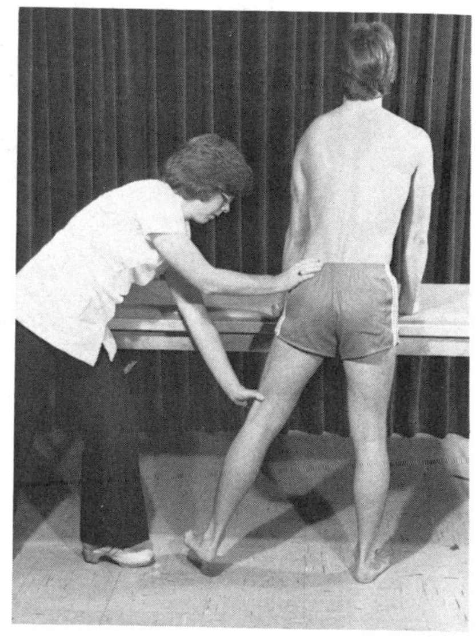

A. Sidewalking.
T. RP.
E. MC pelvis and thigh.

FIGURE 3–74

Clinical Implications and Stages of Motor Control. The assumption of the standing posture from sitting has first a flexor and then an extensor phase. The independent assumption of a posture is considered to be the controlled mobility level of motor control. Many patients may have stability in standing—that is, may be able to maintain the position—before they can assume the posture without assistance.

Initially, stability is promoted in standing, upper extremity support being provided by the parallel bars or other supportive devices. Once trunk stability has been achieved in this manner, upper extremity support can be reduced or eliminated. Manual contacts can be altered to emphasize stability of different body segments: upper trunk, lower trunk, or both. Procedures used in the standing posture while the arms are in contact with the parallel bars not only enhance stability, but also indirectly activate upper extremity musculature. In this position, as in sitting, the shoulder is in the fairly nonstressful and frequently nonpainful range of 0 degrees.

A normal gait pattern requires the correct sequence of pelvic and lower extremity motion and specific timing of movements and muscular contraction (20). These sequential events can be promoted individually, and the therapist can focus on the component movements, and then recombine them into the total pattern.

The determinants of gait that can be emphasized individually with the feet symmetrical are forward, lateral, and rotational movements of the pelvis. As in kneeling, the motion of the total trunk must be monitored to ensure that the movement is confined to the lower trunk and pelvic regions. In a stride position, these three pelvic motions are combined to assist the pelvis in coming up and over the stance leg while the opposite side of the pelvis rotates forward to begin the swing phase of that lower extremity (Figure 3–72). Deliberate walking then follows. Specific pelvic motions can be controlled and guided with manual contacts on the pelvis. When patients have a unilateral problem, moving in and out of the stance phase of gait—which is more similar to the controlled mobility level of control—is emphasized before the swing phase, which demands skilled movement.

Some patients may not have to use this deliberate walking sequence, especially if their major deficit is a decrease in the speed of movement. Deliberate ambulation emphasizing specific aspects of gait makes the patient conscious of this normally automatic activity. Walking independently with minimal assistance at a relatively normal speed may be more appropriate for certain patients than the sequence of deliberate walking. Whether support of the trunk or upper extremities is required depends on the needs of the patient.

Walking backward incorporates hip extension with knee flexion and is especially important if synergistic patterns exist (Figure 3–73). Sidewalking in both directions promotes free abduction of one lower extremity while the other lower extremity supports the trunk laterally (Figure 3–74). Because free abduction without hip hiking is a skilled movement that is difficult for many patients, this movement is usually emphasized toward the end of

TABLE 3–1

	MOBILITY	STABILITY: *Tonic Holding*	STABILITY: *Cocontraction*	CONTROLLED MOBILITY	*Static-Dynamic*	SKILL
Sidelying (rolling)		modified pivot prone	with appropriate techniques to upper and lower body	log rolling	segmental upper and lower trunk movements	trunk counterrotation
Sitting	90° flexion of hips	modified pivot prone	with or without arm support lower trunk stability prerequisite	upper trunk movements with or without UE support	support of one UE	manipulation functional ADL
Pivot Prone	movement into the posture	stretch sensitivity developed in postural extensors	N/A	N/A	N/A	N/A
Prone on Elbows	45° of shoulder flexion full extension of hips	upper trunk tonic holding is a prerequisite	in proximal UE, upper trunk, head	in all directions, especially lateral; head rotation	one UE support	crawling
Quadruped	90° of shoulder flexion; 90° of flexion hips and knees	upper and lower trunk tonic holding is a prerequisite	of upper trunk, lower trunk, and proximal LE	rocking in all directions	each extremity may be lifted	creeping

LTR	minimal ROM hips and knees	holding in shortened range of lower body extensors	hooklying of lower body	smooth reversal movements	N/A	N/A
Bridging	full hip extension	holding shortened range of LTR is a prerequisite	with appropriate techniques, hip and lower trunk	pelvic motions	one LE support	"crab" walking
Kneeling	full hip extension	holding of lower body extensors is a prerequisite	of hips and lower trunk	upper trunk and lower trunk movements	one LE support	kneewalking
Half-Kneeling			of hips and lower trunk with appropriate techniques	rocking	N/A	N/A
Modified Plantigrade			of all proximal and distal joints with appropriate techniques	in all directions	each extremity may be lifted	"cruising"
Standing (walking)			with or without UE support of weight-bearing limbs	pelvic movements in all directions feet symmetrical and in stride	one LE support	walking in all directions

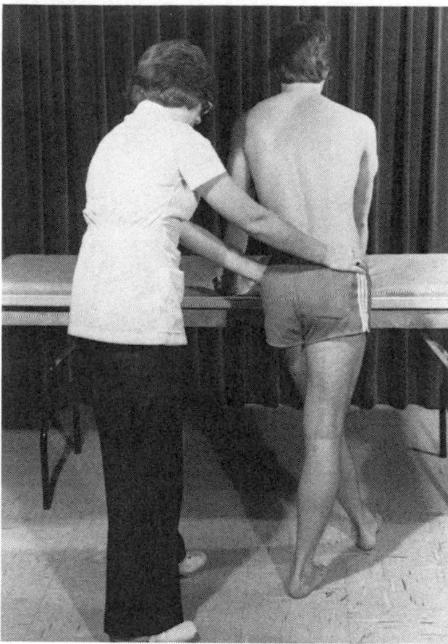

A. Braiding.
T. RP.
E. MC pelvis.

FIGURE 3–75

treatment. In monitoring the position of the feet, the therapist can note whether the movement is occurring in the frontal plane, as desired, or whether the patient is substituting other movements. Braiding (Figure 3–75), the most difficult motion of the walking sequence, incorporates lower trunk rotation, crossing of the midline, and advancement of the dynamic lower extremity both anteriorly and posteriorly to the static supporting limb. During braiding, as in other gait sequences, emphasis can be placed on one phase of the total pattern or on the sequencing of the entire movement (33).

In summary:

- Compared with the other developmental postures, standing and walking have the smallest B of S and the highest C of G, and thus require the greatest amount of motor control.
- The stages of motor control can be promoted to enhance the control needed for functional ambulation.
- Upper extremity activity can be promoted as an indirect approach.

EXTREMITY PATTERNS

Limb patterns can be performed unilaterally or bilaterally, and when used in combination they are termed trunk patterns (17). Motor unit activity of specific shoulder muscles has been shown to be lowest during the performance of trunk patterns and greatest during unilateral patterns (37). Thus, in terms of motor unit facilitation, the greatest demands are placed on a muscle during the performance of unilateral patterns. If the goal of treatment is to gradually increase the challenge of activities for the patient, the order of application of patterns should be trunk to bilateral to unilateral. Each combination may be used to accomplish specific goals, which are discussed in the next sections. For the sake of clarity, the patterns and clinical implications are discussed in the following order: unilateral, bilateral, and trunk patterns.

Unilateral Patterns

Extremity movements are combined into two diagonal patterns arbitrarily termed diagonal 1 (D_1) and diagonal 2 (D_2) (20). Associating the D_1 movement with the initial mobility feeding pattern described by Rood (38) will help the therapist to differentiate between the two diagonals. All diagonal patterns have both a flexor and an extensor direction (D_1F, D_1E, D_2F, D_2E), which is determined by the movement of the shoulder or hip joint.

The movement components of the upper extremity patterns are:

- D_1F (Figure 3–76)—scapula-elevation, abduction, and upward rotation; shoulder flexion, adduction, and external rotation;

(a)

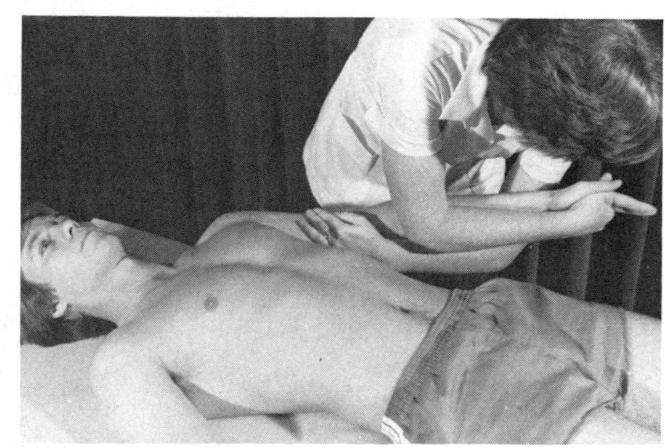

(b)

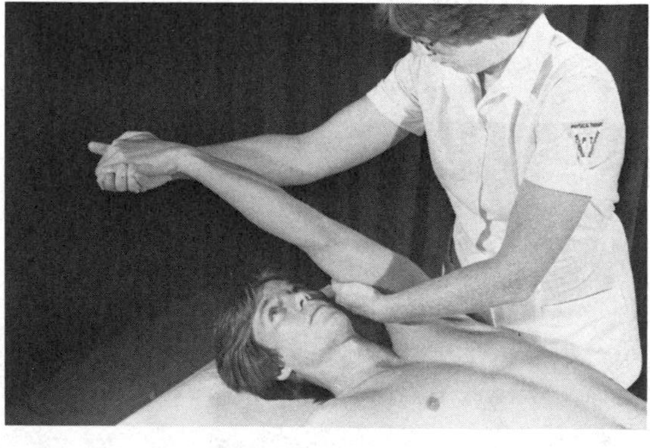

A. D_1F, UE: elbow straight.
E. MC arm and hand.

FIGURE 3–76

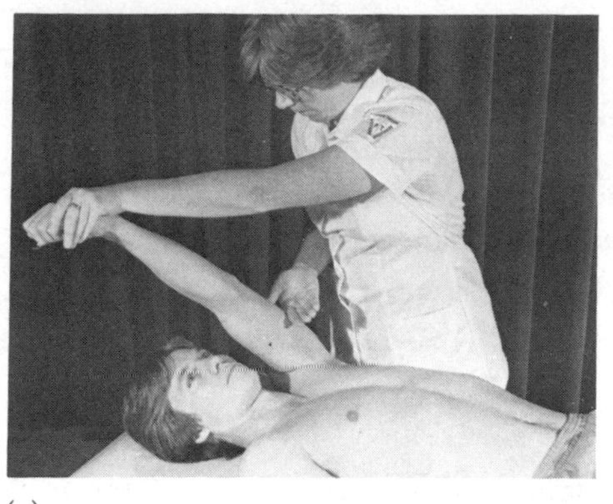

(a)

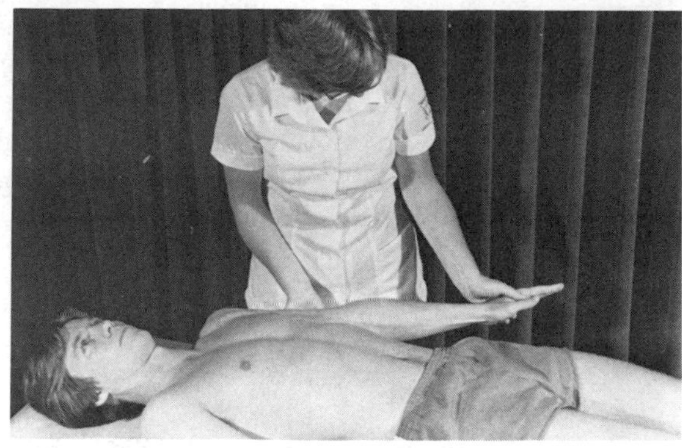

(b)

A. D_1E, UE: elbow straight.
E. MC arm and hand.

FIGURE 3–77

forearm-supination, and wrist and finger flexion to the radial side with the thumb adducting.

- The antagonistic D_1E (Figure 3–77)—scapula-depression, adduction, and downward rotation; shoulder extension, abduction, and internal rotation; forearm-pronation; and wrist and finger extension to the ulnar side with the thumb abducting.
- D_2F (Figure 3–78)—scapula-elevation, adduction and upward rotation; shoulder-flexion, abduction, and external rotation; forearm-supination; wrist and finger extension to the radial side with thumb extension.
- The antagonistic D_2E (Figure 3–79)—scapula depression, abduction, and downward rotation; shoulder extension, adduction with internal rotation; and forearm-pronation, and wrist and finger flexion to the ulnar side, with thumb opposition. (17)

Movements are coupled to reflect biomechanical needs and synkinetic motions (31). Shoulder flexion, for example, is always combined with external rotation, scapula elevation, and upward rotation to allow the greatest freedom of movement; external rotation of the shoulder is combined with supination (both are rotational movements occurring in the same direction); shoulder abduction is coupled with wrist and finger extension.

Thrusting patterns recombine the proximal and distal movements of D_1 and D_2 motions. The D_1 thrust (Figure 3–80) or ulnar thrust combines the proximal scapula and shoulder D_1F movements with the elbow extending and the distal D_1E forearm, wrist, and hand movements. The result is scapula protraction, shoulder flexion, adduction and external rotation, elbow ex-

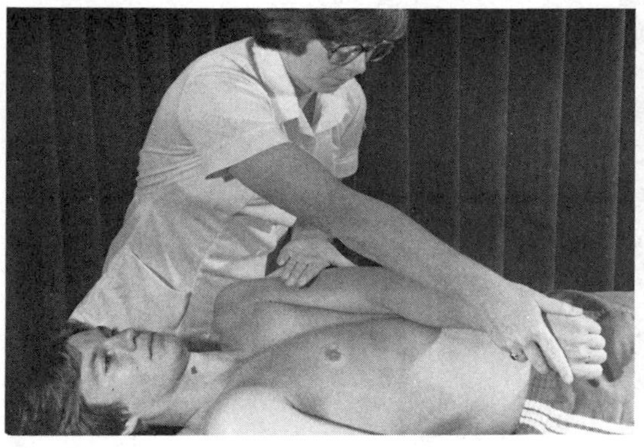

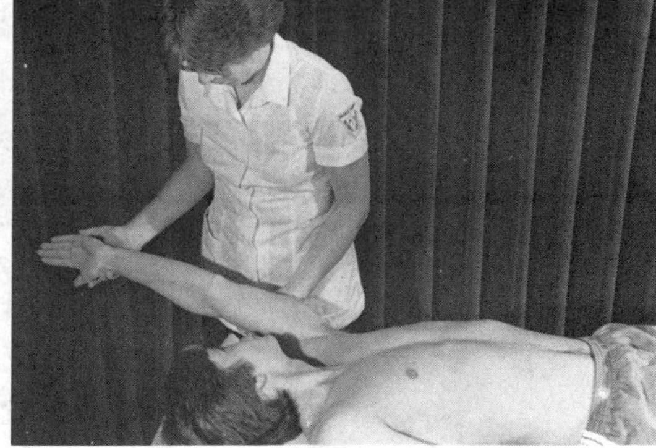

(a) (b)

A. D_2F, UE: elbow straight.
E. MC arm and hand.

FIGURE 3–78

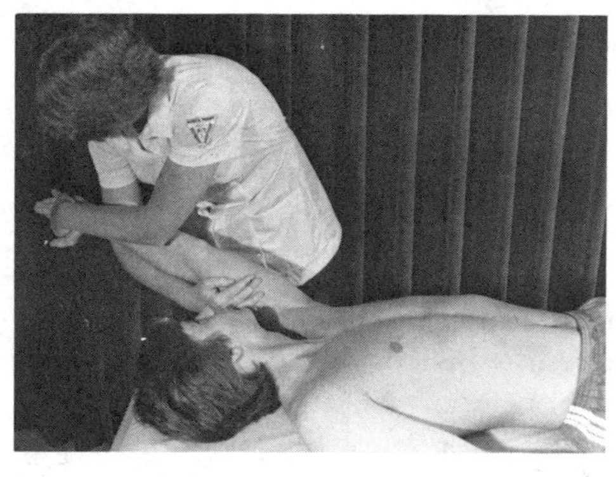

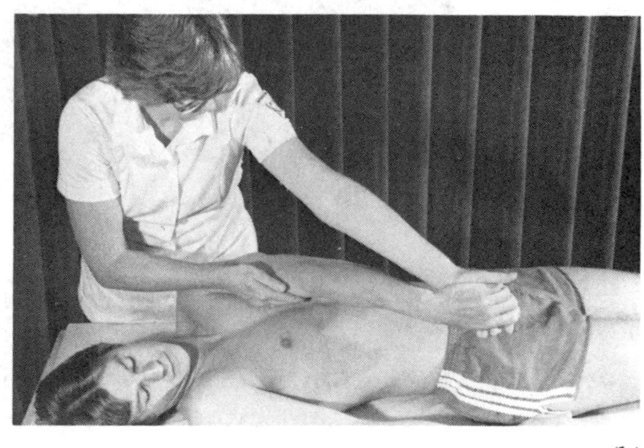

(a) (b)

A. D_2E, UE: elbow straight.
E. MC arm and hand.

FIGURE 3–79

tending, and forearm pronation with hand opening. The reverse of the thrust, a withdrawal pattern, also recombines the proximal and distal components: scapula retraction, shoulder extension, abduction, and internal rotation are combined with elbow, wrist, and hand flexion (17). The thrusting movement can be used advantageously for a variety of orthopedic and neurological disabilities (see chapters 8 and 10). The serratus anterior, anterior

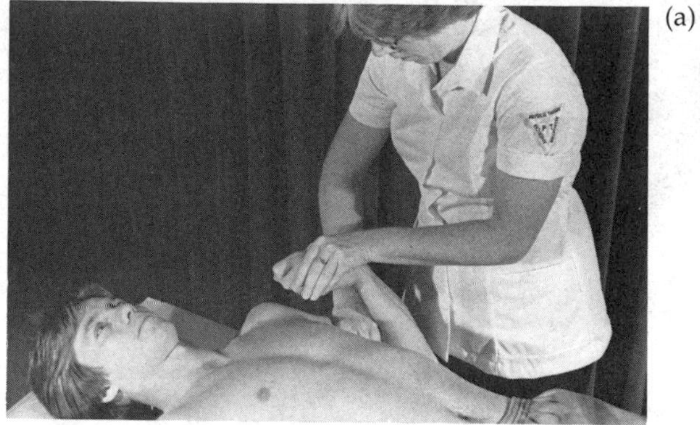
(a)

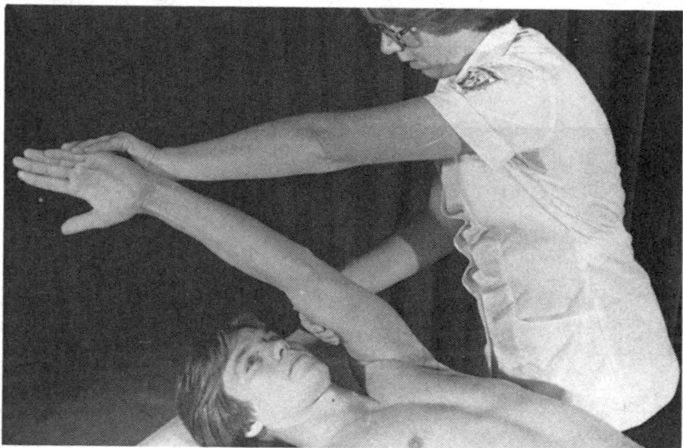
(b)

A. D_1 thrust.
E. MC arm and hand.

FIGURE 3–80

deltoid, triceps, and wrist and finger extensors all can be effectively strengthened in this pattern. The reverse thrust or withdrawal pattern is useful for strengthening the rhomboids, posterior deltoid, biceps, and wrist and finger flexors. Holding in the shortened range of the withdrawal pattern against some form of resistance is similar to a pull pattern described by Rood (38), and can be considered a modified unilateral pivot prone pattern. Movement into shoulder hyperextension can be easily facilitated with a reverse thrust, and is an important goal in the treatment of patients with spinal cord injuries and some shoulder pathologies (see Chapters 9 and 10).

The D_2 thrust (Figure 3–81) and withdrawal patterns are similar to the hemiplegic synergistic pattern (6). If facilitation of synergistic movements is desired, application of these patterns is indicated (see Chapter 8).

Each muscle has an optimal pattern in which it functions. For example, the sternal portion of the pectoralis major (PM) is most active in the D_2E pattern, the anterior deltoid (AD) in D_1F and the antagonistic posterior deltoid (PD) in D_1E. Although muscles are optimally active in one pattern, they may contribute to various movements of other patterns. The middle deltoid (MD) has been found to be most active in the D_2F pattern, but is also active in D_1E, which has an abducting component.

Because of the combination of movements occurring within a pattern, many muscles act synergistically to complete the movement. Some muscles or portions of muscles may be more active during the initiation of the movement, while others show more activity in the shortened range.

Varying the elbow component by maintaining the elbow straight or by flexing or extending it during the movement will alter the activity of certain muscles (Figures 3–82, 3–83, and 3–84). The shoulder muscles already mentioned—the MD, PD, AD, and sternal portion of the PM—are most active in their respective patterns when the elbow is maintained in extension throughout the range. The MD and AD have been shown to be more active when the shoulder flexor patterns are performed with the elbow flexing than when performed with the elbow extending. Conversely, the shoulder extensors—the PD and PM—demonstrate more activity when the elbow is extending, rather than flexing, throughout the pattern (39).

The activity of the biceps and triceps also varies with the many combinations of patterns. Obviously these muscles are most active when the elbow flexes and extends. The biceps is most active in D_1F when the elbow flexes or when it remains straight, and the triceps is most active in D_1E when the elbow extends or remains straight. The length of the lever arm, the muscle length tension relationships of the two joint muscles, and the action of the biceps and triceps at both the shoulder and elbow may all contribute to differences in muscular activity (40).

The above evidence supports the premise that certain muscles function optimally in specific patterns of movement. In total, there are twelve combinations of upper extremity patterns plus the four thrusting patterns. All combine different joint movements and, as we have noted, the muscle response can vary.

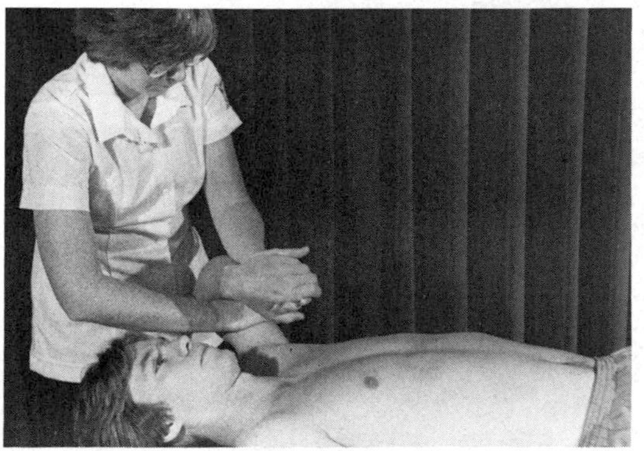
(a)

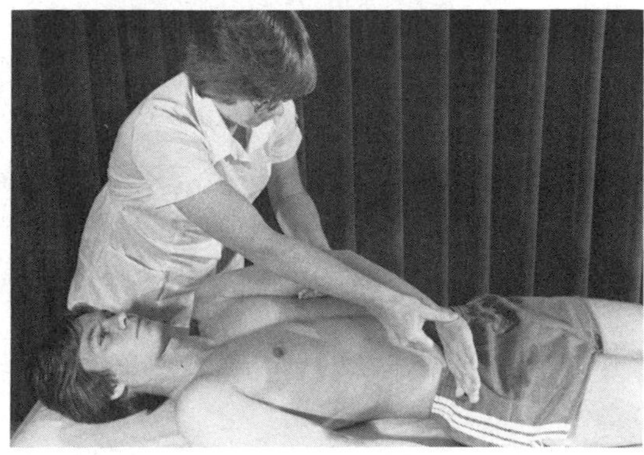
(b)

A. D_2 thrust.
E. MC arm and hand.

FIGURE 3–81

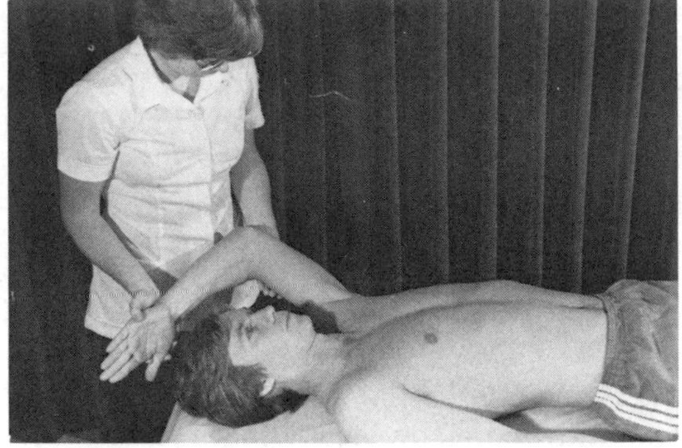

A. D_2F with elbow flexing.
E. MC arm and hand.

FIGURE 3–82

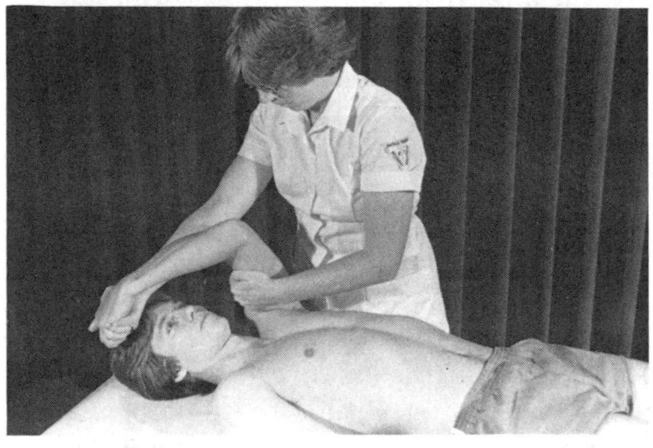

A. D_1F with elbow flexing.
E. MC arm and hand.

FIGURE 3–83

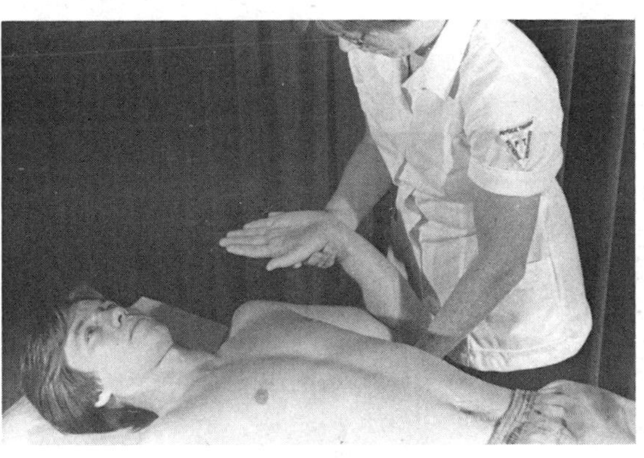

A. D_1E with elbow flexing.
E. MC arm and hand.

FIGURE 3–84

A more extensive description of combining movements of upper extremity patterns appears in chapters 9 and 10. By altering the position of manual contacts, different portions or segments of the pattern can be emphasized. When movement or strengthening of muscles at one joint is the goal, then manual contacts should be positioned just proximally and distally to that joint. If increased range or strengthening of wrist radial flexion is the goal, for example, the manual contacts are positioned on the patient's forearm and hand so that the specific movement of wrist flexion can be enhanced (Figure 3–85). If flexion at the MCP joint is specifically desired, then the proximal contact is in the hand and the distal contact on the fingers (Figure 3–86).

Upper extremity patterns can be performed in many postures such as supine, prone, and sitting. During many of the developmental sequence activities such as quadruped or modified plantigrade, patterns are incorporated into the static-dynamic stage of motor control. (A more complete discussion of the application of patterns in various postures can be found in the following sections.) Various techniques can be superimposed on these patterns according to the desired goals, for example, increased ROM, proximal stability, strengthening, and enhancement of the normal timing of movement. Various means of sensory input, elements, can be added to achieve these goals (see Chapters 4 and 5).

Like the upper extremity patterns, the lower extremity movements are separated into two diagonal patterns, D_1 and D_2. Both patterns have a flexor

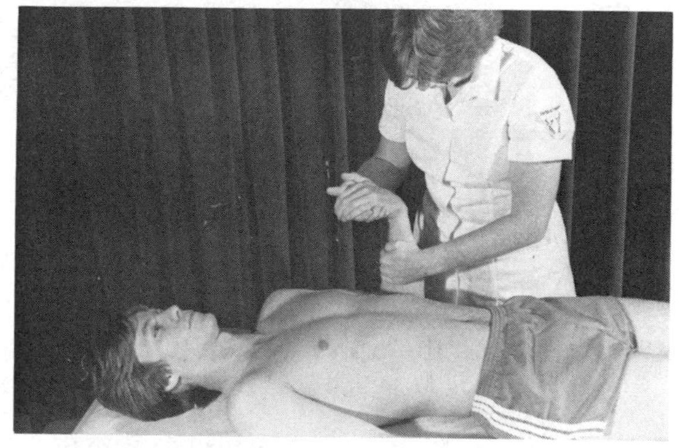

A. D_1 withdrawal: emphasis on wrist flexion.
E. MC forearm and hand.

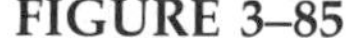

FIGURE 3–85

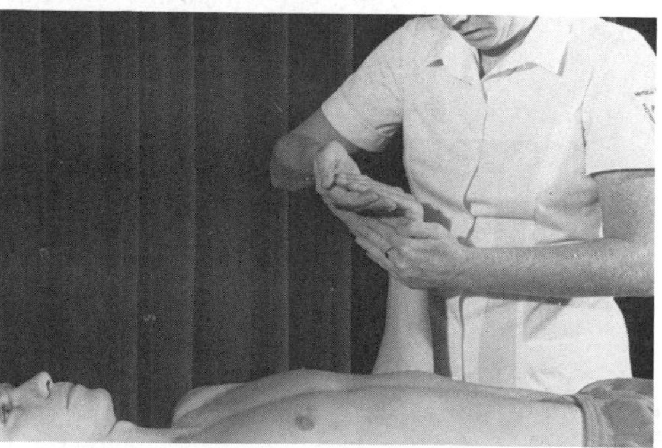

A. D_1 withdrawal: emphasis on MCP flexion.
E. MC hand and fingers.

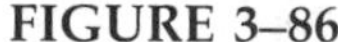

FIGURE 3–86

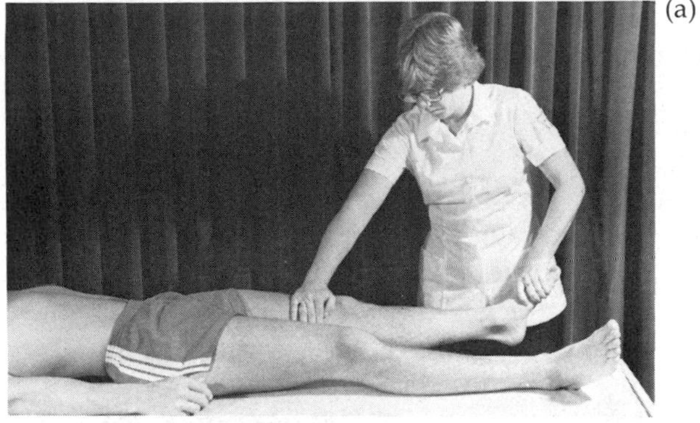
(a)

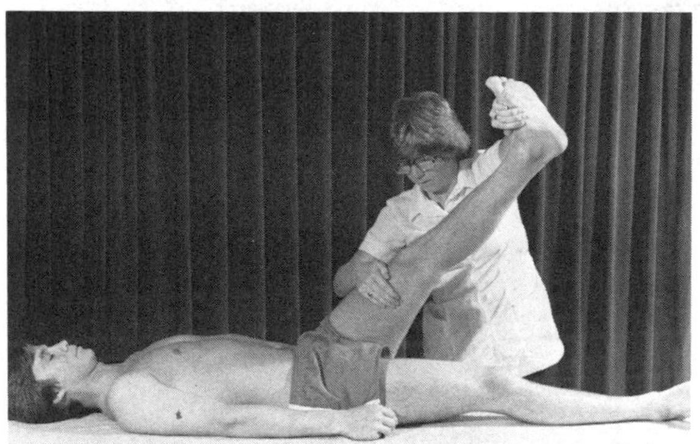
(b)

A. D_1F with knee straight.
E. MC thigh and foot.

FIGURE 3–87

and extensor direction. D_1F and D_1E combine the same proximal movements as the upper extremity patterns.

- D_1F (Figure 3–87) combines pelvic forward rotation or protraction; hip flexion, adduction, external rotation, ankle and foot dorsiflexion with inversion and toe extension.
- D_1E (Figure 3–88) combines pelvic backward rotation or retraction; hip extension, abduction, internal rotation; ankle and foot plantar flexion with eversion and toe flexion.

The D_2F and D_2E patterns differ from the UE patterns in the rotational component.

- D_2F (Figure 3–89) includes pelvic elevation or hip hiking, hip flexion, abduction and *internal* rotation, ankle and foot dorsiflexion with eversion and toe extension.
- D_2E (Figure 3–90) combines pelvic depression, or lateral pelvic downward tilt, hip extension, adduction and *external* rotation, ankle and foot plantar flexion with inversion and toe flexion (17).

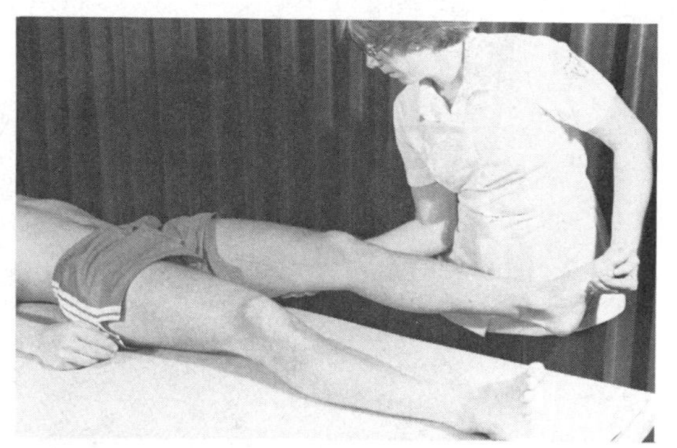

A. D_1E with knee straight.
E. MC thigh and foot

FIGURE 3–88

(a)

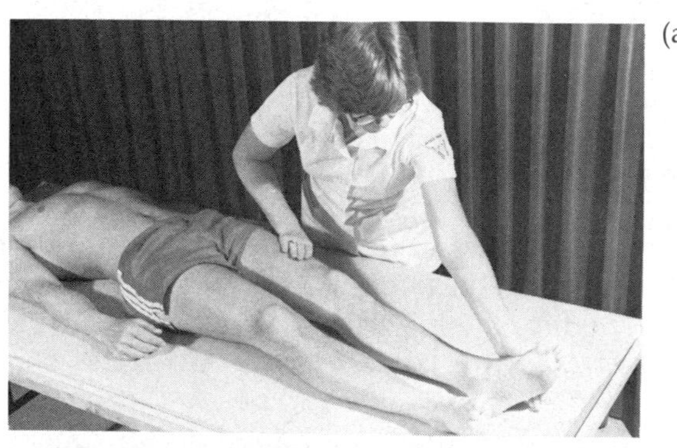

(b)

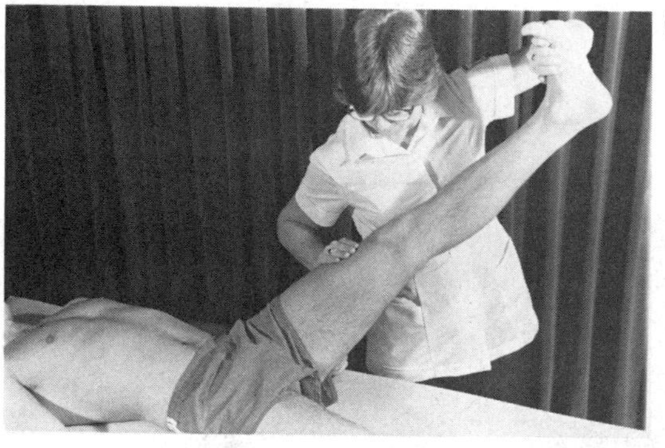

A. D_2F with knee straight.
E. MC thigh and foot.

FIGURE 3–89

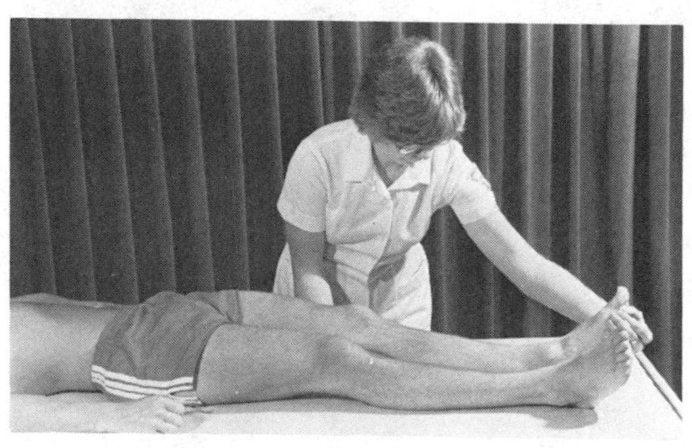

A. D_2E knee straight.
E. MC thigh and foot.

FIGURE 3–90

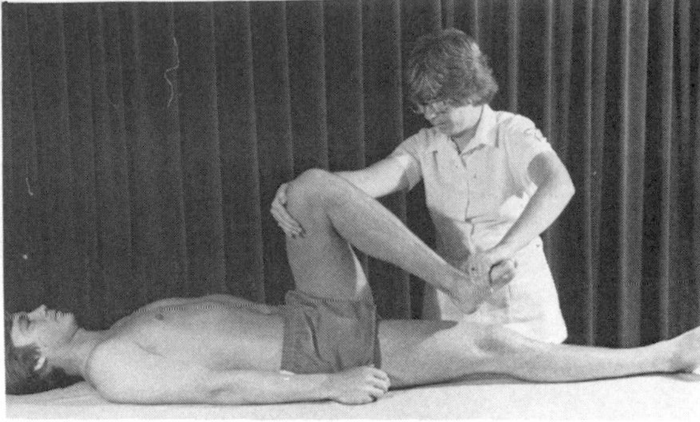

A. D_1F knee flexing.
E. MC thigh and foot.

FIGURE 3–91

As with the upper extremity patterns, the motion of the intermediate joint, the knee, can vary; it can be maintained in extension throughout the movement, or the knee may flex (Figure 3–91) or extend (Figure 3–92) during the pattern. The pattern may be a mass flexion or extension movement or an advanced combination (17) (Figure 3–93). As discussed earlier, mass patterns, which combine hip, knee, and ankle flexion or extension, are used primarily to enhance strength or balance tone. Advanced combinations in which the hip and ankle extend while the knee is flexing, or the hip and ankle flex while the knee is extending, are important for functional activities such as gait.

To choose an appropriate procedure, the therapist must determine the

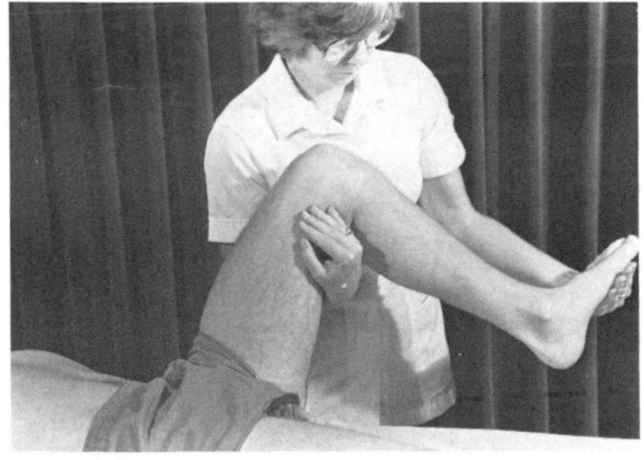

(a)

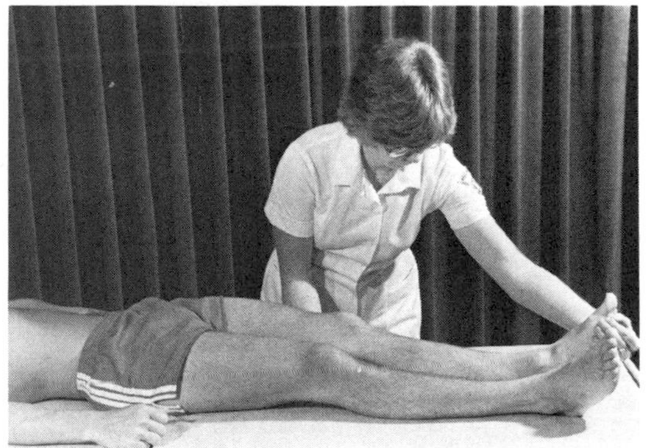

(b)

A. D_2E with knee extending.
E. MC thigh and foot.

FIGURE 3–92

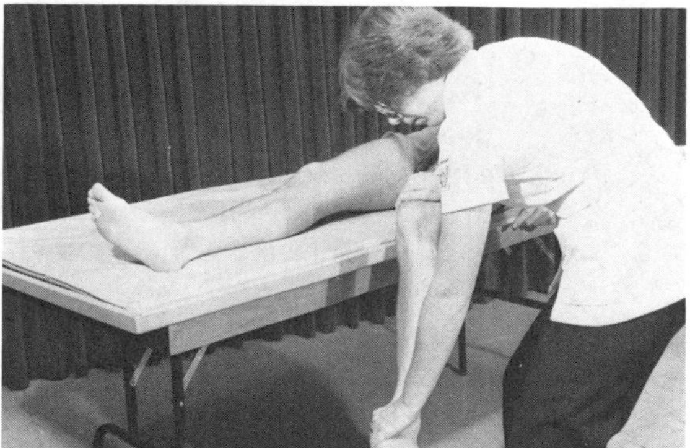

A. D_1F with knee extending.
E. MC thigh and foot.

FIGURE 3–93

muscle or movement to be facilitated, and the optimal diagonal pattern for that muscle. A mass movement combination can be performed if the goal is initiation of activity or strengthening; an advanced combination is indicated if skilled functional movement is the desired outcome. If imbalances of strength exist, a pattern combination is selected that can elicit optimal overflow from the stronger muscles in the limb. If, for example, the anterior tibial muscle is weak because of a peroneal nerve injury, D_1F, which combines the ankle motions of dorsiflexion and inversion, would be the pattern of choice.

A mass flexor pattern combining hip, knee, and ankle flexion may promote overflow from the proximal muscles (Figure 3–94). During gait, how-

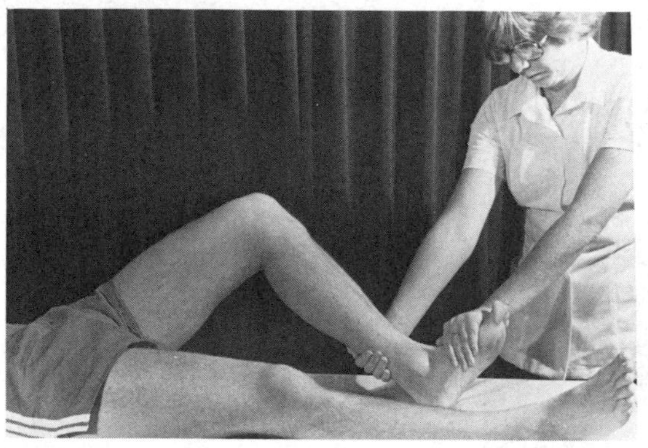

(a)

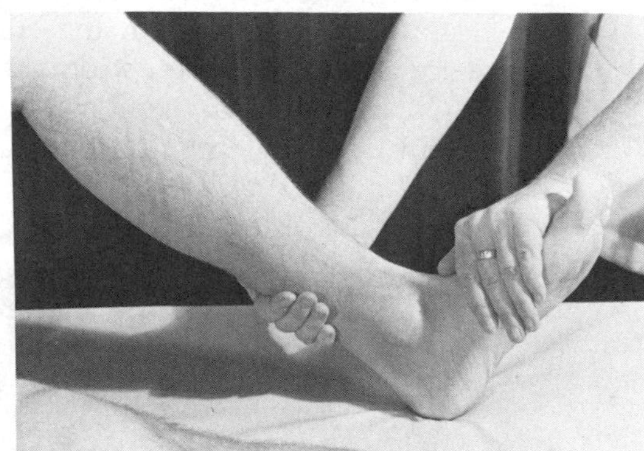

(b)

A. D_1F with knee flexing: emphasis on ankle flexion.
E. MC lower leg and foot.

FIGURE 3–94

ever, the anterior tibial muscle functions with the knee extensors at heel strike. An advanced combination of knee extension with ankle dorsiflexion (Figure 3–93) is used at later stages to promote the segmental combinations needed for ambulation. To enhance muscular activity, the therapist can incorporate techniques for strengthening, normal timing, and eccentric control within these activities, along with elements such as stretch, resistance, manual contacts, vibration, and icing.

Both the upper and lower extremity patterns can be performed in most positions. During the developmental postures the extremity patterns are incorporated into the stability, controlled mobility, static-dynamic, and skill levels of motor control. During stability and controlled mobility procedures, the direction of either the resistive force or the rocking motion will promote diagonal patterns. When the patient performs the static-dynamic level of control, the patterns are incorporated into the movement of the dynamic limb, and may be used to strengthen the dynamic limb or to promote dynamic stability control of the supporting limbs. In prone on elbows, a D_1 thrust (Figure 3–41) and withdrawal are the most easily accomplished patterns, while in quadruped and modified plantigrade both upper and lower D_1 (Figures 3–46 and 3–70) and D_2 (Figure 3–45) patterns can be added to the activity. Resistance can be applied manually or mechanically with pulleys or weights.

The therapist should carefully select the posture in which the patient will be performing movement patterns. As stated earlier in the chapter, when the goal of the procedure is to strengthen an extremity movement or a specific muscle, a stable posture with a large B of S and low C of G should be chosen. Emphasis can then be placed on the involved segment without concern for balance reactions that are required to maintain more advanced positions. The most stable positions are supine, prone, sidelying, and sitting. In each position the effect of gravity and tone will vary, as will the range in which the patterns can be optimally performed.

In supine, all combinations of both upper and lower extremity patterns can be easily accomplished. Gravity will resist flexor motions to midrange,

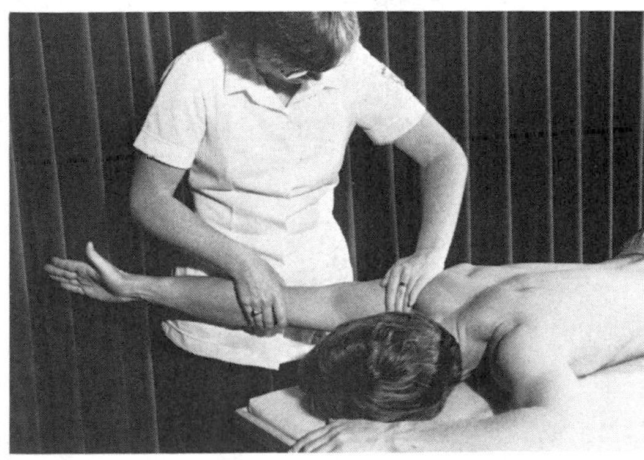

A. D_2F prone.
E. MC scapula and arm.

FIGURE 3–95

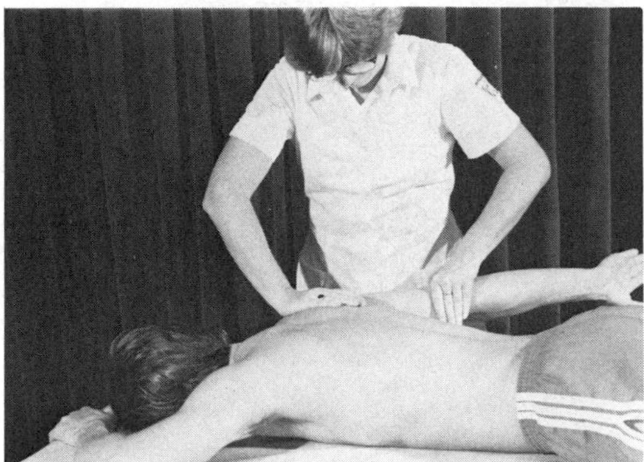

A. D_1E prone.
E. MC scapula and arm.

FIGURE 3–96

and then will assist movement into shortened ranges. In general, reflex effects and gravity assist extension. Although supine is a very stable posture, the motion of the scapula may be restricted by the supporting surface during the performance of extremity patterns.

In the prone position, the upper extremity can be resisted both by manual contacts and by gravity. The patterns most effectively performed are D_2F (Figure 3–95) and D_1E (Figure 3–96). The scapula is free to move and manual contacts can be placed directly on the scapula to emphasize proximal control. The range into the antagonistic D_2E and D_1F patterns is restricted by the supporting surface.

Lower extremity patterns can also be performed both unilaterally and bilaterally (Figure 3–97) in prone. Because the hip is maintained in extension by the supporting surface, emphasis is usually directed toward control at the knee and ankle joints. The extended position of the hip in prone results in a different length-tension relationship of the quadriceps and hamstrings than that which occurs in other postures, such as supine and sitting in which these muscles are frequently facilitated. The hamstrings contracting against the resistance of gravity can be easily facilitated both concentrically and eccentrically in the mid to lengthened range, and thus may improve the control needed for gait. The shortened range of knee flexion in prone is not usually emphasized (see section on "Prone on Elbows"). Procedures for strengthening the quadriceps in prone are appropriate only when gravity-resisted activities are too stressful. Ankle dorsiflexion and plantar flexion motions are combined with the knee patterns either to enhance the activity of the knee musculature or to facilitate specifically more distal activity. Visual feedback is limited in prone. Without this sensory input many patients may have difficulty performing movement in the correct direction.

In sidelying, extremity patterns are limited to movements of the uppermost limbs. A procedure may be designed to emphasize control of the extremities or the extremity movement can be used to improve the rolling activity. When the focus is on extremity control, the goals are usually to balance tone or to initiate a movement. Facilitation of the extremity patterns

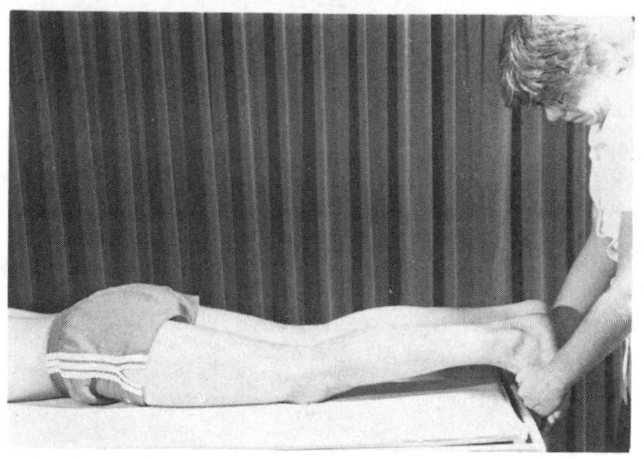

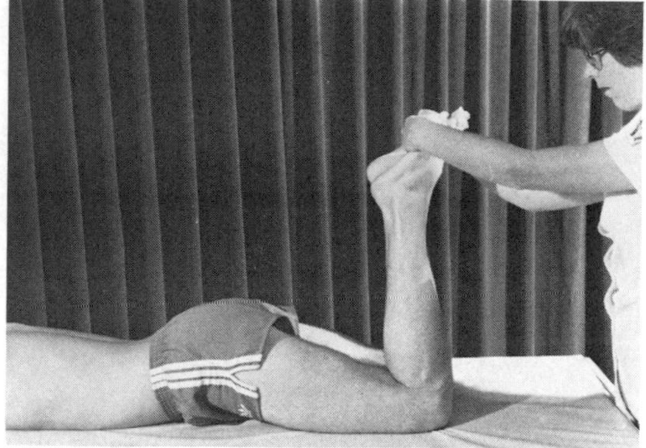

(a) (b)

A. Bilateral lower extremity patterns, prone.
E. MC feet.

FIGURE 3–97

may be separated into separate joint movement before the pattern as a whole is performed. Scapula protraction or retraction, for example, may be emphasized prior to movement of the entire upper extremity. Isometric contraction of the upper extremity postural muscles in the shortened range of D_1E (Figure 3–98) or a withdrawal pattern is important for patients with hypotonia and can be easily accomplished in sidelying. Other extremity movements or positions can be used to promote a balance of tone (see Chapter 8).

Because the B of S is decreased and the C of G raised in sitting, this posture requires either trunk control or support. Resisted extremity patterns

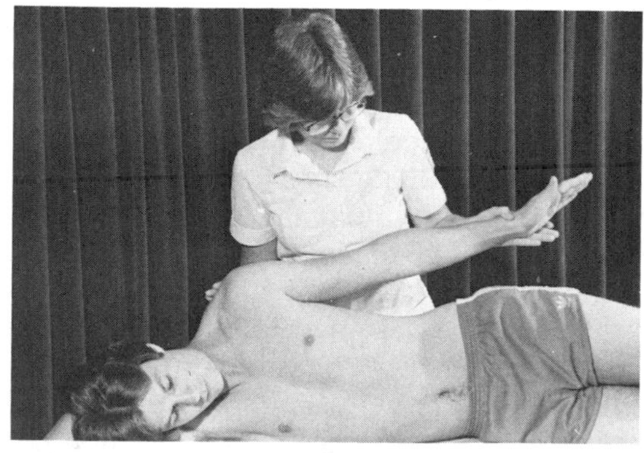

A. Sidelying: D_1E of UE.
T. SHRC.
E. MC scapula and wrist.

FIGURE 3–98

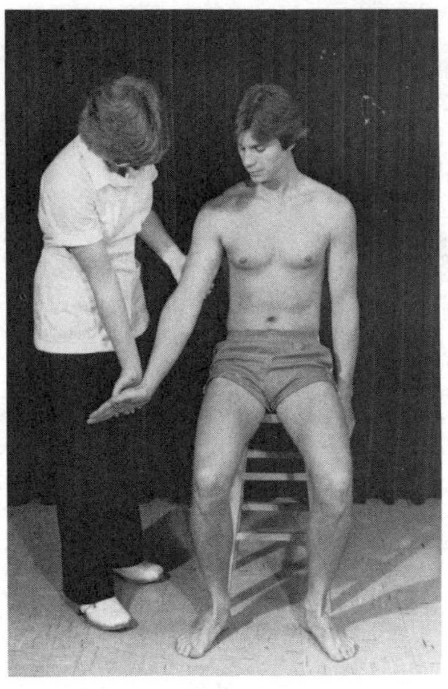

(a)

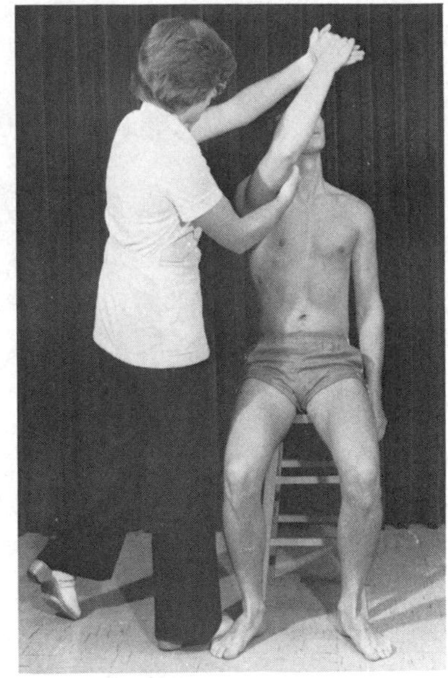

(b)

A. Sitting: UE D_1.
T. SRH.
E. MC arm and hand.

FIGURE 3–99

can be used to indirectly promote or challenge balance reactions in the posture. Gravity resists upper extremity flexor motions through full range and conversely assists extensor motions to neutral range (Figure 3–99). (Because the scapula is not as restricted by the supporting surface in sitting as it is in supine, movements of the scapula are frequently emphasized in the sitting position.) In the lower extremity, gravity resists knee extension and assists knee flexion. Lower extremity patterns are performed with the hip maintained in flexion; thus, in contrast to the prone position, the length-tension relationship of the two joint muscles is altered in this posture. Techniques to promote ROM and strengthening of the knee musculature are frequently performed in sitting.

Bilateral Patterns

The term bilateral patterns implies that both upper or lower extremities are being exercised simultaneously. Four combinations are possible: symmetrical, asymmetrical, reciprocal, and cross-diagonal. A symmetrical pattern

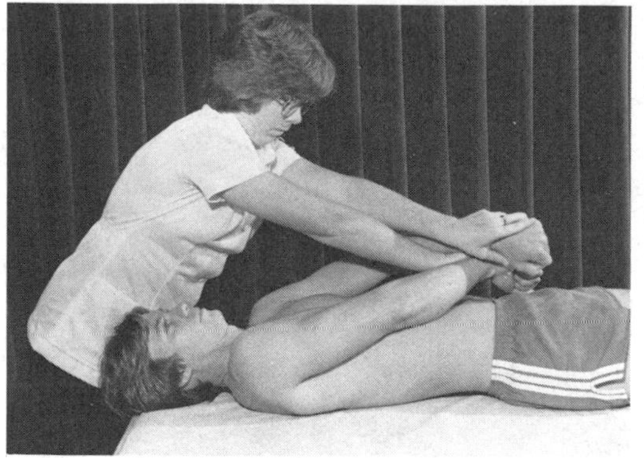

(a)

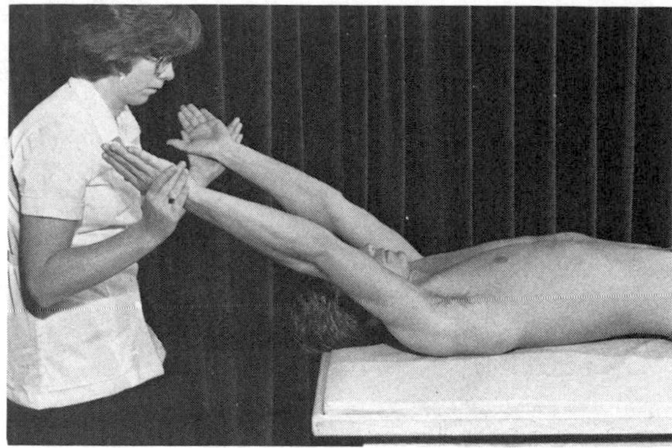

(b)

A. Supine: UE BS D_2F.
E. MC wrists.

FIGURE 3–100

combines the same diagonal pattern in the same direction of movement, for example, bilateral symmetrical BS D_2F (Figure 3–100). Symmetrical patterns can be used to facilitate activity of the trunk flexors or extensors. BS D_2F of the upper extremity reinforces trunk extension; conversely, BS D_2E increases trunk flexion. In the lower extremity the reinforcement pattern is reversed,

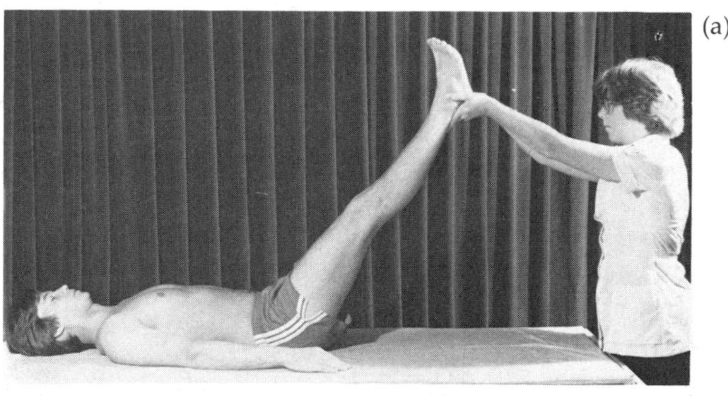

(a)

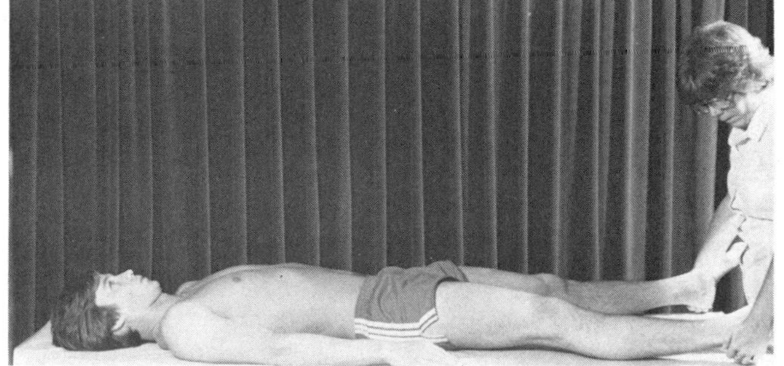

(b)

A. Supine: LE BS D_1.
E. MC heels.

FIGURE 3–101

so that hip flexion facilitates trunk flexion [Figure 3–101(a)] and hip extension augments trunk extension [Figure 3–101(b)].

Asymmetrical patterns combine the two different diagonal patterns moving in the same direction. For example, bilateral asymmetrical (BA) flexion to the left combines D_1F of the right extremity and D_2F of the left extremity (Figure 3–102). Asymmetrical patterns can also be used to promote trunk flexion or extension. Unlike the symmetrical combinations, however, asymmetrical patterns combine trunk movement with rotation.

Reciprocal patterns combine the same pattern moving in opposite directions. During bilateral reciprocal (BR) combinations, one extremity performs D_2F while the other extremity moves into D_2E (Figure 3–103). Rotation is the trunk movement promoted by reciprocal extremity patterns.

Cross-diagonal or reciprocal asymmetrical patterns are the opposite patterns moving in opposite directions. One extremity, for example, performs D_2E while the other moves into D_1F (Figure 3–104). Because the extremity movements of flexion-extension and abduction-adduction are antagonistic, trunk stability is enhanced.

The D_1 thrusting patterns can also be performed bilaterally in either a symmetrical or reciprocal combination (Figures 3–105 and 3–106). A BS D_1 reverse thrust, which is a modified pivot prone activity, can enhance bilateral contractions of the tonic postural muscles of the upper body (17, 32). BS D_2 thrust and reverse when performed in sitting are similar to Brunnstrom's rowing pattern used to facilitate synergistic motions (6).

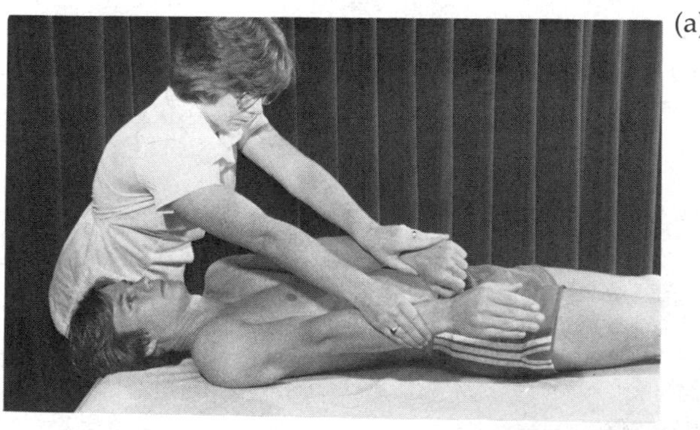
(a)

(b)
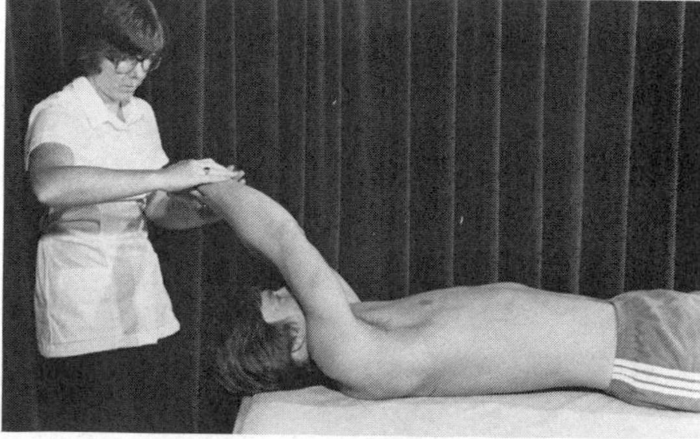

A. Supine: UE BA F to the L.
E. MC wrists.

FIGURE 3–102

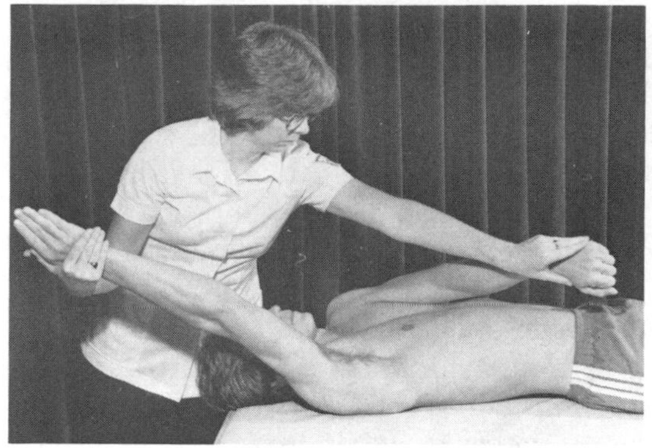

A. Supine: UE BR D_2.
E. MC wrists.

FIGURE 3–103

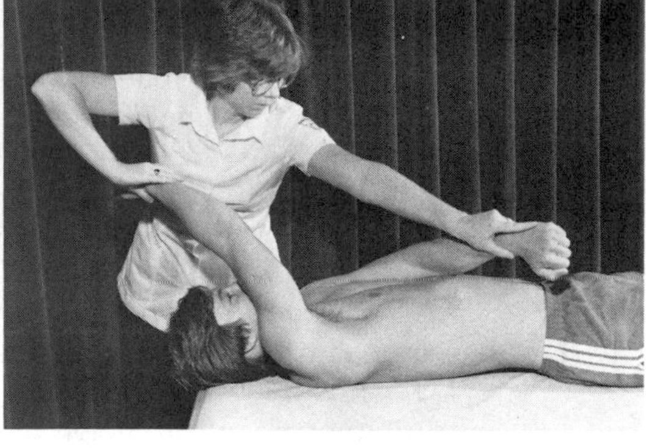

A. Supine: UE cross-diagonal.
E. MC wrists.

FIGURE 3–104

Before an effective treatment program can be implemented, the therapist must determine the movement pattern to be facilitated and the combination of patterns that will best enhance that movement. The following examples will illustrate this point: First, many patients with Parkinsonism may experience decreased trunk extension and respiratory functioning. A BS D_2F combination will facilitate trunk extension and can be coordinated with breathing patterns (17). Trunk rotation and extension can be combined with bilateral asymmetrical flexion of the upper extremities, or trunk rotation can

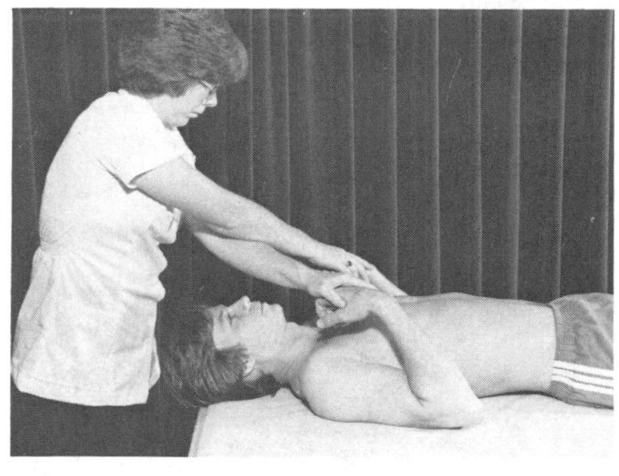

(a)

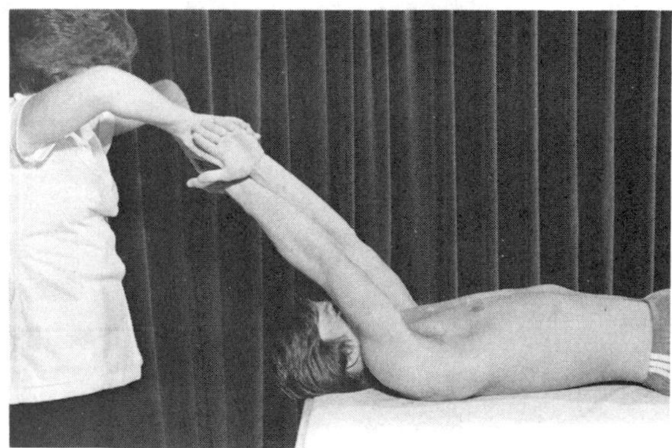

(b)

A. BS D_1 thrust.
E. MC wrists.

FIGURE 3–105

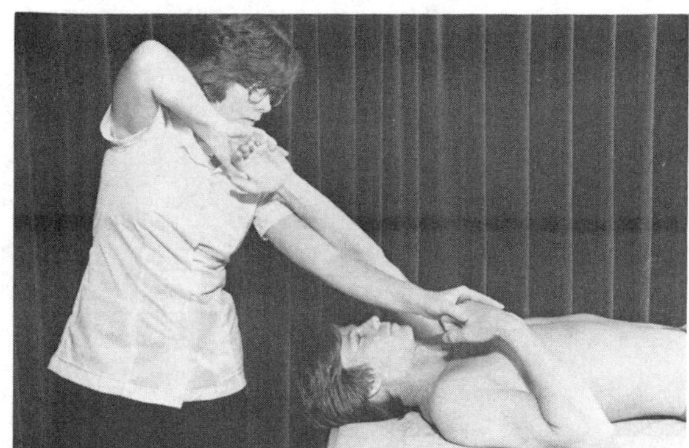

A. BR D_1 thrust.

FIGURE 3–106

be specifically emphasized with BR patterns to improve arm swing in gait. Second, during initial treatment sessions, patients with unilateral weakness may benefit from the application of bilateral patterns. If the right gluteus maximus is weak, for instance, a BS D_2E pattern combined with a strengthening technique may be used to enhance the response of the weakened muscle.

Like unilateral patterns, bilateral patterns can be performed in many positions. All upper extremity bilateral patterns are easily facilitated in supine or sitting. In sitting, however, the therapist's position usually limits the ability to resist the movement through full range (Figure 3–107). Bilateral lower

(a) (b)

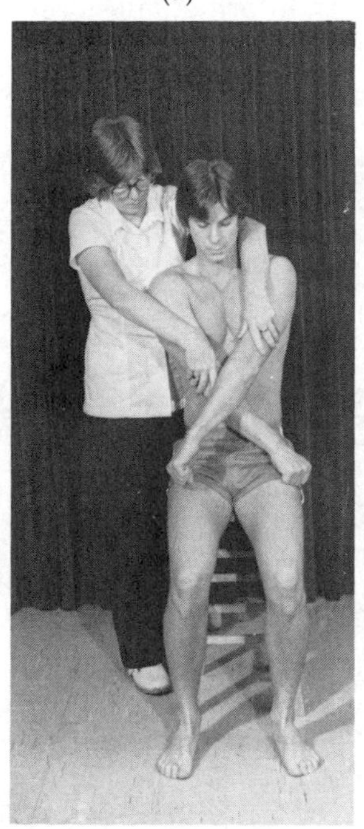

A. Sitting: UE BS D_2F.
E. MC wrists.

FIGURE 3–107

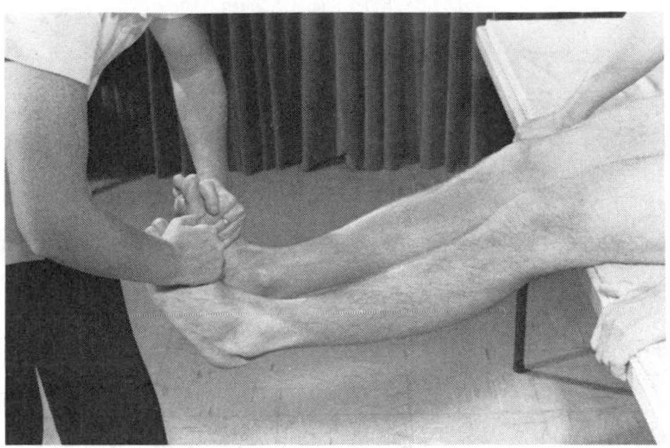

A. Sitting: LE BS D_1F.
E. MC feet.

FIGURE 3–108

extremity patterns can be performed in supine, prone, and sitting. In supine, because the patient may have difficulty coordinating the movement of both lower extremities, patterns are usually limited to symmetrical combinations. Similarly, symmetrical patterns are the movements most frequently applied in prone as the lack of visual input may make other combinations too difficult. In sitting, all lower extremity combinations can be easily applied (Figures 3–108, 3–109, and 3–110). Because the hip is relatively fixed (extension in prone, flexion in sitting), the emphasis in these postures is on knee and ankle control.

With the exception of the lower extremity patterns in the prone and sitting positions, the intermediate joint—the elbow or knee—is usually main-

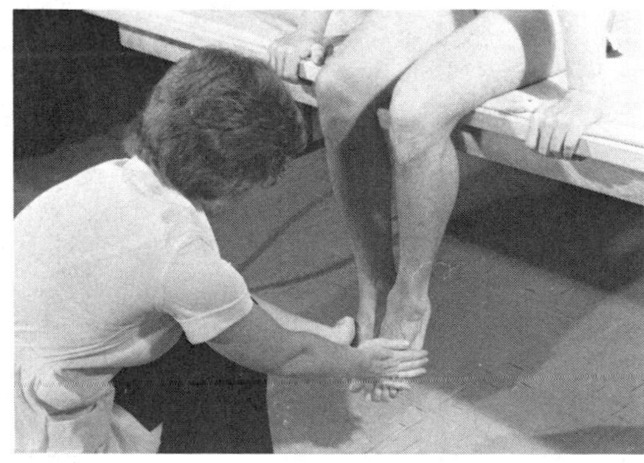

(a)

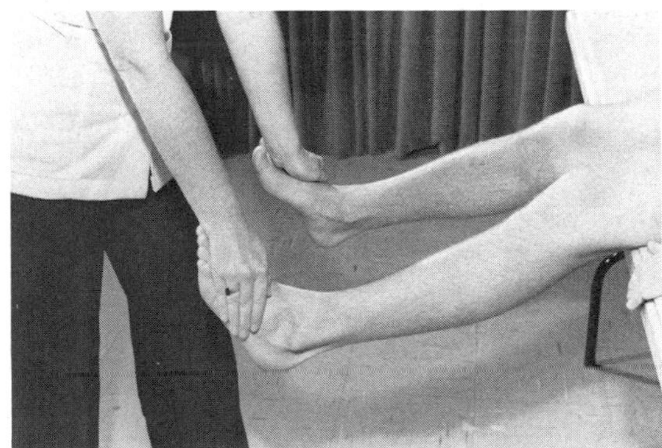

(b)

A. Sitting: LE BS D_2F.
E. MC feet.

FIGURE 3–109

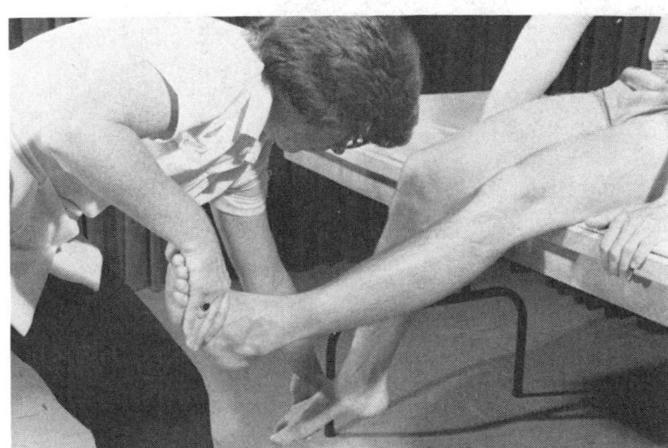

A. Sitting: LE cross-diagonal.
E. MC feet.

FIGURE 3–110

tained straight throughout the application of bilateral patterns to allow the therapist more control of the pattern. Therefore, bilateral patterns are most frequently used to emphasize activity at the shoulder or hip joints or to promote an associated trunk movement. Because there is only one manual contact on each extremity, the fine control that can be gained with unilateral patterns is lost.

■ Trunk Patterns

Trunk patterns are a combination of asymmetrical extremity diagonal patterns. The extremities are in contact with each other; this relationship, termed body-on-body contact, creates a closed kinematic loop (33, 41). Emphasis in the performance of the pattern is usually placed on the trunk and proximal components, rather than on the extremity and distal areas.

1. Upper Trunk Patterns. Upper trunk patterns combine head, neck, and upper trunk movement with asymmetrical upper extremity patterns. Arm contact is made by allowing one hand to grasp the other forearm. Upper trunk patterns are divided into two major activities, a chop and a lift (20). Each pattern has a reversal motion. In a chop and reverse chop the leading upper extremity or free arm, performs a D_1 pattern (Figure 3–111), whereas in the lift and reverse lift the lead arm is in a D_2 pattern (Figure 3–112).

Chopping or trunk flexion with rotation combines head, neck, and upper trunk flexion and rotation with upper extremity asymmetrical extension patterns. The lead upper extremity, the abducting arm, performs a D_1E pattern, while the assisting arm is in a D_2E pattern. The reversing motion, or reverse chop is an asymmetrical flexion motion of the upper extremities; the lead arm moves up and across the face in a D_1F pattern, while the assisting arm is in D_2F. The chopping activity is commonly used to strengthen the

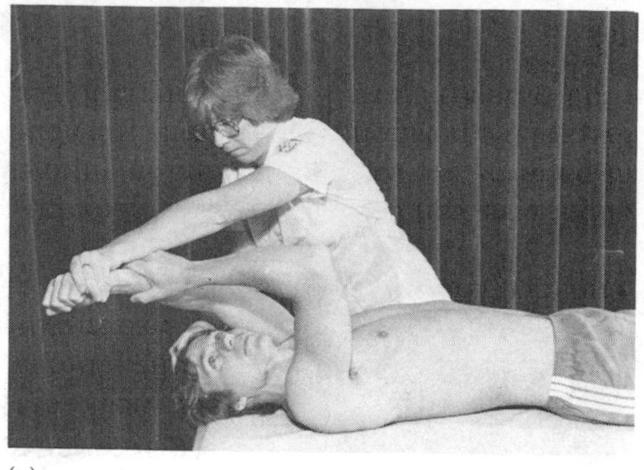
(a)

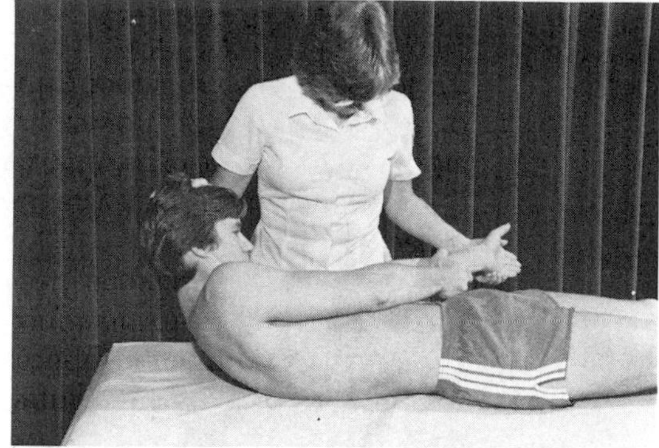
(b)

A. Supine: chop.
E. MC head and wrist.

FIGURE 3–111

oblique abdominals, to enhance overflow to either of the upper extremities, neck, or lower extremities, to improve upper trunk mobility, and to facilitate rolling. The reverse chop is also used to facilitate rolling and in addition to improve upper extremity flexion in the D_1F pattern (20) (see Chapters 8 and 10).

The lifting motion, or trunk extension with rotation, combines head, neck, and upper trunk extension with rotation with asymmetrical upper extremity flexion patterns. The lead upper extremity, the abducting arm, per-

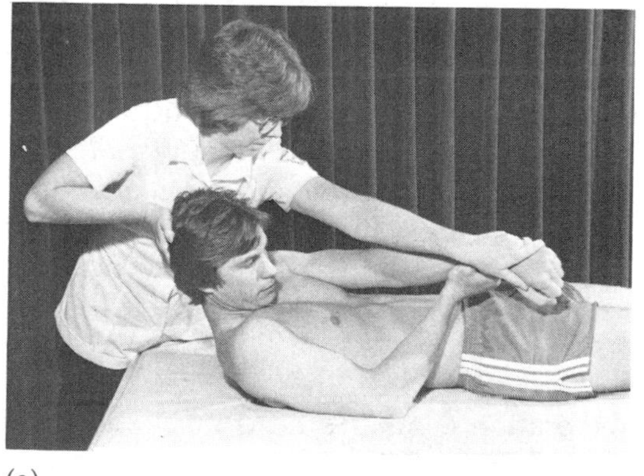
(a)

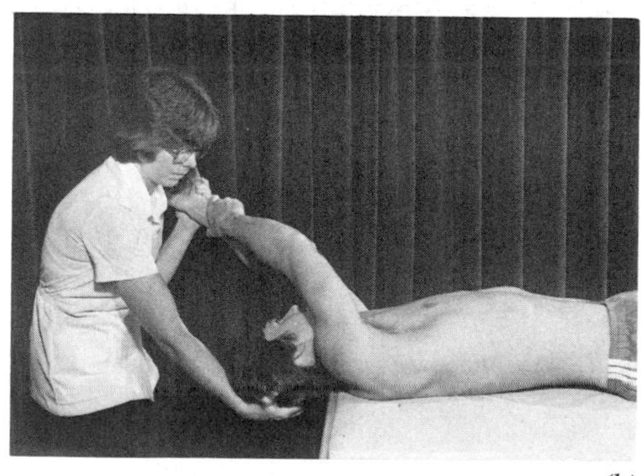
(b)

A. Supine: lift.
E. MC head and wrist.

FIGURE 3–112

forms D_2F pattern, while the assisting extremity is in a D_1F pattern. Clinically, lifting is useful whenever trunk extension with rotation is a goal. A more complete range of shoulder flexion can be accomplished with lifting rather than a reverse chop because the leading arm is moving into D_2F. Lifting can be coordinated effectively with breathing patterns; inspiration is combined with trunk extension and shoulder flexion and expiration with trunk flexion and shoulder extension (20). The reverse lift usually has no particular functional goal other than to promote a reversal of antagonists.

Trunk patterns, which combine proximal dynamic stability and distal mobility, can be considered the beginning of the skill level of extremity movements. The previous stages of motor control—stability and controlled mobility—were promoted in developmental postures. The progression of skilled activities would begin with trunk patterns and proceed to bilateral, then unilateral extremity patterns.

As in the case of unilateral patterns, the placement of manual contacts may vary, depending on the segments to be emphasized. When the emphasis is on the scapula and shoulder motions, both manual contacts can be placed on the scapula or one can be placed proximally on the scapula and one distally on the wrist or hand. If a goal of the procedure is to increase mobility at any of the extremity joints, the manual contacts can be positioned on the forearms (Figure 3–113) or on just one extremity. Sitting and supine are the most common postures in which to perform upper and lower trunk patterns. The effects of gravity and reflexes will differ depending on the posture (Figure 3–114). Lifting can also be performed in prone, but because both gravity and tonic reflex effects can resist lifting in this position, manual resistance must be carefully graded. Lifting in prone is an effective but stressful trunk strengthening activity and as such is best incorporated into advanced treatment progressions.

2. Lower Trunk Patterns. Like upper trunk patterns, lower trunk patterns combine asymmetrical extremity patterns with the lower extremities maintained in contact with each other. They are named by the direction of the motion: lower trunk flexion with rotation to the right and the antago-

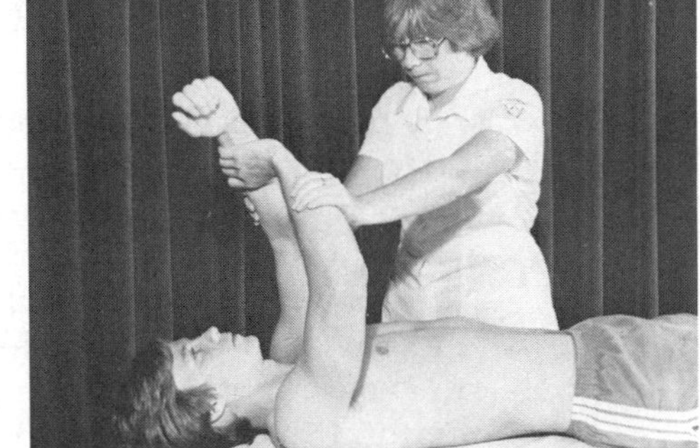

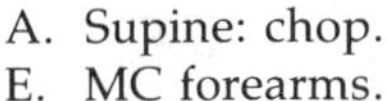
A. Supine: chop.
E. MC forearms.

FIGURE 3–113

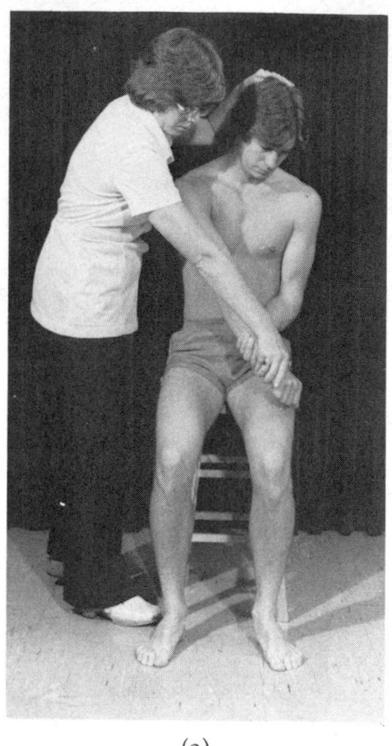

(a)

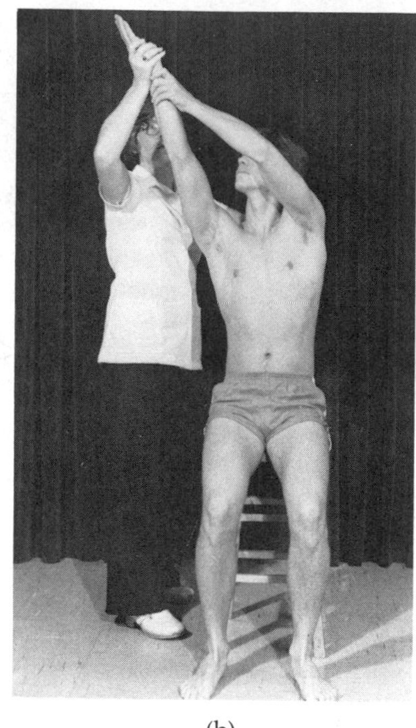

(b)

A. Sitting: lift.
E. MC head and wrist.

FIGURE 3–114

nistic motion of trunk extension with rotation to the left (Figure 3–115). In trunk flexion with rotation to the right, the D_2F leg (R) leads with the D_1F leg (L) following. In trunk extension to the left, the D_1E leg (L) leads and the D_2E leg (R) follows. The other diagonal movement, flexion with rotation to the left and extension to the right, employs the opposite combination of diagonal patterns. As with the chopping and lifting patterns, the abducting limb is considered the leading extremity.

The angle of the knee, the intermediate joint, can be varied during the performance of lower trunk patterns. Mass flexion or extension with the knee flexing and extending in combination with the hip motion is one alternative. The knee can also remain straight when moving to either flexion or extension (Figure 3–116). The advanced combination incorporates knee extension with hip flexion and knee flexion with hip extension (17). Resistance must be carefully applied when performing straight-leg or advanced combinations because of the length of the lever arm. If lower abdominal strength is not sufficient, a lumbar lordosis may occur when these patterns are performed. In such cases, an appropriate amount of assistance must be given during the hip flexor phase of lower trunk flexion to allow the patient to maintain a posterior pelvic tilt. Manual resistance may be indicated during the extensor phase when gravity is assisting. If the goal of treatment is to avoid synergistic lower extremity movements, the involved limb should perform the D_1 pattern. Because D_1 combines flexion with adduction, and

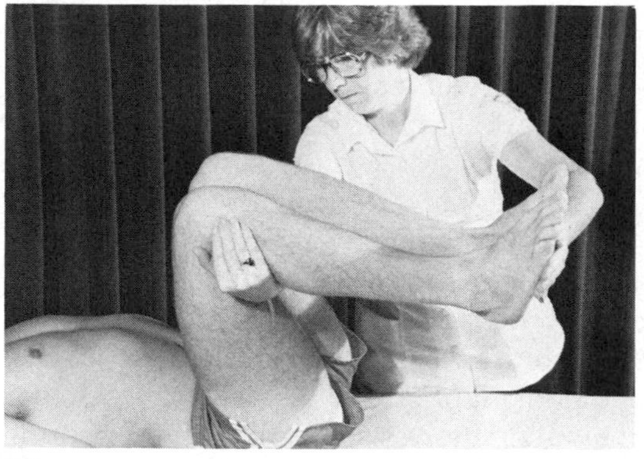

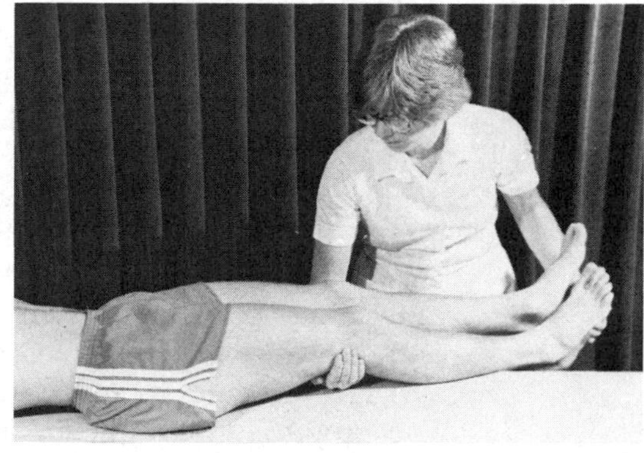

(a) (b)

A. Supine: lower trunk flexion and extension.
E. MC thighs and feet.

FIGURE 3–115

extension with abduction, the synergistic pattern is not reinforced (see Chapter 8).

Lower trunk mass patterns may enhance strengthening of the trunk, hip, or knee muscles by maximizing overflow from the stronger to the weaker areas. These patterns can effectively enhance activity of the internal obliques (34), an important consideration in the treatment of patients with some low back dysfunctions. In such cases, emphasis would not be placed on resistance through range, but rather on isometric contractions in the shortened range. Straight-leg combinations are appropriate when knee motion through range is contraindicated, as it is for patients with chondromalacia or a dislocating patella. The advanced combination of trunk patterns has been found to be the most difficult of the lower trunk movements and

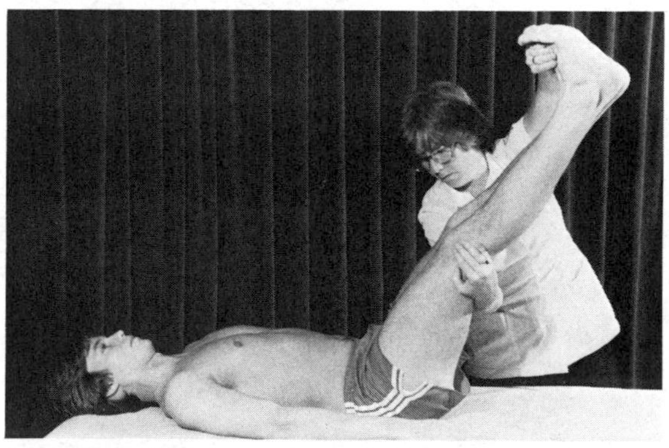

A. Supine: lower trunk flexion, knee straight.
E. MC thighs and feet.

FIGURE 3–116

is usually appropriate only for enhancing the hip and knee movements needed for gait.

For both upper and lower extremity combinations, the sequencing of trunk, bilateral, and unilateral patterns is determined by the evaluative findings and the treatment goals. Activities for a weak gluteus medius, for example, might begin with a lower trunk extensor pattern with the right lower extremity moving into D_1E. This pattern promotes overflow from the trunk and uninvolved lower extremity and enhances the response of the weakened hip abductor. BS D_1E patterns follow, progressing to a unilateral D_1E pattern, which requires the most muscle control. Developmental activities such as LTR, bridging, quadruped, modified plantigrade, and standing should also progress in a sequence that will alter the resistance of weight bearing and the amount of stretch on the muscle.

Clinically, trunk patterns have been used to treat a variety of patients and to promote many goals. Because the extremities move asymmetrically, trunk rotation is a component of each pattern. Rotation has been empirically found to decrease tone when hypertonia or rigidity is present (16). Trunk rotation also can promote righting reactions that may result in a decrease in the dominance of symmetrical tonic reflexes. Crossing of the midline, which occurs during this asymmetrical extremity combination, is an essential goal for patients with perceptual or denial problems or who are dominated by the ATNR. When performed as a reversing motion, that is, alternating directions of flexion and extension, a reciprocation of antagonistic muscle groups occurs that is particularly important when spasticity or weakness is present (17).

Trunk patterns may be clinically effective in reaching the following goals:

1. **To strengthen trunk musculature.** If both upper or lower extremities are in the good to normal ranges, they may be combined to produce overflow to the weaker trunk musculature. Patients with paraplegia, for example, may use the stronger upper extremities to promote trunk activity.
2. **To strengthen or reinforce extremity musculature.** If weakness is present in one extremity but the trunk and contralateral extremity are of good to normal strength, resisted trunk patterns may result in overflow to the area of weakness. Facilitation of the weakened extremity also may be due to body-on-body contact, which is termed the tracking of the involved side with the uninvolved side.
3. **To promote movement that is limited by pain.** Patients with pain can frequently move into more range when they are contacting and supporting their involved limb with the uninvolved pain-free limb. If one upper extremity is painful, especially at the proximal joints, upper trunk patterns may promote more freedom of move-

ment than unilateral patterns. The addition of appropriate relaxation techniques can further enhance this movement.

4. **To enhance functional activities.** Rolling with upper trunk patterns can be used when weakness of one extremity or unilateral neglect is a problem, as in the case of hemiplegic patients. Other patients, typically those with spinal cord injury, will use their stronger upper extremities to assist with rolling activities.
5. **To promote a balance of tone.** When imbalances of tone exist in the trunk, trunk patterns can be used to enhance one direction of motion and thus can help restore a balance of antagonists. A patient demonstrating an increase in trunk extensor tone, for example, would benefit from a trunk pattern emphasizing flexion.

This chapter discusses activities as being only one component of any given procedure selected to help a patient attain short-term goals. The therapist can choose from a multitude of activities that include developmental postures, and trunk, bilateral, and unilateral extremity patterns. Biomechanical, tonal, and neurophysiological factors can influence the maintenance of a posture or movement within a posture. With these considerations in mind, a sequence of activities can be designed to achieve or reinforce the necessary stages of motor control for each patient.

REFERENCES

1. Shaltenbrand G: The development of human motility and motor disturbances. Arch Neurol Psychiat 20:720–730, 1928
2. Sherrington CS: The Integrative Action of the Nervous System. New Haven, Yale University Press, 1922
3. Hirt S: The tonic neck reflex mechanism in the normal human adult. Amer J Phys Med 46:362–369, 1966
4. Hellebrandt FA, Houtz SJ, Partridge MJ, et al: Tonic neck reflexes in exercises of stress in man. Amer J Phys Med 35:144–159, 1956
5. Voss DE: Proprioceptive neuromuscular facilitation. Amer J Phys Med 46:838–898, 1966
6. Brunnstrom S: Movement Therapy in Hemiplegia. New York, Harper & Row, 1970
7. Bobath B: Adult Hemiplegia: Evaluation and Treatment. London, Heinemann Medical Books Ltd, 1978
8. Weisz S: Studies in equilibrium reactions. J Nerv Ment Dis 88:150–162, 1938
9. Kabat H: Studies on neuromuscular dysfunction. In Payton OD, Hirt

S, Newton RA (eds): Neurophysiologic Approaches to Therapeutic Exercise. Philadelphia, FA Davis, 1977

10. Burg D, Szumski AJ, Struppler A, et al: Influence of a voluntary innervation on human muscle spindle sensitivity. In Shahani M(ed): The Motor System: Neurophysiology and muscle mechanisms. New York, Elsevier, Publisher, 1976
11. Cheney PD, Preston JB: Classification of fusimotor fibers in the primate. J Neurophysiol 39:9–19, 1976
12. Granit R: The functional role of the muscle spindles—facts and hypothesis. Brain 98:531–556, 1975
13. Stockmeyer SA: An interpretation of the approach of Rood to the treatment of neuromuscular dysfunction. Amer J Phys Med 46:900–956, 1966
14. Urbscheit N: Reflexes evoked by group II afferent fibers from muscle spindles. Phys Ther 59:1083–1087, 1979
15. Stockmeyer SA: Analysis of procedures to improve motor control. Unpublished notes from Boston University PT 710, 1979
16. Semans S: The Bobath concept in treatment of neurological disorders. Amer J Phys Med 46:732–785, 1966
17. Knott M, Voss DE: Proprioceptive Neuromuscular Facilitation, ed 2. New York, Harper & Row, 1968
18. Hagbarth KE: Excitatory and inhibitory skin areas for flexor and extensor motoneurons. ACTA Physical Scand 26, suppl 94:5
19. Eldred E, Hagbarth KE: Facilitation and inhibition of gamma efferents by stimulation of certain skin areas. J Neurophysiol 17:59–65, 1954
20. Voss DE: Proprioceptive neuromuscular facilitation. Amer J Phys Med. 46:838–898, 1966
21. Partridge MJ: Electromyographic demonstration of facilitation. Phys Ther Rev 34:227–232, 1954
22. Fiorentino M: Normal and Abnormal Development. Springfield, IL, Charles C Thomas, 1972
23. McGraw MB: The Neuromuscular Maturation of the Human Infant. New York, Columbia University Press, 1943. Reprinted edition, New York, Hafner Publishing Co, 1962
24. Ter Vrugt D, Pederson DR: The effects of vertical rocking frequencies on the arousal level of two-month-old infants. Child Dev 44:205 209, 1973
25. Knott M: Report of a case of Parkinsonism treated with proprioceptive facilitation technics. Phys Ther Rev 37:229, 1957
26. Voss DE, Knott M, Kabat H: Application of neuromuscular facilitation in the treatment of shoulder disabilities. Phys Ther Rev 33:536–537, 1953

27. Jensen GM: Biomechanics of the lumbar intervertebral disc: A review. Phys Ther 60:765–773, 1980
28. Peiper A: Cerebral Function in Infancy and Childhood. New York, Consultant's Bureau, 1963
29. Dee R: Structure and function of hip joint innervation. Ann Roy Coll Surg Engl 45:357–374, 1969
30. Seeger MA, Perry J, Hislop HJ: Electromyographic Study of Weight Bearing Upper Extremity Postural Reactions of Adults with Hemiplegia. Read at the Annual Conference of the American Physical Therapy Association, Phoenix, 1980
31. Poland JL, Hobart DJ, Payton OD: The Musculoskeletal System. Flushing, NY, Medical Examination Publishing Co, 1977
32. Stockmeyer SA: A sensorimotor approach to treatment. In Pearson PH, Williams CE (eds): Physical Therapy Services in the Developmental Disabilities. Springfield, IL, Charles C Thomas, 1972
33. Voss DE: Therapeutic exercise. Unpublished notes from Northwestern University, 1974
34. Konecky C: An EMG Study of Abdominals and Back Extensors During Lower Trunk Rotation. Thesis. Boston, MA, Boston University Sargent College of Allied Health Professions, 1980
35. Knott M, Voss DE: Proprioceptive Neuromuscular Facilitation. New York, Harper & Row, 1956
36. Saunders JB, Inman VT, Eberhart HD: The major determinants in normal and pathological gait. J Bone Joint Surg 35–A:543–558, 1953
37. Francis N: EMG Analysis of Unilateral and Bilateral PNF Patterns. Thesis. Boston, MA, Boston University Sargent College of Allied Health Professions, 1980
38. Rood M: Treatment of Neuromuscular Dysfunction: Rood Approach. Read at Conference sponsored by Massachusetts Chapter American Physical Therapy Association, Boston, 1976
39. Sullivan PE, Portney LG: Electromyographic activity of shoulder muscles during unilateral upper extremity proprioceptive neuromuscular facilitation patterns. Phys Ther 60:283–288, 1980
40. Portney LG, Sullivan PE: EMG Analysis of Ipsilateral and Contralateral Shoulder and Elbow Muscles During the Performance of PNF Patterns. Read at the Annual Conference of the Society for Behavioral Kinesiology, Boston, 1979
41. Steindler A: Kinesiology. Springfield, IL, Charles C Thomas, 1955

chapter 4

Techniques

INTRODUCTION

This chapter describes various PNF techniques and explains how they may be used to progress through the four stages of motor control (mobility, stability, controlled mobility, and skill). In addition, it examines some of the underlying neurophysiological mechanisms that may be responsible for the efficacy of these techniques. Most neurophysiological research has been conducted on isolated animal motor units or muscle spindles. Extrapolation of these findings to the complex human condition is extremely difficult. Both facilitatory and inhibitory central and peripheral influences constantly bombard the final common pathway. Exactly which of these influences may predominate in a given set of circumstances for different individuals with varying conditions is unknown. The rationales presented in this chapter are by no means conclusive. Using present information, we have suggested various neurophysiological mechanisms that may contribute to facilitatory and inhibitory responses when a technique is applied. Certainly, much more research is needed to verify or discredit these suggestions.

The techniques described are employed to promote desired types of muscular contractions for the attainment of short-term goals. They may combine isotonic (concentric and eccentric) and isometric contractions and may emphasize either movement in one direction or reversing movements (1). Techniques may be applied throughout a movement pattern or they may be restricted to the lengthened, mid-, or shortened ranges, depending on the treatment objectives.

MULTI-FACETED TECHNIQUES

Although many PNF techniques are used specifically to attain one of the four levels of motor control, others are more versatile. Slow reversal (SR), slow reversal hold (SRH), repeated contractions (RC), timing for emphasis (TE), and agonistic reversals (AR) can be combined with other techniques to promote several stages of motor control. In the following sections each of these five techniques is first explained in detail and then its application in conjunction with other techniques is discussed in relation to mobility, stability, controlled mobility, and skill.

■ Slow Reversal and Slow Reversal Hold (SR, SRH)

The slow reversal technique, also referred to as reversal of antagonists, involves alternate, slow, rhythmical concentric contractions of all the components of agonistic and antagonistic patterns without relaxation between reversals (1). In cases of muscle imbalance around a joint, resistance should first be applied to the stronger pattern, because it may have a facilitatory effect on weaker antagonistic musculature. Resistance is always graded to allow the patient to move through as much active range as possible. At the same time, the resistance should be sufficient to elicit maximal motoneuron recruitment. Slow reversal hold varies from SR in that a gradually applied isometric contraction is introduced at the end of the range of the movement pattern.

Neurophysiological rationale:

- The effects of slow reversal may be explained by Sherrington's law of successive induction, which maintains that a pattern of movement is facilitated by the immediate preceding contraction of its antagonist (2). The rationale underlying this phenomenon is unclear. One explanation could be that as the stronger pattern actively approaches the shortened range and as the external stretch of the muscles in this pattern diminishes, the unloading of the muscle spindle reduces the spindle afferent input from these receptors to higher centers. Unless resistance, particularly isometric resistance, is emphasized in the shortened range to facilitate the fusimotor system and subsequent spindle afferent firing, the inhibitory influences of Golgi tendon organs (GTOs) and Renshaw cells on agonistic anterior horn cells could predominate. The result, therefore, could be one of inhibition of the contracting pattern and reciprocal facilitation to the antagonist (3).

- The simultaneous stretching of the antagonistic muscles at the end of the range can result in autogenetic facilitation to those muscles via the primary afferents of the muscle spindles.
- Recent electromyographic studies have shown that under certain conditions the onset of antagonistic activity occurs prior to the time when the antagonistic muscle groups are stretched. This evidence strongly suggests that facilitation to the antagonistic pattern may be a result of central programming rather than influences from peripheral mechanisms (4–5).
- When an isometric contraction is introduced, as with SRH, the neurophysiological response may change. A gradually applied isometric contraction should recruit more gamma static motoneurons than an isotonic contraction (6–8). Because of the increased gamma motoneuron activity, the muscle spindles are less likely to become slack at the end of the range, as may be the case for SR. Therefore the spindle afferent endings may continue to fire, and thus may cause motor unit facilitation (9). Although both GTO and Renshaw cell inhibition may still occur, both central and peripheral facilitatory effects may predominate. It appears, then, that the introduction of an isometric contraction enhances the contraction of muscle groups, whereas a simple isotonic contraction during a pattern of movement may possibly produce more inhibitory effects toward the end of the range (3). The repeated use of SR and SRH should lead to facilitation of the muscles in both directions of movement.

Repeated Contractions (RC)

Repeated contractions differ from a slow reversal in that the emphasis of the movement occurs only on one side of the joint. Repeated contractions to the weakened muscles in a pattern may, however, be preceded by an isotonic contraction of the muscles of the stronger antagonistic pattern to facilitate the weakened musculature by successive induction. This technique is particularly effective in three instances of muscle weakness and is applied somewhat differently in each case:

1. If the muscles in a movement pattern are in the trace to poor range, as assessed by a manual muscle test, voluntary initiation of the pattern will be difficult, if not impossible. In such instances, the muscles in the pattern are quickly stretched in the lengthened range to initiate a reflex response (1). Because a trace to poor muscle lacks adequate stretch sensitivity, the external stretch imposed by the therapist may have to be repeated several times along with strong verbal commands before any significant visible response will occur. Once the muscles do respond, they must be immediately resisted in order to perpetuate the isotonic contraction. RC should be concluded with an isometric contraction at the end of the gained range to enhance the gamma or spindle bias [Figure 4–1(a)]. Caution must also be taken when the muscle group(s) repeatedly stretched are postural extensors (see Chapter 5).

2. Repeated contractions can be applied throughout a movement pattern

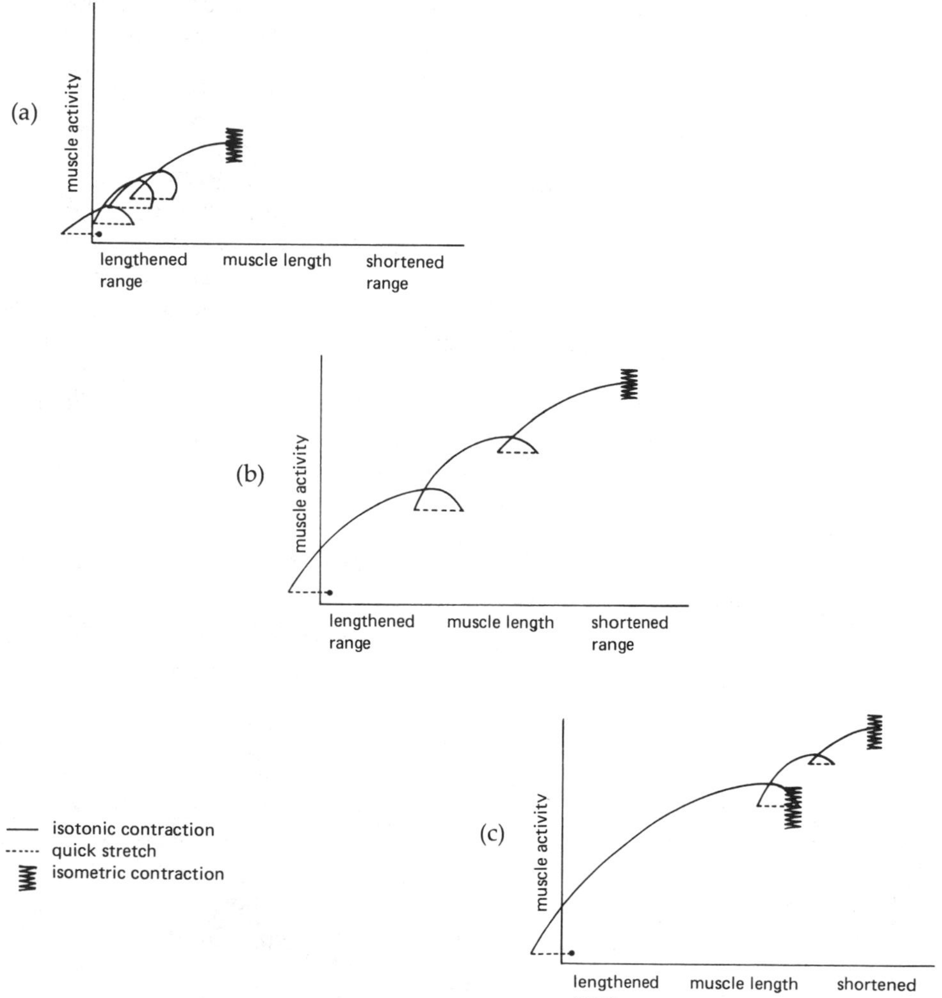

FIGURE 4–1
Three types of repeated contractions.

when the muscle grades are in the fair range and the weakness is consistent throughout the range. Quick stretches resulting in a reflex contraction can be superimposed on the voluntary isotonic contractions at varied points in the range for purposes of enhancing the response. Because a muscle with a fair grade does not completely lack stretch sensitivity, the magnitude of the manually applied stretch does not have to be as great as that cited in the first example [Figure 4–1(b)].

3. When the muscles active in a given movement pattern do not have equal strength throughout the range, RC are applied at the particular point in the range at which the response begins to diminish. At this point of weakness an isometric contraction is elicited, followed immediately by a series of small superimposed manual stretches and resisted isotonic movement further into the range (1) [Figure 4–1(c)].

Neurophysiological rationale:

- If the internal stretch of intrafusal fibers of muscle spindles by the gamma motoneurons is deficient, the primary afferents of the spindles can be activated by rapid and substantial external stretches of the entire muscle (10–12). However, resistance even of a very slight amount is then necessary to facilitate the gamma system; such resistance keeps the spindles loaded or taut and thus responsive to stimulation. Stretch without subsequent resistance can result in unloaded or slack intrafusal fibers of the muscle spindle and a subsequent decrease in spindle afferent firing (13). Terminating the technique with a maintained isometric contraction in as shortened a range as possible is a particularly effective means of facilitating the static gamma motoneurons and enhancing spindle bias (3). Strong verbal commands will enhance the response through the reticular activating system (14–15).
- Quick stretches superimposed on an isotonic contraction should increase spindle primary afferent firing and contribute to alpha motor neuron recruitment (8, 16).
- As already stated, an isometric contraction at the point of weakness will increase gamma motoneuron activity and thus increase spindle bias or stretch sensitivity. The longer the contraction is held, the more this gamma activity will be increased. Consequently, the spindles should become more biased (3). The primary afferents of the spindles should then be responsive to subsequent quick stretches, which will lead to alpha motoneuron recruitment.
- Resistance to the antagonistic pattern will reduce fatigue of the weakened muscles and through successive induction enhance subsequent contractions of the weakened pattern.

■ Timing for Emphasis (TE)

Timing for emphasis is an effective technique when the weakness in a movement pattern is restricted to only one component of the pattern, such as the wrist, elbow, or shoulder. This technique is used to elicit a strong contraction of the more normal components of the pattern in order to produce an overflow effect into the weaker components (1). Overflow is produced by allowing the entire pattern to contract isotonically to a point in the range at which the stronger components can contract isometrically with the greatest efficiency. Although this point of optimal isometric contraction varies, it is often in the mid range of the movement for flexor muscles, and the more shortened range for extensor muscles. Since no norms have been established, the isometric contraction is always elicited in that part of the range which, in the therapist's judgment, the patient can hold best. At that point, the hold of the stronger musculature is sustained while the weaker musculature simultaneously performs an isotonic contraction with quick stretch superimposed (1). Basically what takes place is that the stronger muscles hold while a repeated contraction coupled with dynamic verbal commands to push or pull is performed by the weaker muscle group. As noted under RC, the stretch and isotonic movement of the weak component should be followed, whenever possible, by an isometric contraction of that same component in the shortened range of the movement.

TE also may be applied to bilateral patterns to elicit overflow from one limb to another or to trunk patterns to elicit overflow from both extremities into trunk musculature. When used in this manner, the stronger limb(s) isometrically contract(s) against manual resistance at a point in the range which appears to be optimal as the weaker limb or trunk musculature performs a repeated contraction toward the shortened range. The bilateral pattern is chosen to optimize overflow from the stronger limb or to enhance the patient's normal reinforcing pattern.

Neurophysiological rationale:

- A maintained isometric contraction of strong muscle groups is capable of producing overflow facilitation effects to the weaker musculature (6, 17–19).
- Increased alpha and gamma motoneuron recruitment should occur.
- By simultaneously superimposing quick external stretches on the isotonically contracting weak muscles, the patient should be able to enhance the firing of the primary afferents of the spindles and obtain a greater response (see rationale following "Repeated Contractions").

Agonistic Reversals (AR)

Agonistic reversals is a technique that promotes both concentric and eccentric contractions of a movement pattern. In order to attain normal function, a patient must be able to control his body weight through the full range of a lengthening contraction. For example, to descend stairs and to sit from a standing position, eccentric control of lower extremity extensors is necessary. Like RC and TE, AR emphasizes either the flexor or extensor component of one movement pattern at a time. The patient is instructed to move isotonically through a range of motion with resistance to tolerance. At the end of the concentric range, instead of reversing the antagonists, the patient undertakes a slow, controlled, rhythmical sequence of eccentric, concentric, eccentric contractions of the same muscle(s), which are repeated a number of times. The verbal commands would be, for example, "Make me work at pulling your limb down or pushing your limb up," as the therapist slowly resists the eccentric contraction of the agonistic muscle groups. AR can be performed through increments of range to promote optimal control.

Patients with spasticity commonly have a great deal of difficulty performing an eccentric contraction throughout a range of motion. The ability to control both shortening and lengthening contractions in a slow, controlled, rhythmical manner appears to preclude the triggering of spastic movement patterns (20). To accomplish this goal AR is performed through increments of range.

AR may be applied to individual patterns or to activities in developmental postures such as bridging or kneeling to promote eccentric control specifically of hip and knee extensors (see Chapters 3, 8, and 11).

Neurophysiological rationale:

- When a muscle contracts against resistance eccentrically, both external and internal stretch occur simultaneously. External stretch refers to the gradual lengthening of the extrafusal and intrafusal muscle fibers, while internal stretch refers to the biasing of the intrafusal fibers by the gamma system.
- The combination of both external and internal stretch of the intrafusal fibers of the spindles should enhance firing of the spindle afferents (21). Weak postural extensors, however, may have more difficulty with eccentric contractions than more phasic muscle groups. As the postural muscle further contracts eccentrically into its lengthened ranges, more stimulus will be provided for secondary spindle afferent firing, and consequently muscle inhibitory influences may be increased.
- Care must be taken to first establish adequate gamma bias of muscle spindles in shortened ranges so that when the gradual external stretch is applied, the primary afferents can respond. Primary afferent firing should then provide enough facilitation at the an-

terior horn cell pool to predominate over any inhibition that may occur.

This section concludes the general description of SR, SRH, RC, TE, and AR. The techniques discussed in the remainder of this chapter can be directed to specific stages of motor control. One or more of the five techniques already described are included under each of the stages of control whenever they can be used appropriately to enhance a particular stage.

APPLICATION OF TECHNIQUES TO PROMOTE MOTOR CONTROL

■ Mobility

Mobility is defined as: the ability to initiate movement, and the availability of a functional range of motion through which to move. The inability to initiate movement can be due to either hyper- or hypotonia. Two techniques are particularly effective in dealing with these two circumstances.

Rhythmic Initiation. Rhythmic initiation (RI) is indicated when a patient is unable to initiate movement or is limited in range because of hypertonus. With this technique, movement of a body part progresses from completely passive to active assisted to slightly resisted as the patient relaxes and is capable of exerting increased control over the movement. The goal is to promote relaxation and consequently increase the range of motion through which the patient can be moved, first passively, then more actively. The verbal commands are "Relax and let me move you," followed by "Now you do it with me" (1). It is important that the verbal commands be soothing and the movements repetitive, slow, and rhythmic. Facilitatory quick stretch to any muscle groups that are to be relaxed must be avoided.

RI is an effective technique for patients such as those with Parkinsonism who have difficulty initiating movement. Rolling, a total body pattern that is important both developmentally and functionally, should be one of the first activities included in a treatment program for this type of patient. The patient is asked to lie on one side and the manual contacts of the therapist are firmly maintained on scapula and pelvis. The patient is then instructed to relax while being passively moved toward prone and then supine. This passive stage is repeated until the therapist feels that the patient has relaxed and can thereby be moved more easily through increments of range. At the same time, the patient may be able to exert some active control through the range. When this occurs, slight resistance is added so that in effect RI may become SR. In the case of a patient with Parkinsonism, the resistance would be applied primarily to the movement of rolling toward supine because the extensor musculature of this patient should be emphasized. Conversely, if a patient were to exhibit extensor spasticity, resisted rolling toward prone would be preferable for facilitation of flexor tone.

RI is also of benefit when a motor learning or communications problem exists instead of, or in addition to, hypertonia. Allowing the patient both to feel and look at either the extremity or trunk movement as the pattern is passively performed facilitates subsequent active or resisted contractions with minimal frustration on the part of both patient and therapist.

Neurophysiological rationale:

- The vestibular system may accommodate to the repetitive rhythmic movements and calming verbal commands associated with RI. Decreased input to the reticular formation may result and thereby may minimize arousal effects (22–23).
- Although the mechanism has not been discussed in the literature, the calming effects of rocking have been attributed to reflexive autonomic changes (22).
- While the agonist contracts, the antagonist receives inhibitory influences from the primary afferents of agonistic muscle spindles, which will allow for increased movement in one direction (24–25). These influences would not occur until the patient began to participate actively in the movement.
- Because verbal commands order the patient to relax, cortical inhibition may be a contributing factor in decreasing tone (26–31).
- At the end of the range of an active contraction, the antagonistic muscle groups may be facilitated (successive induction).

Hold Relax Active Movement (HRAM). Hold relax active movement can be applied in cases of hypotonia when movement in one direction cannot be initiated because of weakness. During the initial aspects of the treatment progression the technique may also be used to promote a balance of tone (32).

The patient is first asked to hold a graded, manually resisted isometric contraction in the mid- to shortened ranges of a pattern into which he has been placed. When the therapist thinks that the contraction is optimal, the patient is given a command to relax. The therapist then quickly moves the patient to the lengthened range of the pattern of weakness and applies a quick stretch or repeated stretches (RC) to the same pattern. With dynamic verbal commands the patient is instructed to return to the more shortened range. The therapist may assist, track, or resist the isotonic movement, depending on the amount of activation elicited. This technique can be used, for example, to help a patient with weakness to initiate rolling toward prone. With manual contacts on pelvis and scapula, the therapist can position the patient in a sidelying to semiprone posture [Figure 4–2(a)] and ask for a maintained hold. When the hold is deemed maximal, the patient is

(a)

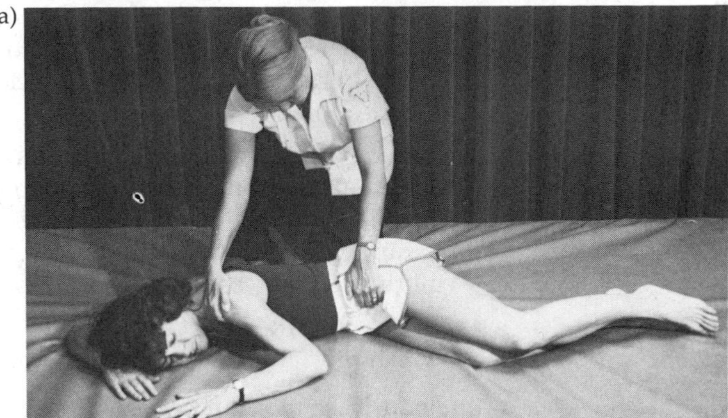

A. Rolling: supine to prone, shortened range.
T. HRAM.
E. MC pelvis, scapula.

(b)

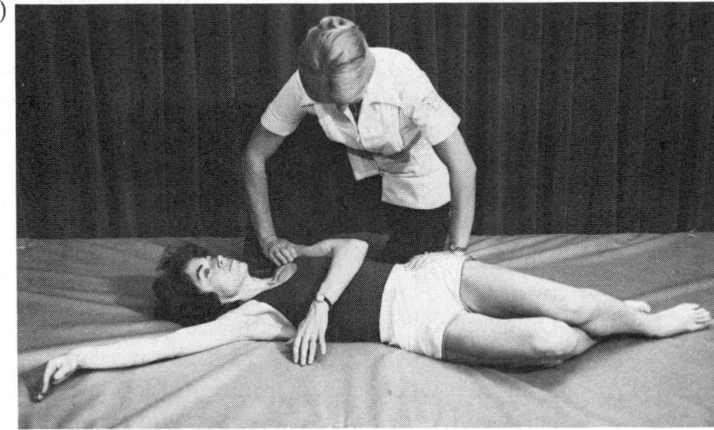

A. Rolling: supine to prone, lengthened range.
T. HRAM.
E. MC pelvis, scapula.

FIGURE 4–2

instructed to relax and is quickly moved back to supine [Figure 4–2(b)], where a stretch to the abdominals is applied. The patient is immediately instructed to roll back toward prone against resistance. Although abdominals have been used in this example, HRAM would certainly be indicated for weak extensor muscles. Emphasis should, perhaps, first be placed on holding of the extensor muscles in their shortened ranges as a preliminary step to developing cocontraction around proximal joints (33). Because the stretch applied in the lengthened range of the muscle with HRAM is dynamic and not prolonged, any danger of tonic muscle inhibition via secondary fibers of muscle spindles is minimized.

Neurophysiological rationale:

- Resisted isometric contractions in shortened ranges should facilitate coactivation, that is, simultaneous facilitation of alpha and gamma motoneurons. As already noted, static gamma motoneurons are particularly sensitive to maintained isometric contractions. When facilitated, these motoneurons can reduce the slack in the intrafusal fibers of the muscle spindles that occurs when a muscle is passively shortened.

- The longer the isometric contraction is held against resistance, the more taut the spindles should become, thus rendering their afferent fibers more sensitive to stretch. Therefore, when the muscle is quickly lengthened, the primary afferents of the spindles are more likely to respond and produce autogenetic facilitation (34).
- Unlike RI, HRAM is characterized by dynamic verbal commands, which may arouse the reticular system.

As previously stated, the other aspect of mobility is the availability of range of motion through which the patient can move. In addition to RI, which can also be used to increase range of motion, four relaxation techniques can be used to accomplish this goal.

Hold-Relax (HR). Hold-relax is an isometric technique that is effective when range of motion has decreased because of muscle tightness on one side of a joint. It is particularly effective when pain either accompanies the limitation of movement or is the primary cause of the immobility. The technique is applied in the following manner: An isometric contraction of all of the components of the range limiting or antagonistic pattern is elicited usually at the point of limitation of the available ROM. If the hamstrings are tight, for example, the isometric resistance would be applied to the D_1 and D_2 extensor patterns with the patient supine and the knee extended.The isometric contraction is gradually maximized over a period of seconds, then it is followed by a command to relax slowly. Once relaxation has been achieved, the limb actively moves against minimal resistance through the newly gained range to the new point of limitation. The technique is then reapplied and the cycle continued until no further increase in range can be accomplished for that treatment period. This combination of active movement following HR may be referred to as slow reversal hold-relax (1). If the agonistic muscles are too weak to move the part into the gained range, passive movement is an alternative.

Hold-relax may be applied to the agonistic pattern instead of the antagonistic or range-limiting pattern. During this variation, the manual contacts of the therapist are placed to resist the agonistic musculature and slight resistance is applied into the nonpainful range to reduce the anxiety of the patient. If a patient were limited in the Diagonal 2 flexor pattern of the upper extremity by a tight pectoralis major, for example, he would actively move to the point of limitation in that pattern. The verbal commands at this point would be "Hold, don't let me push your arm *down*," as resistance is applied to the middle deltoid (Figure 4–3). HR to the agonist appears to be effective, especially during initial treatment sessions when gaining the pa-

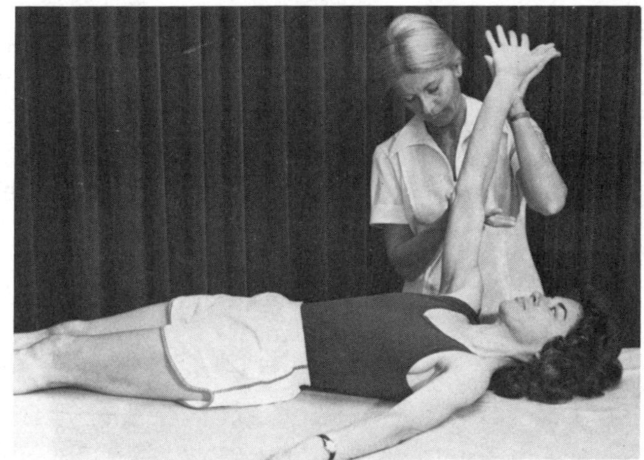

A. Supine: D_2F UE.
T. HR to agonist.
E. MC upper arm, hand.

FIGURE 4–3

tient's confidence is important. In addition, a hold applied to a weak agonist, particularly to a postural muscle that has undergone adaptive lengthening, will facilitate restoration of normal spindle bias (see Chapter 11).

Neurophysiological rationale:

- Depending on the length of time of application of HR to the antagonist and the number of repetitions during one treatment session, fatigue of motor units occurring at the neuromuscular junction may contribute to dampening of muscle tension (35–36).
- Golgi tendon organs (GTOs) are extremely sensitive to active muscle tension and when activated provide the anterior horn cells of the spinal cord with autogenetic inhibitory impulses (24–25). Increases in range of motion that occur seconds after the application of the technique directly to the antagonist may be affected by GTO activation. The inhibitory influence on the motoneurons pool by GTOs is not long lasting, however (it is only milliseconds) (37). As a result, it is difficult to attribute range of motion increments solely to these peripheral receptors.
- Discharge of Renshaw cells inhibits previously discharging alpha motoneurons. This recurrent inhibition appears to be most predominant on the low-threshold tonic motor units (8, 38). The active muscle tension produced by HR is submaximal, except during the last few seconds of contraction. According to normal motoneuron recruitment order (39), it appears likely, then, that the majority of motor units recruited during the application of HR to the antagonist would be more tonic in composition.
- If the tight muscle to which HR is applied is a postural extensor,

any inhibitory effects of muscle spindle secondary afferents reacting to the resistance or stretch may predominate (3).

- Low-threshold, slowly adapting joint receptors can be stimulated by changes in isotonic or isometric muscle tension. Inhibitory influences to the muscles surrounding a joint can result (40).
- Suprasegmental inhibition must be considered a factor as the patient is instructed to relax.
- Relaxation that occurs as a result of the application of HR to *agonistic* musculature may be attributed to reciprocal inhibition of the tight muscles through the primary afferents of agonistic muscle spindles (24–25).

Contract-Relax (CR). Contract-relax, a combination of both isotonic and isometric contractions, is also applicable when there is decreased range of motion on one side of the joint. The difference between CR and HR is in the verbal commands and the type of muscle contraction. With the joint at the point of limitation, the subject is asked not to hold, but to turn and pull or turn and push as much as possible. The result is an isotonic contraction of the rotatory component and an isometric contraction of the other two components of the antagonistic pattern (1). As with HR, a change in joint angle of flexion-extension, abduction-adduction is not allowed to occur. Unlike HR, however, the rotation is allowed; the buildup in tension is immediate, not gradual, and the release is abrupt. For this reason, CR is not an appropriate choice in cases of pain. It has been shown, however, to yield greater increases in motion than HR on two joint muscles in normal subjects (41). In contrast to HR, CR is always applied to the antagonistic, range limiting pattern or muscle group.

Neurophysiological rationale (review rationale under HR for similarities and differences):

- Fatigue may play a greater role in CR than in HR. The maximal effort elicited throughout the entire application of the CR technique may result in the recruitment of more phasic motor units that are quick to fatigue (42–44).
- In comparison with HR, sustained maximal tension may serve to increase GTO recruitment or the rate of firing (45–47).
- Renshaw cell discharge inhibits previously discharging alpha motoneurons.
- Secondary muscle-spindle afferent inhibition may contribute to the increases in ROM if the activated muscle is a postural extensor (48, 49).
- Joint receptors may contribute inhibitory influences to alpha motoneuron pools.
- Suprasegmental inhibition may occur as the result of the verbal commands to relax.

- Empirical evidence indicates that rotation unlocks or relaxes muscle tightness.

Traditionally, both HR and CR are applied at the point of limitation of the available range of movement. It has been demonstrated, however, that the techniques can be applied at other points in the available range with equivalent gains in motion (50, 51). The optimal time of application of one contraction or the number of contractions necessary to gain ROM has been minimally investigated. One study on normal subjects has indicated a positive relationship between the length of time of application of HR and immediate increases in motion (52). Regardless of the technique applied, the therapist should allow adequate time for the patient to relax before movement into a newly gained range is attempted. Further research must be conducted, however, to establish normal parameters relating to any of the relaxation techniques.

Rhythmic Stabilization (RS). Rhythmic stabilization is another isometric technique that can be used to increase ROM (1, 53). It is most beneficial when limitation of movement is caused by splinting around a joint or by pain as occurs, for example, in patients with burns. When isometric contractions of both agonistic and antagonistic patterns are simultaneously and then alternately elicited by the therapist, the result is cocontraction. Relaxation is not allowed to occur between alterations in manual contacts from agonist to antagonist. The strength of the contractions is gradually increased during the entire sequence. When it appears that the patient is contracting maximally, he is instructed to relax slowly. To gain range of motion at the elbow joint, for example, the proximal hand of the therapist would resist a D_1E pattern (triceps at the shoulder), while the distal hand resisted a D_1F pattern (biceps at the elbow). When both patterns are contracting optimally and simultaneously (approximately 5 seconds), manual contacts are changed to opposite surfaces without allowing relaxation to occur. The proximal

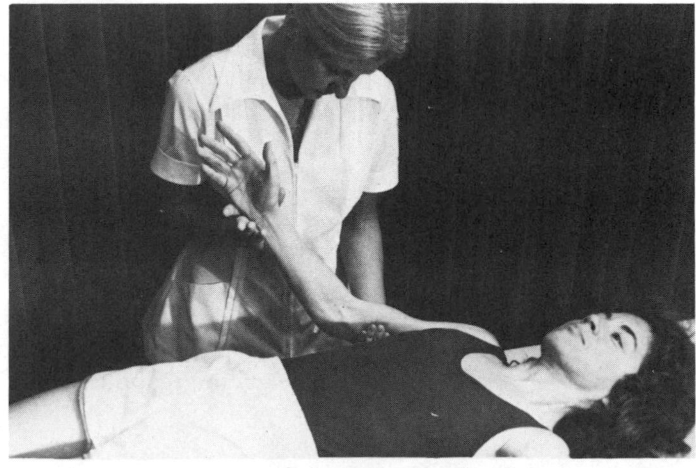

A. Supine: D_1 UE.
T. RS.
E. MC arm, wrist.

FIGURE 4–4

hand would then resist D_1F (biceps at the shoulder) while the distal hand resisted D_1E (triceps at the elbow) (see Figure 4–4). The verbal command is simply "Hold and don't let me move you." The end result of the application of these counter-rotatory forces should be simultaneous contraction around the joint, followed by gradual relaxation (20). In addition to eliciting muscle relaxation, the intermittent muscle contractions may cause an increase in local circulation owing to muscle-pumping action (1). Although it is extremely effective in gaining ROM, RS requires manual dexterity by the therapist and voluntary control by the patient to a greater degree than either HR or CR.

Because the verbal commands associated with RS instruct the patient to "hold," care must be taken to maintain a proper breathing pattern during the application of the technique, particularly with patients having cardiovascular, neurological, or respiratory complications.

Neurophysiological rationale:

- The rationale for HR, which elicits a completely isometric contraction, can be applied to RS.

Rhythmical Rotation (RR). Unlike HR, CR, and RS, rhythmical rotation (RR) involves completely passive movement (20). Although it can be used for many disabilities, it is particularly effective for patients who have hypertonia with no active motion, as often occurs with spinal cord injury, or for those patients whose hypertonia markedly increases with voluntary contraction. RR should be avoided when there is pain on rotational movement. The therapist supports the limb or body segment and rotates it alternately in both directions in a slow rhythmical manner around the longitudinal axis for approximately 10 seconds (Figure 4–5). The verbal command is "Relax and let me move you." Once relaxation is achieved, the limb is moved passively or actively, if active movement is possible, into the newly gained range. There has been some question regarding the most effective means of gaining motion with this technique. Should the rotation and counterrotation of the limb be applied at the joint angle of the limb's resting posture or, is it better to move the limb simultaneously through range while the rotation is occurring? Interestingly, a study performed on normal subjects with tight hamstrings indicated that increases in range of motion are not dependent on changes in the joint angle but rather on the rotation alone (54).

Neurophysiological rationale:

- GTOs are particularly sensitive to active contractile tension (55–56), but have been shown to respond to passive tension (57). On this basis, it can be hypothesized that these receptors contribute to inhibition at the motoneuron pool during the application of RR. However, the responses of GTOs to passive changes in muscle length are comparatively small in the absence of active muscle contractions (57–58).

- Suprasegmental inhibition may occur but cannot be considered a significant factor for patients with complete spinal cord transections.
- Rotation appears to relax hypertonic muscles (59).
- It is probable that the efficacy of rythmical rotation results from the firing of mechanoreceptors located in ligaments or capsules of proximal joints. Different classifications of joint receptors exist (40, 60). The exact relationship of this technique to specific joint receptors and resulting increases in movement is not known.

(a)

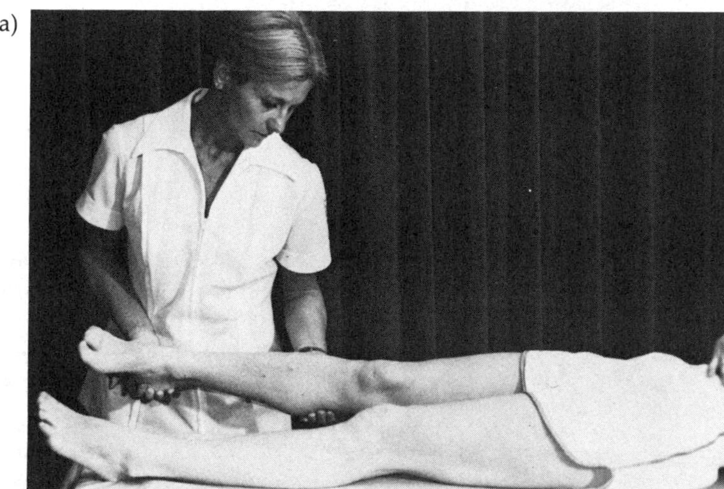

A. Supine: D_1E lower extremity.
T. RR.
E. MC lower leg, foot.

(b)

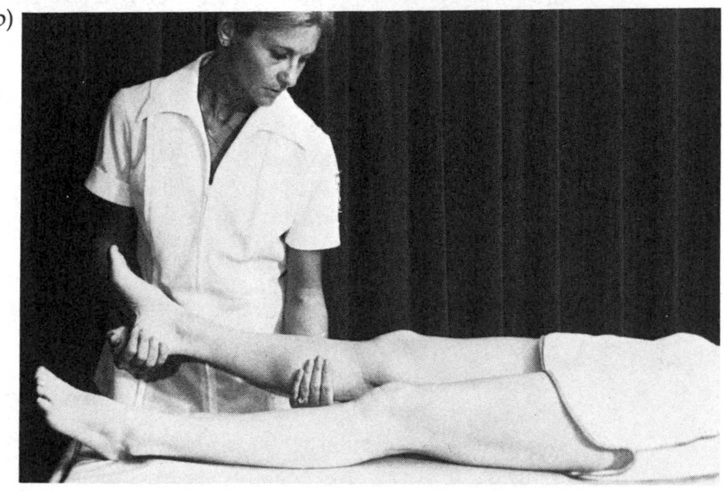

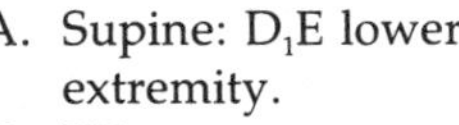

A. Supine: D_1E lower extremity.
T. RR.
E. MC lower leg, foot.

FIGURE 4–5

The relaxation techniques of HR, CR, RS, and RR have one important common denominator. Once relaxation has been achieved, it is followed by active movement with some resistance into the newly gained range, whenever such active movement is possible. At this point and at subsequent points in the range, the sequencing of technique followed by active movement is repeated until it is evident that no more range will be gained in that treatment session.

Why should active resisted contractions always be the preferred means of movement into the desired ranges? There are two basic reasons: First, active movement of the agonistic pattern may perpetuate the inhibition to the tight antagonist via the primary afferents of the agonistic muscle spindles. Secondly, slight resistance, be it gravity or minimal manual, will serve to strengthen the agonistic pattern, a most important treatment goal. If this goal is not achieved, the antagonistic muscle may quickly return to its contracted or tight position. A patient who has had his elbow flexed at a 90 degree angle for a period of weeks, for example, has two major problems: adaptive shortening of elbow flexors and adaptive lengthening of elbow extensors. The extensors have not functioned in their shortened range for a period of time and have thus become weak in this range. Neurophysiologically, this means that their muscle spindles have become biased at a new resting length of 90 degrees of elbow flexion. Consequently, when the elbow is extended after relaxation of flexors has occurred, the extensor spindles are unloaded—that is, on slack—and gamma bias of the extensors then must be restored with the muscle at this new length. If gamma bias is not restored, the primary spindle afferents of the extensors will lack stretch sensitivity, that is, will be unresponsive to stretch in shortened ranges; the result will be a lack of facilitatory impulses from the Ia fibers at the anterior horn cell pool. As noted, resistance, particularly isometric resistance, is facilitatory to static gamma motoneurons and spindle afferent firing. A treatment session, therefore, should always be concluded with an isometric contraction to the agonistic pattern in the most shortened range possible. The length of time of the contraction and not necessarily the amount of resistance appears to be the key factor in establishing the gamma bias. The longer the isometric contraction is maintained, the more static gamma motoneurons may be programmed by the higher centers to increase the bias of the muscle spindles (3). Once the stretch sensitivity of the extensors has been reestablished, the time of the hold can be decreased in subsequent treatments and the amount of resistance increased to enhance muscle-fiber hypertrophy, if that is a goal. Resistance must always be applied cautiously. Heavy resistance applied prematurely, particularly to a hypotonic postural muscle (61), may result in a predominance of inhibition at synapses at anterior horn cell pools.

Resistance to the agonist should follow the relaxation techniques whether the agonist to be strengthened is a flexor or an extensor. However, isometric holding in shortened ranges to extensors may be more important. These muscles function more commonly in a holding capacity, and are usually required to do so in more shortened ranges than the flexors.

Assist to Position. Until controlled mobility and adequate trunk rotation are achieved, the therapist may have to assist the patient into a posture. Assist to position, therefore, is an appropriate technique when the posture cannot be assumed independently. If the patient has the available ROM to be moved into that posture, he is considered to be at the mobility level of motor control and is then ready to progress to developing stability in that particular position.

■ Stability

The primary goal of the mobility techniques is to establish range of motion and to develop the ability to initiate movement. Once mobility has been established, the ultimate purpose of the stability techniques is to improve the patient's ability to maintain both weight-bearing and nonweight-bearing postures and midline positions. Many patients with both orthopedic and neurological problems have difficulty achieving this level of motor control. The next section presents a progression of techniques that the authors have found to be effective in helping a patient stabilize in various postures.

Stability can be defined as cocontractions or simultaneous contractions of muscles around a joint (61). Before cocontraction can be attained during treatment, stretch sensitivity of muscles, particularly the postural extensors is required (13, 61). Stretch sensitivity can be developed most easily in nonweight-bearing postures such as pivot prone or in sidelying by resisting isometric contractions in shortened ranges. Holding in this range is termed a shortened held resisted contraction or SHRC (3, 61) (Figure 4–6). If the patient has difficulty contracting the tonic muscles isometrically in this shortened range, the technique of SR along with the gradual introduction of an isometric contraction (SRH) in or approaching the shortened range can be used to achieve this goal. Once isometric or postural holding of tonic muscles has been achieved, attempts can be made to elicit cocontraction of the

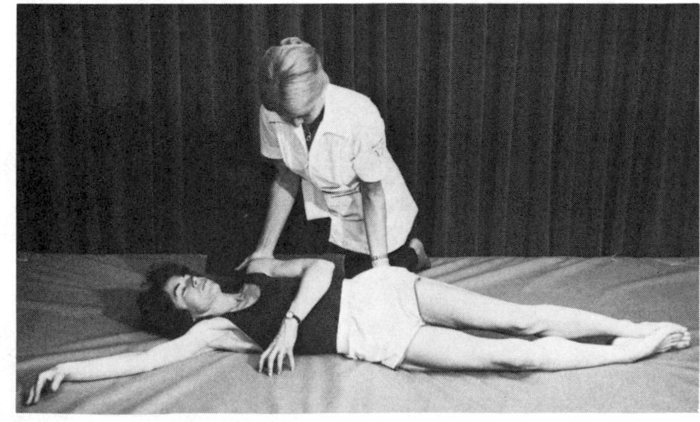

A. Sidelying to supine.
T. SHRC.
E. MC shoulder, pelvis.

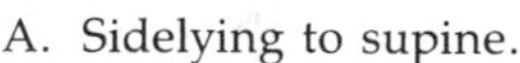

FIGURE 4–6

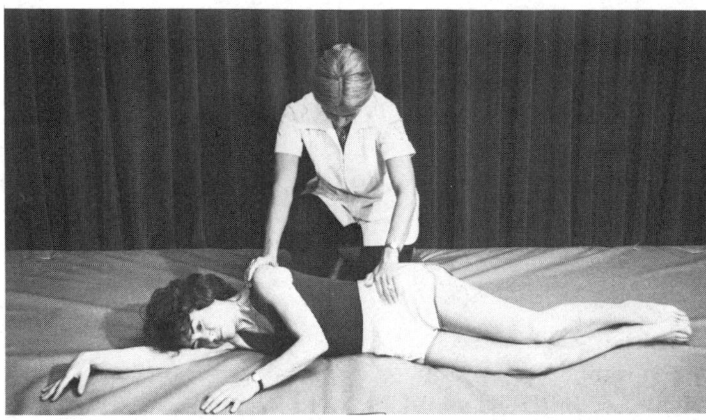

(a)

A. Sidelying.
T. RS.
E. MC posterior shoulder, anterior pelvis.

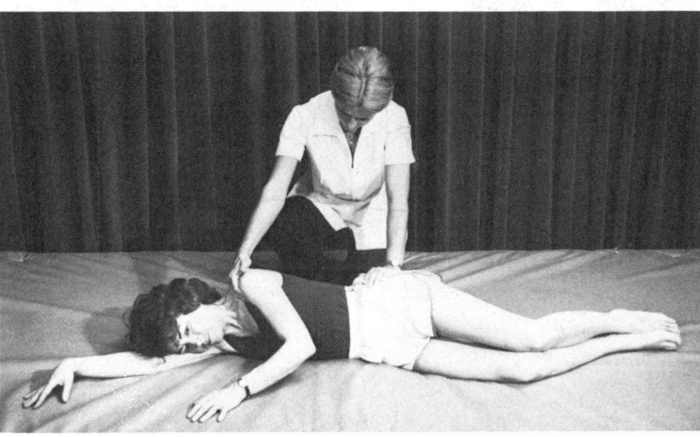

(b)

A. Sidelying.
T. RS.
E. MC anterior shoulder, posterior pelvis.

FIGURE 4–7

proximal musculature with the technique of RS (1). In sidelying, for example, with one hand on the posterior shoulder to facilitate both shoulder and upper trunk extensors and the other hand on the anterior pelvis to facilitate both hip and lower trunk flexors, the therapist gives the command to hold as resistance is applied (20) [Figure 4–7(a)]. Without allowing relaxation to occur, manual contacts are then gradually altered to the opposite sides of the joints and the hold is repeated [Figure 4–7(b)]. If, however, the patient has difficulty making the transition from SHRC and tonic holding of the postural muscles to RS and cocontraction, an intermediate step can be interposed. Alternating isometrics (AI), as the name implies, facilitates holding of the musculature on one side of a joint followed immediately by holding of antagonistic musculature (Figure 4–8). RS is the more difficult of the two techniques because it appears to facilitate simultaneous contractions of all of the muscles surrounding a joint, including the rotators. In order of difficulty, therefore, the techniques that can be used to achieve cocontraction in nonweight-bearing postures are:

(SRH)→SHRC→(AI)→RS.

When a patient can perform SHRC of postural extensors and can cocontract proximal musculature in a nonweight-bearing posture, progression to a weight-bearing position is indicated. When stretch-sensitive or biased postural muscles are placed on prolonged stretch or are resisted, as occurs in weight bearing, cocontraction theoretically occurs through the excitation of the spindle afferent fibers of those muscles (13, 61–63). The physical therapist can enhance the cocontraction produced in positions such as quadruped with the application of RS. However, because quadruped compared with sidelying has a raised C of G and a decreased B of S, the patient may have difficulty coping with the demands of RS in this posture. If this inability is evident, the therapist may begin, as in sidelying, with a technique to which the patient can favorably respond. SRH applied through decrements of range (SRH ↓ range) is one such technique (1). This is performed by assisting the patient through rocking movements in a backward and forward direction with holds superimposed at the beginning and end of the movement. The application of SRH ↓ range is particularly beneficial for pa-

(a)

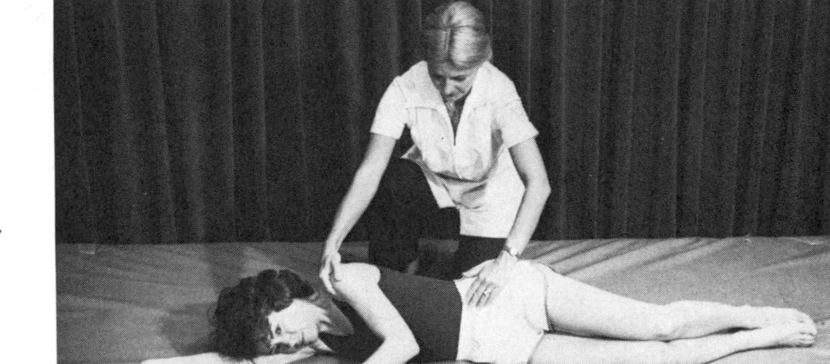

A. Sidelying.
T. AI.
E. MC anterior shoulder, pelvis.

(b)

A. Sidelying.
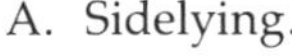
T. AI.
E. MC posterior shoulder, pelvis.

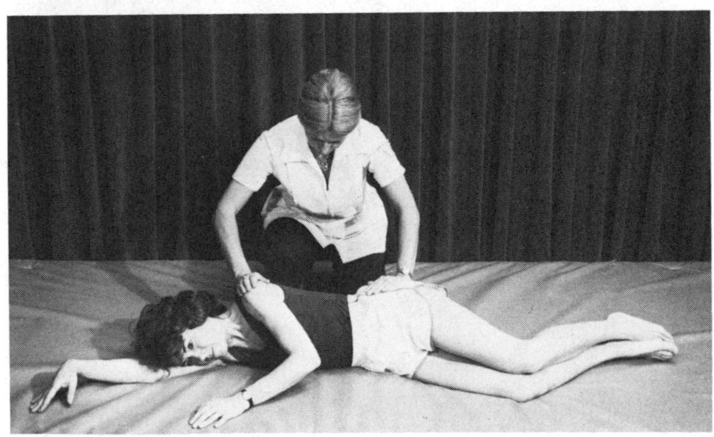

FIGURE 4–8

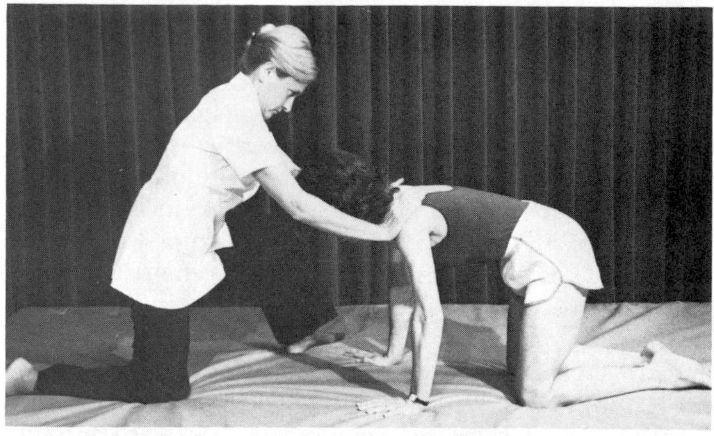

(a)

A. Quadruped.
T. AI.
E. MC anterior shoulders.

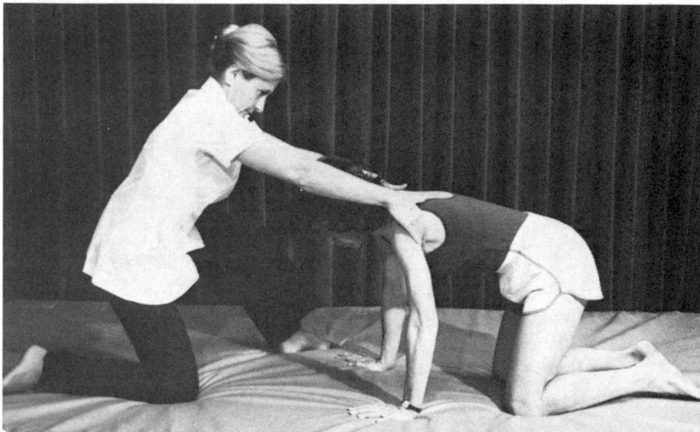

(b)

A. Quadruped.
T. AI.
E. Posterior shoulders.

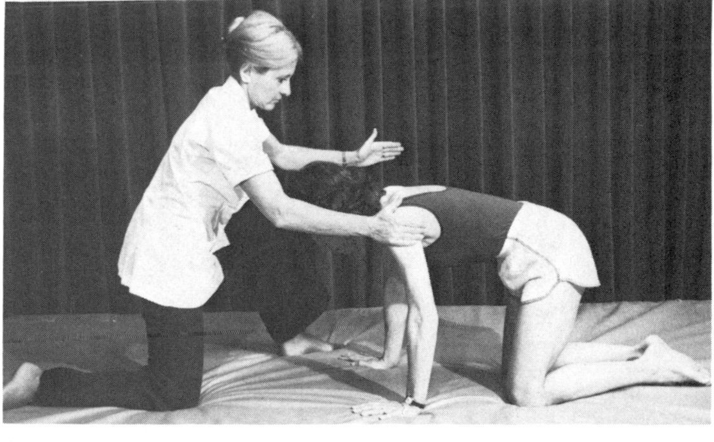

(c)

A. Quadruped.
T. AI.
E. MC lateral shoulders.

FIGURE 4–9

tients who demonstrate obvious instability in weight bearing such as patients with athetosis and ataxia (1). By gradually decreasing the range of motion through which the patient moves, the patient can develop the ability to alternately isometrically contract (AI) proximal flexors, extensors, abduc-

(d)

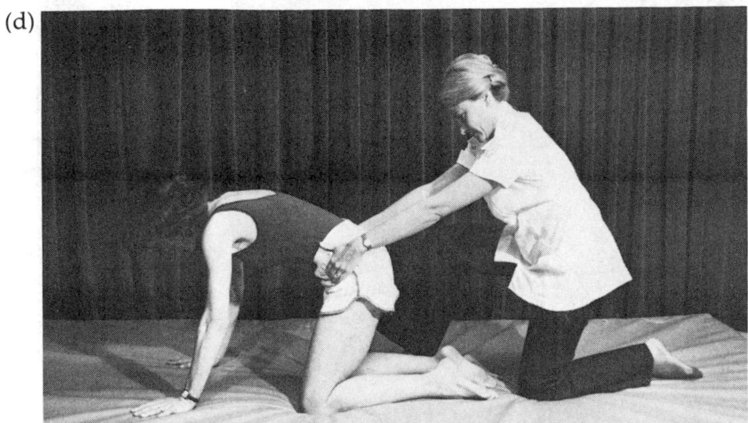

A. Quadruped.
T. AI.
E. MC anterior pelvis.

(e)

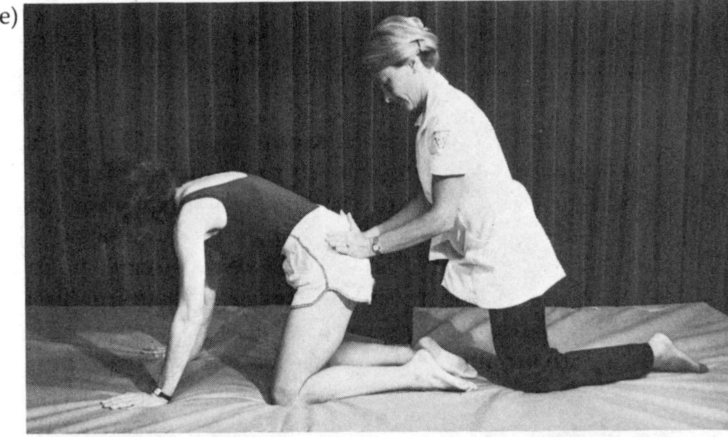

A. Quadruped.
T. AI.
E. MC posterior pelvis.

(f)

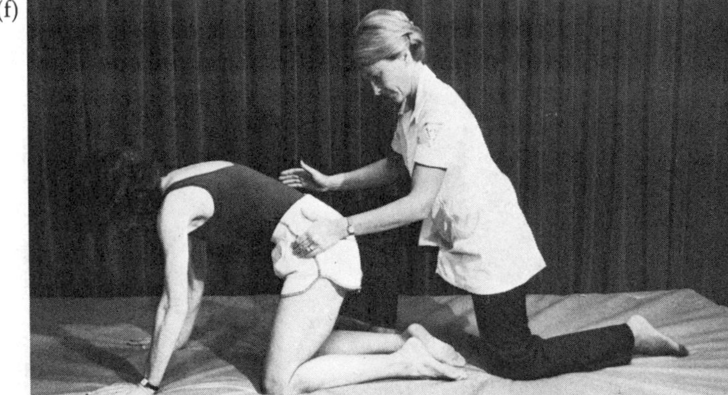

A. Quadruped.
T. AI.
E. MC lateral pelvis.

FIGURE 4–9 (Cont'd.)

tors, and adductors with the shoulder and hip at 90 degrees (Figure 4–9). Finally, cocontraction of all muscle groups around shoulders, hip, or entire trunk can be promoted with RS (Figure 4–10). The sequence therefore, is SRH ↓ range→AI→RS. Approximation is an integral component of both AI

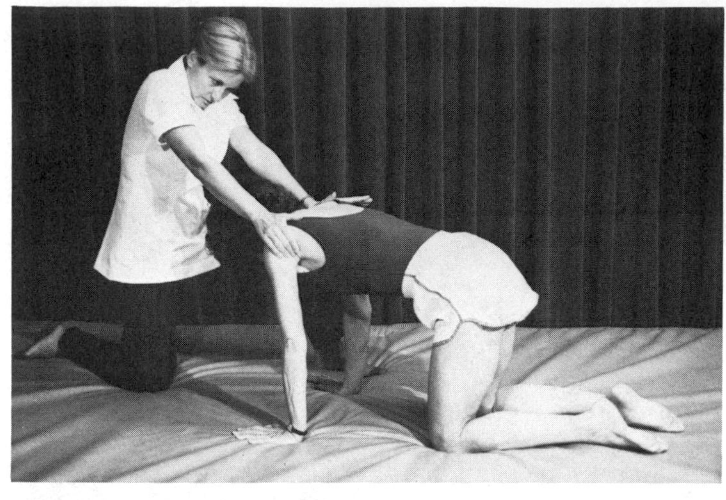

(a)

A. Quadruped.
T. RS.
E. MC shoulders.

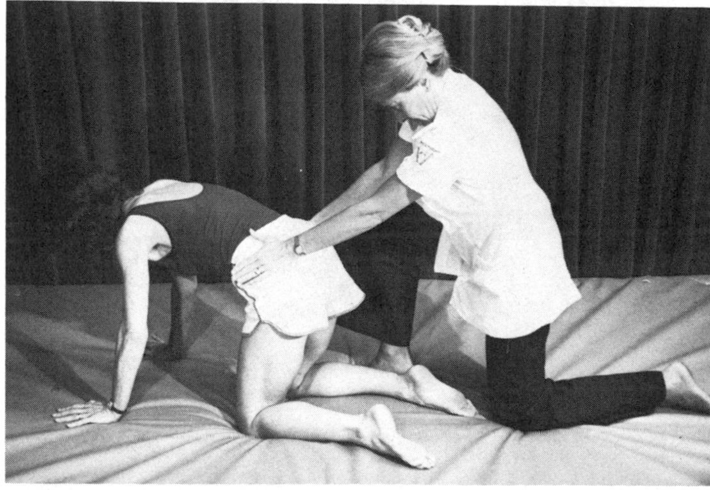

(b)

A. Quadruped.
T. RS.
E. MC pelvis.

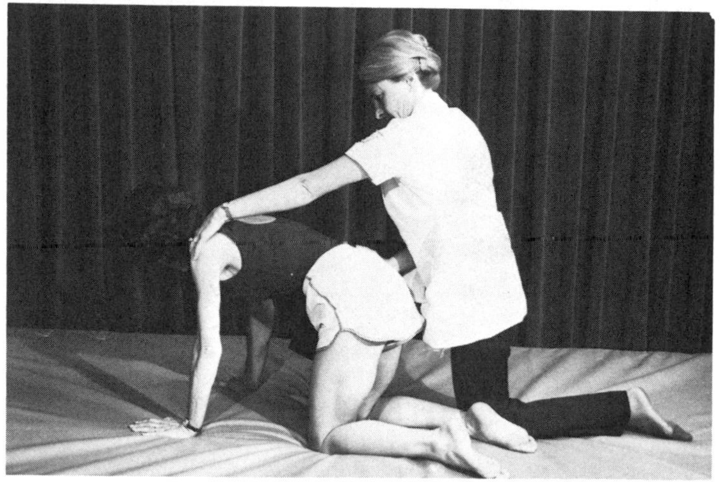

(c)

A. Quadruped.
T. RS.
E. MC shoulder, pelvis.

FIGURE 4–10

and RS and is maintained throughout the application of the techniques to enhance stability in the posture (see Chapter 5). If the patient is capable of responding initially to RS in any weight-bearing position, the preliminary steps of SRH ↓ range and AI may be omitted.

RS can also be applied to bilateral or trunk patterns to indirectly promote stability of the trunk or can be applied to unilateral patterns to promote stability of an extremity (20, 53) (Figure 4–11). Such application of RS is of particular benefit when one or both of the extremities is of good to normal strength and can be used to produce overflow effects.

Neurophysiological rationale:

- Isometric contractions applied on either side of a joint as occurs with SRH ↓ range, AI, and RS, should result in facilitation of alpha and gamma motoneurons and motor-unit recruitment.
- Cocontraction that occurs around a joint when resistance is applied or during weight-bearing postures when biased postural muscles are lengthened may be a result of muscle-spindle afferent firing in the tonic postural extensors. Not to be discounted, however, are the reciprocal facilitatory effects of GTOs that can occur from tonic to phasic muscle groups (24). Inhibition of inhibitory interneurons (disinhibition) to phasic muscles from more tonic groups by Renshaw cells may also play a role in the cocontraction phenomenon (8, 38).
- Although the pathways are unclear, it is possible that joint receptors responding to the approximation of joint surfaces may contribute to stability in weight-bearing postures (see Chapter 5).
- RS is applied identically whether the goal is stability or relaxation. Why two such seemingly different results can occur regardless of the goal is difficult to explain given our present body of knowledge.

Controlled Mobility

The ability to move within any weight-bearing posture with the distal component fixed or head or trunk rotation around the long axis is characteristic of the third stage of motor control. The goals accomplished may be:

1. Strengthening within the available range of motion
2. Promoting balance reactions
3. Increasing the patient's ability to use range of motion functionally at both distal and proximal joints
4. Enhancing the ability to assume a posture independently
5. Developing proximal dynamic stability in preparation for skill

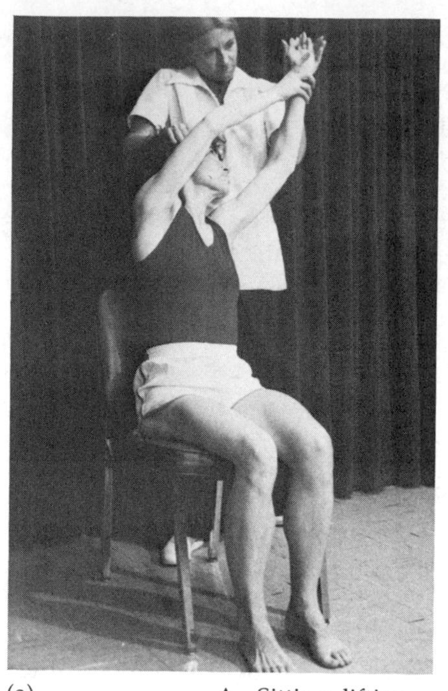

(a)
A. Sitting: lifting.
T. RS.
E. MC head, hand.

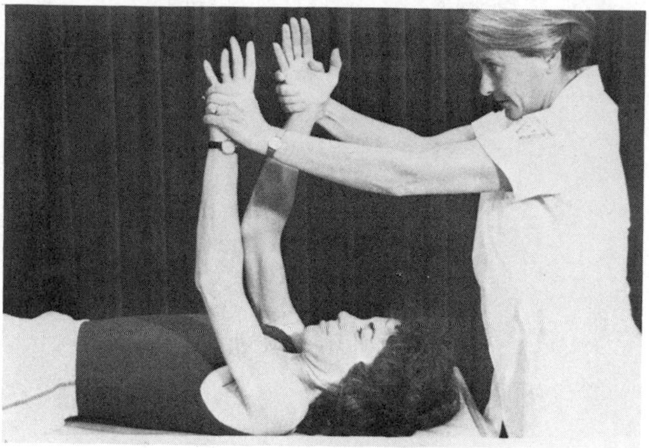

(b)
A. Supine: reciprocal D_2.
T. RS.
E. MC hands.

FIGURE 4–11

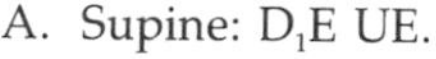

A. Supine: D_1E UE.
T. RS.
E. MC hand.
(c)

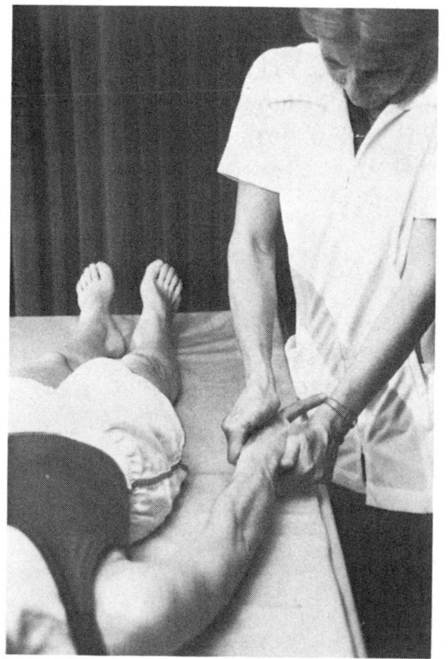

(d)
A. Hooklying.
T. RS.
E. MC knees.

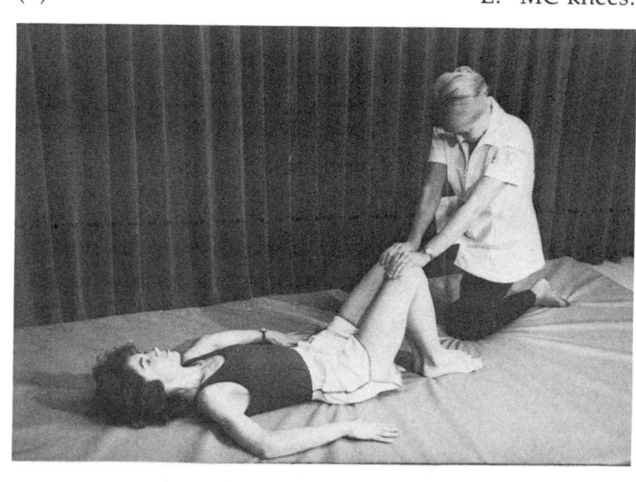

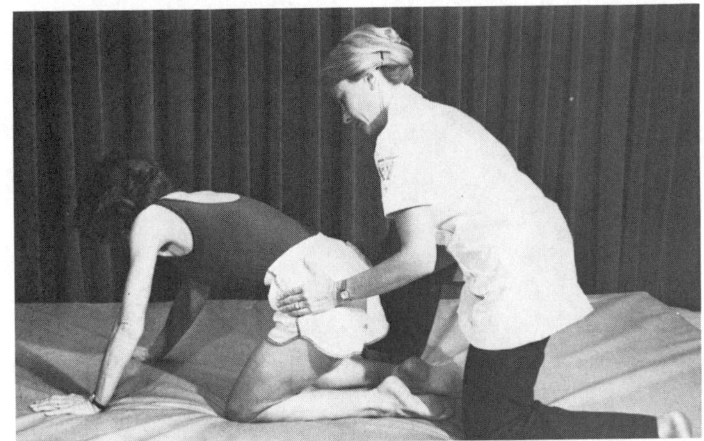

A. Quadruped: rocking back to left.
T. SRH.
E. MC pelvis.

FIGURE 4–12

SR, SRH, RC, TE, and AR applied through increments of range can be used to help achieve any of these goals. Regardless of the techniques used, the manual contacts of the therapist are always placed on the area that needs the most facilitation or support.

Weight bearing on either one of the upper and lower extremities will be increased if the patient is required to move in a diagonal direction. If the patient in quadruped rocks diagonally backward toward the left and forward toward the right, for example, body weight will be shifted toward the left lower and right upper extremities, respectively (Figure 4–12). If a hold is superimposed at either end of the range, further demands will be placed on the limb toward which the patient is rocking. If the patient can cope with the weight-bearing demands that occur during movement within the posture, static-dynamic activities for the purpose of developing unilateral control may follow (see Chapter 3).

During static-dynamic activities the more resistance that is applied to the dynamic or moving extremity, the more dynamic holding should be required of the proximal musculature of the static limb. Techniques, such as SR, SRH, RC, or AR may be easily applied to the movement of the dynamic extremity while RS or AI to the static limb will enhance its stability.

■ Skill

Once proximal dynamic stability has been developed adequately and the patient can move within a particular posture, the patient can progress to the skill level of motor control. Skill is characterized by the ability to move out of a posture (locomotion) and manipulate the environment with the extremities while the trunk maintains an upright posture.

AR, which promotes eccentric control, can be used effectively for the

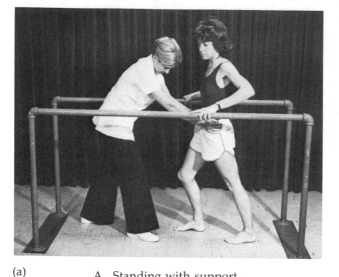

(a)

A. Standing with support.
T. RP.
E. MC pelvis.

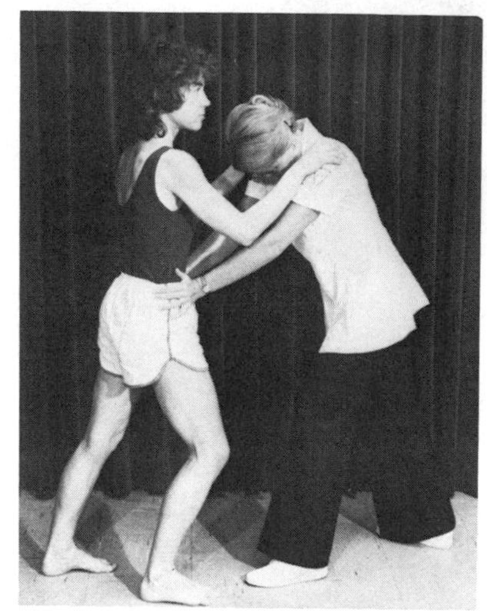

(b)

A. Standing without support.
T. RP.
E. MC pelvis.

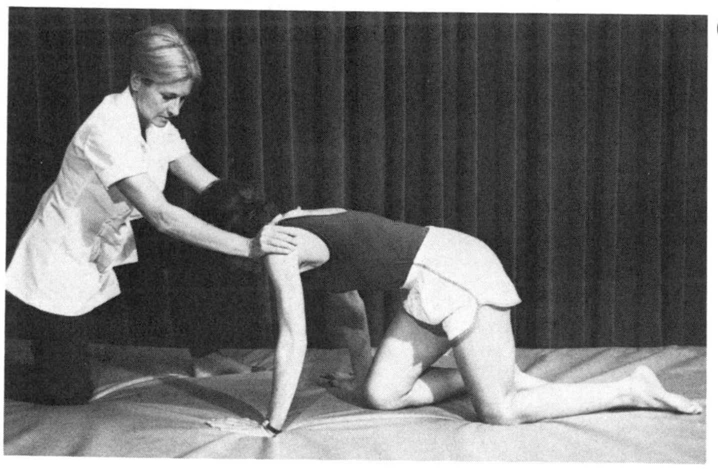

(c)

A. Quadruped.
T. RP.
E. MC shoulders.

FIGURE 4–13

attainment of advanced or skill activities. It can be applied to free distal components in several developmental postures, for example, a D_2F upper extremity pattern in sitting or an advanced pattern of the lower extremity in an upright posture.

Resisted Progression (RP). Resisted progression is, as the name implies, simply resistance to locomotion either in upright or prone postures for purposes of further increasing strength and endurance or enhancing the normal timing of movement (Figure 4–13). As with controlled mobility, the manual contacts of the therapist are determined by the part of the body to be emphasized, be it scapula, pelvis, or limbs. RP also helps to promote motor learning.

Neurophysiological rationale:

- Resistance, as previously discussed, can be used to facilitate muscle spindle afferent firing with alpha motoneuron recruitment of agonistic musculature. If the resistance is prolonged or of sufficient magnitude, overflow of impulses to other muscles may be promoted. Because of the difficulty of the activity, the amount of resistance is usually minimal but of a sufficient amount to sustain the contraction.
- Sensory input to the CNS produced by manual contacts and verbal commands will provide the system with more feedback than the use of verbal commands alone (1).

Normal Timing (NT). Normal timing is used to develop coordination of the components of a movement pattern when there is adequate strength to control a pattern but the sequencing of the movements is not normal (1). NT should proceed from a distal to a proximal direction (1). During treatment, a movement pattern is initiated but all proximal motion is delayed

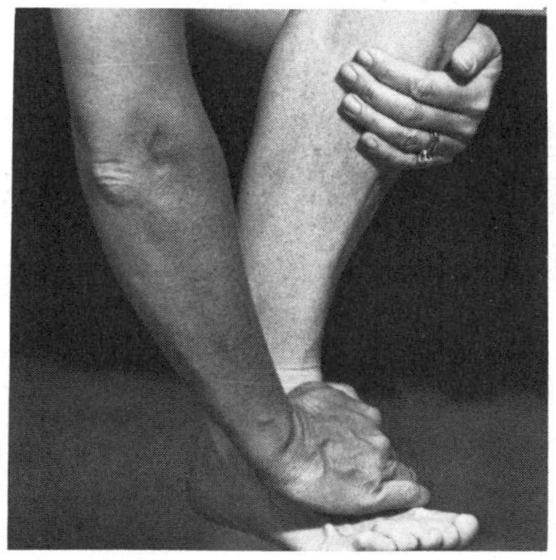

(a)

A. Supine: D_1F, knee extending, LE.
T. NT.
E. MC anterior lower leg, dorsum of foot.

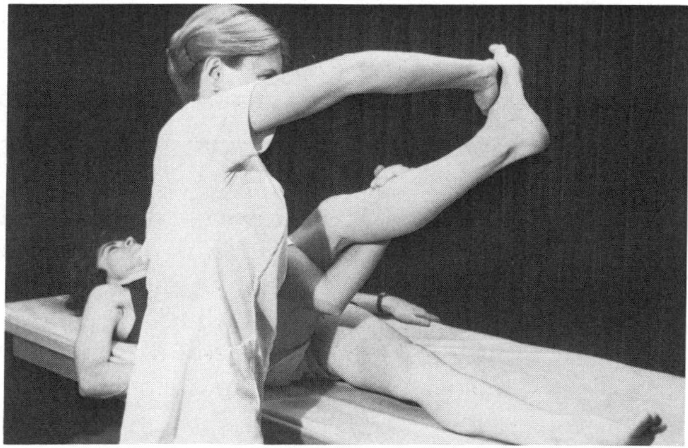

(b)

A. Supine: D_1F, knee extending, LE.
T. NT.
E. MC anterior lower leg, dorsum of foot.

FIGURE 4–14

TABLE 4–1
Summary of Techniques as They Relate to the Stages of Motor Control

MOBILITY *Initiate Movement* Rhythmic initiation (RI) Hold relax active movement (HRAM) Repeated contractions (RC) *Increase ROM* Rhythmic initiation (RI) Hold-relax (HR) Contract-relax (CR) Rhythmic stabilization (RS) Rhythmical rotation (RR)	CONTROLLED MOBILITY (Distal Component Fixed) Slow reversal (SR) Slow reversal hold (SRH) Repeated contractions (RC) Timing for emphasis (TE) Agonistic reversals (AR) } All can be applied through increments of range
STABILITY *Holding of Postural Muscles nonweight-bearing* Slow reversal hold (SRH)→alternating isometrics (AI) *Tonic Holding of Postural Muscles and Cocontraction in Nonweight-bearing* (SRH) → SHRC → (AI) → RS *Cocontraction in Weight-bearing* SRH ↓ Range ⟶ AI ⟶ RS	SKILL (Distal Component Free) Slow reversal (SR) Slow reversal hold (SRH) Repeated contractions (RC) Timing for emphasis (TE) Agonistic reversals (AR) Resisted progression (RP) Normal timing (NT)

until the distal component approaches full range [Figure 4–14(a)]. RC or TE to the lagging component may be used. When movement through distal range is satisfactory, the entire pattern is allowed to occur [Figure 4–14(b)]. Once NT has been attained, repetition will reinforce the coordinated movement. A properly timed SR would be the ultimate goal of treatment since this is a prerequisite for the performance of all activities of daily living (1).

Neurophysiological rationale:

- Repetition is an important principle in motor learning. If impulses constantly travel over the same pathways, transmission of those impulses will become easier (64–65). Therefore a movement may first be initiated cortically but with repetition and then may be relegated to subcortical levels yielding more automatic responses. (Table 4–1 presents a summary of the techniques as they relate to the development of motor control.)

REFERENCES

1. Knott M, Voss DE: Proprioceptive Neuromuscular Facilitation, ed 2. New York, Harper & Row, 1968
2. Kabat H: Proprioceptive facilitation in therapeutic exercise. In Licht S(ed): Therapeutic Exercise, ed 2. New Haven, CT, Elizabeth Licht, Publisher, 1961
3. Stockmeyer SA: Procedures for improvement of motor control. Unpublished notes from Boston University, PT 710, 1978.
4. Angel RW: Antagonistic muscle activity during rapid arm movements: Central versus proprioceptive influences. J Neurol Neurosurg Psych 40:683–686, 1977
5. Wannstedt G, Mayer N, Rosenholtz H: Electromyographic Features of an Antagonistic Muscle. Read at the 4th Congress of the International Society of Electrophysiological Kinesiology, Boston, 1979
6. Burg D, Szumski AJ, Struppler A, et al: Influence of a voluntary innervation on human muscle spindle sensitivity. In Shahani M(ed): The Motor System: Neurophysiology and Muscle Mechanisms. New York, Elsevier, Publisher, 1976
7. Cheney PD, Preston JB: Classification of fusimotor fibers in the primate. J Neurophysiol 39:9–19, 1976
8. Granit R: The functional role of the muscle spindles—facts and hypotheses. Brain 98:531–556, 1975
9. Vallbo AB: Discharge patterns in human muscle spindle afferents, during isometric voluntary contractions. ACTA Physiol Scand 80:552–556, 1970
10. Schmidt RF: Fundamentals of Neurophysiology, ed 2. New York, Springer-Verlag, 1978
11. Lance JW, McLeod JG: A Physiological Approach to Clinical Neurology, ed 2. Boston, Butterworth, 1975
12. Ralston HJ: Some considerations of the neurophysiological basis of therapeutic exercise. Phys Ther Rev 38:465–468, 1958
13. Crutchfield CA, Barnes MR: The Neurophysiological Basis of Patient Treatment, ed 2. Atlanta, GA, Stokesville Publishing Co, 1975, vol 1
14. Burg D, Szumski AJ, Struppler A, et al: Afferent and efferent activation of human muscle receptors involved in reflex and voluntary contraction. Exp Neurol 41:754–769, 1973
15. McCandless GA, Rose DE: Evoked cortical response to stimulus change. J Speech Hear Res 13:624–634, 1970
16. Ashworth B, Grimby L, Kugelberg E: Comparison of voluntary and reflex activation of motor units. J Neurol Neurosurg Psychiat 30:91–98, 1967

17. Partridge M: Electromyographic demonstration of facilitation. Phys Ther Rev 34:227–232, 1954
18. Wellock L: Development of bilateral muscle strength through ipsilateral exercise. Phys Ther Rev 34:227–232, 1954
19. Portney LG, Sullivan PE: Electromyographic Analysis of Ipsilateral and Contralateral Shoulder and Elbow Muscles during the Performance of PNF Patterns. Read at the Annual Conference of The Society for Behavioral Kinesiology, Boston, 1979
20. Voss, DE: Therapeutic exercise. Unpublished notes from Northwestern University, 1974.
21. Trombly CA, Scott AD: Occupational Therapy for Physical Dysfunction. Baltimore, Williams & Wilkins, 1977
22. Ter Vrugt D, Pederson DR: The effects of vertical rocking frequencies on the arousal level of two-month-old infants. Child Dev 44:205–209, 1973
23. Pederson DR: The soothing effect of rocking as determined by the direction and frequency of movement. Can J Behav Sci 7:237–243, 1975
24. Matthews PBS: Mammalian Muscle Receptors and Their Central Connections. London, Edward Arnold Ltd, 1972
25. Granit R: The Basis of Motor Control. New York, Academic Press, 1970
26. Basmajian JV: Control of individual motor units. Amer J Phys Med 49:480–486, 1966
27. Basmajian JV: Neuromuscular control of voluntary movement. In Buerger AA and Tobis JS(eds): Neurophysiologic Aspects of Rehabilitation Medicine. Springfield, IL, Charles C Thomas, Publisher, 1976
28. Jacobson E: Progressive Relaxation. Chicago, University of Chicago Press, 1959
29. Kottke FJ: Facilitation and inhibition as fundamental characteristics of neuromuscular organization. In Buerger AA, Tobis JS(eds): Neurophysiologic Aspects of Rehabilitation Medicine. Springfield, IL, Charles C Thomas, Publisher, 1976
30. Grzesiak RC: Relaxation techniques in the treatment of chronic pain. Arch Phys Med Rehabil 58:270–272, 1974
31. Coursey RD: Electromyograph feedback as a relaxation technique. J Consult Clin Psychol 43:825–834, 1975
32. Knott M, Voss DE: Proprioceptive Neuromuscular Facilitation. New York, Harper & Row, 1956
33. Stockmeyer SA: A Sensorimotor approach to treatment. In Pearson PH and Williams CE(eds): Physical Therapy Services in the Developmental Disabilities. Springfield, IL, Charles C Thomas, Publisher, 1976
34. Harris FA: Facilitation techniques in therapeutic exercise. In Basmajian JV(ed): Therapeutic Exercise, ed 3. Baltimore, Williams & Wilkins, 1978

35. Darling RC: Fatigue. In Downey JA and Darling RC(eds.): The Physiological Basis of Rehabilitation Medicine. Philadelphia, WB Saunders, Publisher, 1971

36. Stephens JA, Taylor A: Fatigue of maintained voluntary muscle contraction in man. J Physiol (London) 220:1–18, 1972

37. Burg D, Szumski AJ, Struppler A, et al: Afferent and efferent activation of human muscle receptors involved in reflex and voluntary contraction. Exp Neurol 41:754–768, 1973

38. Eyzaguirre C, Fidone SJ: Physiology of the Nervous System, ed 2. Chicago, Year Book Medical Publishers, 1975

39. Henneman E: Peripheral mechanisms involved in the control of muscle. In Mountcastle VB(ed): Medical Physiology. St Louis, CV Mosby, Publisher, 1974, vol 1

40. Wyke B: Neurology of joints. Ann Roy Coll Surg Engl 41:25–49, 1967

41. Markos PD: Ipsilateral and contralateral effects of proprioceptive neuromuscular techniques on hip motion and electromyographic activity. Phys Ther 59:1366–1373, 1979

42. Burke RE, Rymer WZ, Walsh JV: Functional specialization in the motor unit population of cat medial gastrocnemius muscle. In Stein RB, Pearson KA, Smith RS, et al(eds): Control of Posture and Locomotion. New York, Plenum Press, 1973

43. Structure and function of skeletal muscle. A discussion, The Physician and Sportsmedicine, May 1977

44. Thorstensson A: Muscle strength, fiber types and enzyme activities in man. ACTA Physiol Scand Suppl 443, 1976

45. Reinking RM, Stephens JA, Stuart DG: The tendon organs of cat medial gastrocnemius: Significance of motor unit type and size for the activation of Ib afferents. J Physiol (London) 250:491–512, 1975

46. Stephens JA, Reinking RM, Stuart DG: Tendon organs of cat medial gastrocnemius: Responses to active and passive forces as a function of muscle length. J Neurophysiol 38:1217–1231, 1975

47. Stuart DG, Stephens JA: The recruitment order of motor units and its significance for the behavior of tendon organs during normal muscle activity. In Shahani M(ed): The Motor System: Neurophysiology and Muscle Mechanisms. New York, Elsevier, Publisher, 1976

48. Eccles RM, Lundberg A: Synaptic actions in motoneurons by afferents which may evoke the flexion reflex. Arch Ital Biol 97:199–221, 1959

49. Bishop, B: Spasticity: Its physiology and management. Phys Ther 57:385–395, 1977

50. Shapiro CH: Effects of Hold-Relax at Different Muscle Lengths. Thesis. Boston, MA, Boston University Sargent College of Allied Health Professions, 1978

51. Bernier S: Effects of Contract-Relax at Different Muscle Lengths. Thesis. Boston, MA, Boston University Sargent College of Allied Health Professions, 1980

52. Cole D, Cooper L, Murphy M, et al: Hold-relax effects over time. Unpublished study, Boston, MA, Boston University Sargent College of Allied Health Professions, 1978

53. Knott, M: Unpublished notes from Vallejo, CA, 1966

54. Crowley J, Dupois AM, Greenberg C: Rhythmical rotation and position effects. Unpublished study, Boston, MA, Boston University Sargent College of Allied Health Professions, 1978

55. Houk J, Henneman E: Responses of Golgi tendon organs to active contractions of the soleus muscle of the cat. J Neurophysiol 30:466–481, 1967

56. Jansen JKS, Rudjord T: On the silent period and Golgi tendon organs of the soleus muscle of the cat. Acta Physiol Scand 62:364–379, 1964

57. Houk J, Singer J, Henneman E: Adequate stimulus for tendon organs with observations on mechanics of ankle joint. J Neurophysiol 34:1051–1065, 1971

58. Stuart DG, Mosher CG, Gerlach RL: Properties and central connections of Golgi tendon organs with special reference to locomotion. In Banker BQ, Przybylski RJ, Van der Meulen JP, and Victor M(eds): Research in Muscle Development and Muscle Spindle, part 2. Amsterdam, Exerpta Medica, 1972

59. Semans S: The Bobath concept in treatment of neurological disorders. Amer J Phys Med 46:732–785, 1966

60. Wyke BD: Articular neurology: A review. Physiotherapy 58:94–99, 1972

61. Stockmeyer SA: An interpretation of the approach of Rood to the treatment of neuromuscular dysfunction. Amer J Phys Med 46:950–956, 1966

62. Burke D, Lance JW: Studies of the reflex effects of primary and secondary spindle endings in spasticity. In Desmedt JE(ed): New Developments in Electromyography and Clinical Neurophysiology, vol 3. Basel, Karger, 1973

63. Patton NJ, Mortensen OA: An electromyographic study of reciprocal activity of muscles. Anat Rec 170:255–268, 1971

64. Fisher E: Physiological basis of volitional movements. Phys Ther Rev 38:405–412, 1958

65. Fisher E: Physiological basis of methods to elicit, reinforce, and coordinate muscular movements. Phys Ther Rev 38:468–473, 1958

chapter 5

Elements

INTRODUCTION

Elements provide sensory input for purposes of either facilitating or inhibiting a response (1). Many elements may be incorporated into one procedure. They may be applied prior to or in conjunction with various techniques (see Chapter 5). Once a desired response is obtained, the goal is to gradually withdraw the sensory input until the patient can perform the task independently.

For certain patients, a given element may produce a localized phasic or tonic response. Given a different set of circumstances, the same stimulus may result in a widespread or more generalized reaction. Parameters controlling the response are: rate, duration, and frequency of application, along with the age of the patient and the state of the central nervous system. Elements that are effective for one person may not only be ineffective for another, but may result in unwanted responses. For this reason, elements should not be applied indiscriminately. Because the neurophysiological rationale underlying the effectiveness of many elements is vague, and there are also individual differences to consider, a predictable result is not always feasible. Present information indicates that rational choices of treatment are possible, but careful monitoring of the patient's response is essential.

The elements presented in this chapter are grouped on the basis of the systems through which they are primarily monitored. Each element is discussed in terms of receptors, afferent and efferent pathways, the neurophysiological response produced, and indications and contraindications.

PROPRIOCEPTIVE ELEMENTS

■ Stretch

1. Quick stretch is commonly used either to facilitate or enhance movement. It can be applied by rapidly tapping over individual muscle bellies or tendons. It can also be applied to a pattern of movement in any part of its range. Most frequently a quick stretch is applied in the lengthened range to initiate movement or is superimposed on a contraction to enhance muscle activity (see "Repeated Contractions" and "Slow Reversals" in Chapter 4). Quick stretch is thought to be mediated by the primary afferent fiber of the muscle spindle; this fiber monosynaptically connects with anterior horn cells of agonistic and synergistic muscles and provides them with facilitatory impulses. At the same time, through an interneuron, inhibitory influences are provided to antagonistic muscle groups (2–3). If muscle activation occurs as a result of the quick stretch, the response should be resisted in order to perpetuate the contraction.

2. Although quick stretch is useful for facilitation, **prolonged stretch** or lengthening may be effective in inhibiting or dampening a muscle response. Why this dampening effect occurs is not clear, although it appears to be related to muscle classification (flexor or extensor). Some peripheral receptors that may contribute to inhibition of certain muscles during lengthening are the joint receptors, Golgi tendon organs (GTOs), and muscle spindle secondary afferents.

Studies on cats have demonstrated that passive knee flexion results in stimulation of mechanoreceptors of the joint capsule with resultant diminution in quadriceps tension (4). Although the effect of joint receptors in humans during active or passive movement of various muscle groups has not been clearly defined (5), we can speculate as to their contribution to muscle inhibition during muscle lengthening.

GTOs are highly responsive to active tension created by motor unit contraction, but may also respond to passive tension (6–8). When excited, the Ib afferent fiber from these receptors contributes inhibitory impulses to synapses at anterior horn cells of agonists and synergists and facilitatory impulses to synapses of antagonistic muscle groups. The result is autogenetic inhibition and reciprocal facilitation (2–3). As GTOs appear to be more prevalent in tonic muscles (9–10), their inhibitory effects, when exerted, are likely to be more predominant in tonic as opposed to phasic muscle groups.

Considerable controversy exists in the literature regarding the role of the secondary afferent receptors of the muscle spindle (11). Current investigations have revealed the complex nature of these endings and suggest that their role may be primarily one of both flexor and extensor facilitation (12–14). Another theory on which certain exercise regimens are based is that when excited, the afferent fibers arising from the secondary endings are primarily facilitatory to flexor muscles and inhibitory to extensors, regardless of whether they are stimulated in the flexor or the extensor muscle group (15–16). Considering the possible inhibitory effects of secondary afferents, GTOs, and joint receptors, it is easy to understand how a muscle that is more tonic in composition could be inhibited by slowly applied maintained stretch. On the basis of these peripheral mechanisms, however, inhibition of a phasic muscle is more difficult to comprehend. In contrast to a tonic muscle, maintained stretch to a phasic muscle appears to result in a predominance of the facilitatory effects produced by the excitation of both the primary and secondary spindle afferents. Clinical evidence indicates that for an inhibitory element to be effective, stretch must be applied to phasic muscles for longer periods (days) than is necessary for more tonic groups. This inhibition to phasic groups resulting from stretch may be caused by adaptation of both spindle afferent and cutaneous receptors over time. The length of time necessary for adaptation of these receptors to occur, if indeed it does occur during prolonged positioning, is unknown and undoubtedly may vary from patient to patient.

Adaptation of spindle afferent receptors may be one of the multiple factors underlying various splinting or bracing procedures. To be effective, however, the stretch provided by the device should be constantly maintained. An improperly fitting splint can precipitate intermittent quick stretches to hypertonic muscles and thus lead to even further muscle facilitation.

Although the rationale is not clear, prolonged stretch to intrinsic musculature of the foot or to the ulnar side of the hand appears to enhance proximal stability (16–17). Forceful grasp of a firm object that elicits stretch of the intrinsics can thus be incorporated into both upper and lower extremity weight bearing postures; the holding of proximal musculature is crucial to the maintenance of these postures and may be augmented by this distal stimulation.

Precautions and contraindications:

- Prolonged stretch can be used effectively to dampen muscle tone. Caution must be taken, however, to avoid this type of sensory input to weak postural extensors in which inhibition or decreased muscle tone is not a goal of treatment.

In summary:

- Quick stretch can be used to initiate or strengthen a muscle response regardless of the classification of the muscle. Prolonged stretch to muscle in its lengthened ranges may result in dampening of tone of that muscle, particularly if the muscle is an extensor. Exactly why this phenomenon occurs is unclear, although it appears to be a result of many convergent inhibitory influences on anterior horn cell pools.

Resistance

Resistance can be used to augment alpha and gamma motoneuron recruitment. It also provides the CNS with sensory feedback from the periphery (18). Muscle activation without resistance of some type (manual, gravitational, mechanical, body weight) can result in the unloading or shortening of muscle spindles and subsequent cessation of movement. The amount of resistance given and the duration of its application should be determined by the classification of the muscle and the quality of the existing tone, as discussed in the following paragraphs.

The tone of hypotonic postural muscles can be dampened by high loads of resistance. Decreases in tone, or control, is most apparent, however, when the two stimuli of stretch and resistance are combined; for example, kneebuckling during stair descent as body weight is superimposed on a flexing knee. This collapse of the quadriceps may be due to the predominance of inhibitory impulses at motoneuron pools caused by the excitation of muscle spindle secondary afferent fibers. In order to prevent this predominance of muscle inhibition, stretch sensitivity of lax muscle spindles needs to be restored so that the facilitatory influences of the primary afferent fibers will take precedence over any inhibitory impulses that may arise from secondary fibers when stretch and resistance of body weight are provided. The optimal way to restore spindle stretch sensitivity of tonic muscles appears to be through the application of low-load isometric contractions in shortened ranges or shortened held resisted contractions (1, 16, 19). As pointed out in Chapter 4, static gamma motoneurons that are facilitated by isometric contractions are responsible for taking up the slack, that is, for internally stretching the intrafusal fibers of the spindles (20–22). The longer the contraction is held, the more the spindles should become biased or stretch sensitive. A stretch-sensitive tonic muscle that is subsequently placed on a prolonged stretch or heavily resisted should respond with both primary and secondary afferent fiber excitation. Thus, any inhibitory impulses that may be produced at anterior horn cells by stimulation of secondary endings or other peripheral receptors should be counterbalanced by facilitatory impulses from the primary afferents.

Maximal resistance may be appropriately applied to hypertrophy the extrafusal fibers of weakened muscles. When applied to muscles of good strength, resistance can result in an irradiation of impulses to either ipsilateral or contralateral muscle groups (23).

Overflow is of obvious benefit when the recipients of the effects are hypotonic muscles. Conversely, when hypertonia is present, resistance to an uninvolved segment can result in enhancement of synergistic movement patterns. Depending on treatment philosophy, this may or may not be consistent with established goals. If it is not, resistance should be kept to a minimum and the total body monitored for unwanted effects.

Precautions and contraindications:

- Caution must be taken when resisting weakened muscles, particularly postural extensors. Phasic muscle groups, however, do not appear to be as "fragile." This may be partly due to the facilitatory effects of the secondary endings in phasic muscles (review discussion of stretch).

In summary:

- Graded resistance, particularly isometric, is necessary to enhance gamma efferent activity to muscle spindles and thus render the muscle sensitive to any type of externally applied stretch. This graded isometric resistance appears to be particularly critical for postural extensors. Maximal resistance applied to strong musculature can create overflow to weaker groups and may be used to strengthen and hypertrophy hypotonic muscles. Resistance may increase hypertonia and must be altered or eliminated if enhancement of synergistic patterns is not a goal.

Vibration

Vibration is a therapeutic tool that has been used with increasing frequency in recent years. The tonic vibration reflex (TVR) has been elicited in all skeletal muscles except those of the face and tongue (24). The effect of the TVR is one of autogenetic facilitation to the muscle being vibrated and reciprocal inhibition to the antagonist. The response, although similar to that produced by quick stretch, is elicited via a more complex pathway.

Like the stretch reflex, the TVR is mediated by the primary afferents of the vibrated muscle spindles; however, the similarity between the TVR and the monosynaptic stretch reflex ends with the afferent limb of the reflex arc. Unlike a simple stretch reflex, the pathway of the TVR is composed of reverberating polysynaptic pathways and is supported by higher centers. The efferent pathway of the TVR inhibits or dampens the monosynaptic stretch reflex when both vibration and quick stretch are applied simultaneously (25). Although controversy once existed regarding the rationale underlying this dampening of stretch reflexes by the TVR, evidence strongly points to presynaptic inhibition at anterior horn cell pools as the primary mechanism (25–27). The precise role of cutaneous receptors that are stimulated by vibration is not clear. The effect may only be one of contributing to conscious awareness of the vibratory stimulus (25). If gamma motoneurons are susceptible to influences from cutaneous receptors, however, vibration—particularly over muscle bellies—could conceivably affect the recruitment of gamma motoneurons and intrafusal fiber contraction (28).

Several parameters influence the response of the TVR. Beside the excitatory state of the CNS, the most important parameter seems to be the frequency of the vibrator. In order to elicit a facilitatory response, the frequency should be 100–200 Hz (cycles per second) (29). Within this range, the higher the frequency, the stronger the response appears to become. Caution must be taken when purchasing a vibrator as many of the battery-operated facial massagers are below 100 Hz. Electric vibrators with higher frequencies seem to be more reliable and effective. Not only do the low-frequency vibrators appear to be less effective, they may in some instances actually cause muscle inhibition. Studies on humans have shown that the spindle secondary afferents and GTOs can respond to lower vibratory frequencies (30–31). Consequently, the elicitation of a TVR in a hypotonic postural extensor with a low-frequency vibrator could result in an unwanted predominance of inhibitory impulses at anterior horn cell pools.

Vibration may be applied to muscle bellies or tendons (29, 32). The response from either area may vary from person to person, but intraindividual reliability for a particular muscle exists—that is, an optimal response once elicited from one person's biceps tendon will continue to be elicited at the same location. The amount of pressure with which the vibrator is applied does not appear to significantly affect the magnitude of the response (33).

Lengthening of a muscle—that is, putting it on external stretch, and positioning of the head of the patient—are two other factors that appear to influence the vibratory response of a weak muscle (25, 29). The TVR of the biceps, for example, may be enhanced by turning the head away from the side being stimulated. Although the use of tonic neck reflexes may be a means of facilitation, the therapist must decide if and when visual input may be of greater benefit. Caution should also be exerted when the muscle externally stretched is a postural extensor.

Clinical Applications. Vibration appears to be an effective tool for the facilitation of hypotonic musculature. If a muscle is extremely weak, a visible response may not be produced. The simultaneous addition of other elements, however, should result in summation and muscle activation. Once activation does occur, the addition of resistance and voluntary input to the reflexive contraction is important; this is necessary to engage the tonic or static gamma system, to establish spindle bias, and to provide the CNS with appropriate feedback.

Because vibration results in reciprocal inhibition to antagonists, it may be used to decrease muscle tension on one side of the joint (34), particularly when such tension is the result of localized muscle tightness or spasm and not due to an upper motor neuron lesion. Because reciprocal inhibitory mechanisms may not be operative in patients with spasticity (35), the use of vibration in such cases may not always yield successful results.

Precautions and contraindications:

- The response to vibration peaks after approximately 30 seconds. As long as the stimulus is applied, the response is maintained. Caution should be taken, however, not to prolong the stimulus in one spot, as a burning or itching sensation or even hives may develop after 60 seconds.
- The use of vibration over time has been shown to result in a decreased muscle response. Although a recent investigation has not corroborated this finding (36), therapists should guard against frequent use of vibration on the same muscle over a period of days.
- When applying a vibrator, bony prominences should be avoided. Bone may act as a conductor and transmit vibratory impulses directly to antagonistic muscle groups (1). In addition, vibration on or near bone may be uncomfortable or actually painful.
- Cryotherapy procedures appear to have a dampening effect on the response of the TVR. Studies on the biceps brachii have shown an increase in latency time of muscle activation and a decrease in range of motion of elbow flexion when vibration has been applied following application of a cold pack. These effects were immediately evident and were also documented over time (37–38).
- Vibration may enhance abnormal movement patterns—for example, ataxia and athetosis (29)—and may trigger seizures in patients who are prone to seizure (1). Spreading of impulses may occur and clonus may be induced in neighboring muscles in patients with spasticity.
- Clinical evidence indicates that vibration applied to a young child can produce unwanted effects. For this reason, artificially produced high-frequency stimuli should be avoided and replaced by stimuli that provide the CNS with more natural types of input (1).

In summary:

- When vibration is applied at a frequency of approximately 100 Hz for 60 seconds, it appears to be effective in eliciting or enhancing the response of a hypotonic muscle. Once the response is elicited, it should be resisted. Vibration on patients with an immature central nervous system, a history of seizures, or abnormal movements patterns is contraindicated.

Approximation

The element of approximation, or telescoping, refers to the heavy compression of joint surfaces for purposes of increasing postural muscle holding (1, 39). The approximation may be applied by positioning the patient in a weight-bearing posture [Figure 5–1(a)] or may be manually applied with firm maintained pressure by the therapist in that part of the range in which tonic holding is a goal, for example, shortened ranges of D_1 extension for the gluteus medius [Figure 5–1 (b)]. Approximation may also be superimposed on a weight-bearing posture to further enhance stability in that posture [Figure 5–1(c)].

Nerve endings are distributed through the tissues of all synovial joints. These endings are particularly prevalent in the joint capsules and ligaments and have been classified into groups according to function, distribution, and morphology (40). Relatively few studies on humans have clearly defined the role of these different mechanoreceptors in the various joints during weight bearing activities. One study has shown that the gluteus medius, a postural muscle, is indeed facilitated during weight bearing and remains active as long as joint compression is maintained (41). This reflex activation is attributed to the nerve endings in the ligamentum capitis femoris. The more phasic muscles surrounding the hip joint are also inhibited. Whether these findings in the hip can be generalized to other joints is open to speculation. Certainly further studies need to be conducted before approximation can be validated as an effective element for the enhancement of specific muscle groups.

Precautions and contraindications:

- Approximation of joint surfaces that are inflamed should be applied with caution and indeed avoided if such stimulation enhances pain.

Traction

Although approximation can be used to promote stability, traction is often combined with external stretch to enhance movement through range (39) (Figure 5–2). Slowly applied, traction to individual painful joints often provides effective relief and is commonly employed in conjunction with joint mobilization techniques (42). Although clinical experience indicates that traction helps to produce movement, the literature is vague regarding the basis of its effectiveness. If joint receptors contribute to the facilitation of

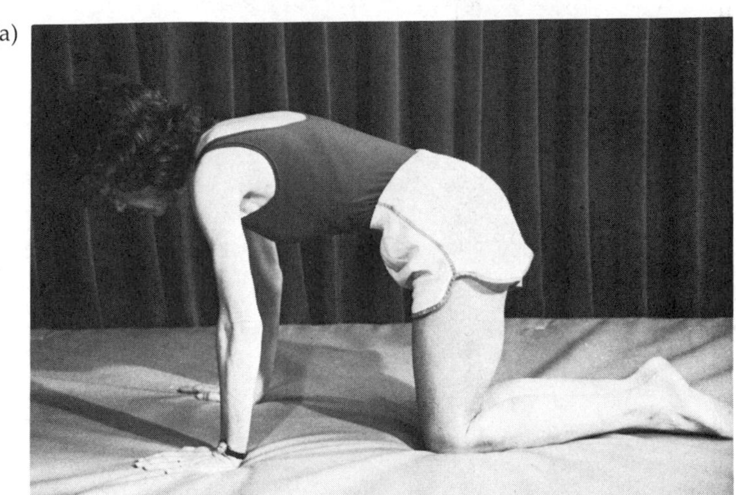
(a)

A. Quadruped.
E. Approximation.

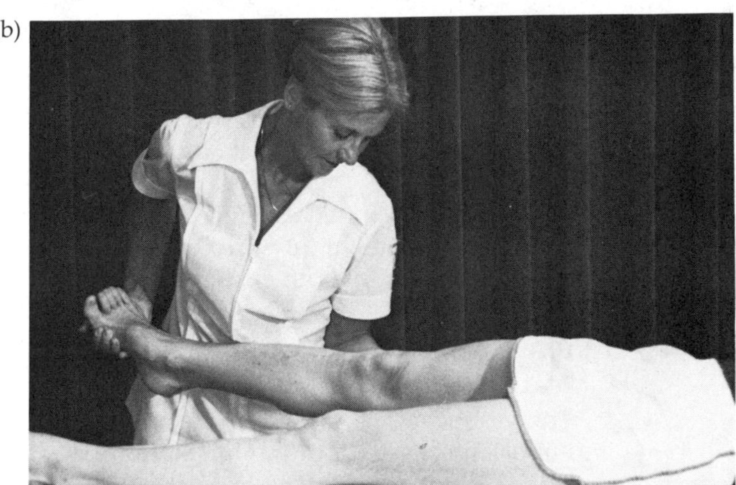
(b)

A. Supine: D_1E LE.
E. Manual approximation, MC thigh and foot.

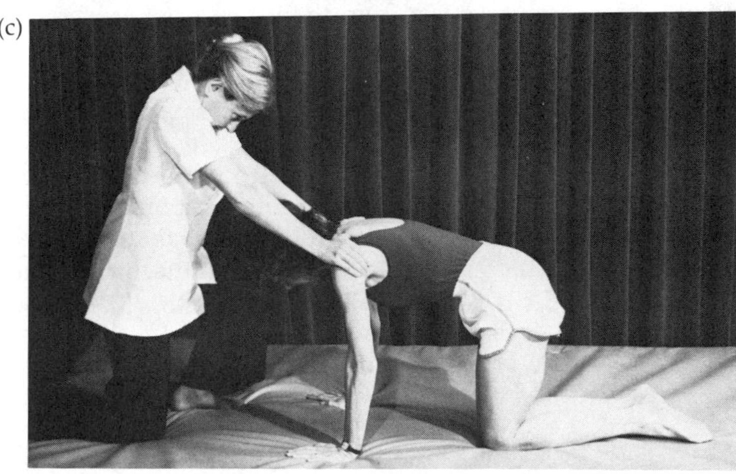
(c)

A. Quadruped.
E. Manual approximation, MC shoulders.

FIGURE 5–1

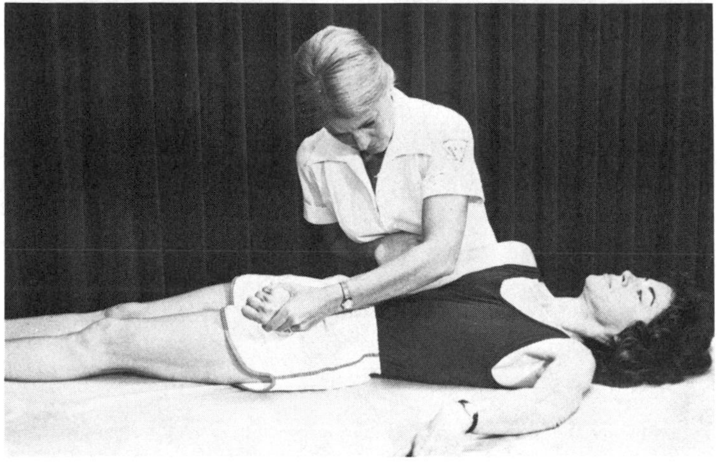

A. Supine: D_2F UE
E. Traction, stretch, MC arm and wrist.

FIGURE 5–2

holding of postural muscles when joint surfaces are compressed, could they also contribute to the facilitation of movement when joint surfaces are separated?

Because it is often difficult during treatment to separate traction of joint surfaces from stretch of surrounding muscle groups, the same precautions apply to the use of both elements.

Angular and Linear Acceleration

The vestibular system, which functions before birth (43), appears to play an important role both in the integration of sensory information and the control of motor output. The two groups of receptors that make up the vestibular apparatus are the semicircular canals (SSC) and the otolith organs. Afferent signals from these receptors are processed in the vestibular nucleii, from which the lateral vestibular spinal tract (LVST) and medial vestibular spinal tract (MVST) originate and transmit the information to the spinal cord. The LVST receives information primarily from the otoliths and appears to be excitatory to extensor motoneurons, particularly of the limb musculature. The MVST receives input from both labyrinthine receptors, but appears to have a predilection for signals from the SSC. The MVST transmits both excitatory and inhibitory messages to axial musculature (44).

Because of its extensive connections with motor pathways of the CNS (45), it is obvious that stimulation of the vestibular apparatus can result in an increase or a decrease of motor responses of the trunk and extremities. The type of motor response produced appears to be related to the manner in which the labyrinthine mechanisms are stimulated. SSC are believed to be affected primarily by changes in angular acceleration of the head and are associated with phasic responses. Otolith organs respond to both maintained linear acceleration and head positioning by producing more tonic responses (44). For years Ayres has advocated the use of activities which incorporate both angular and linear acceleration to increase muscle tone of children with certain types of sensory integrative dysfunction (17). More recently, this type of vestibular stimulation was found to be effective in increasing the motor skills of adult hemiplegics (46), children with cerebral palsy (47), Down's syndrome (48), and mental retardation (49–50). Although a positive relationship between vestibular facilitation and improved function is becoming more evident, exactly how these improvements are attained is uncertain.

■ Rolling

Rolling, an important activity in the developmental sequence, appears to affect the arousal state of an individual, depending on its manner of application. Studies have shown that repetitive rocking can have a soothing effect on infants, regardless of whether it is performed in a vertical or horizontal plane (51). To date, however, the efficacy of this stimulus has not been satisfactorily explained. That repetitive stimulation of the vestibular system directly affects the output of the reticular activating system is one theory; that it influences reflexive autonomic changes is another (52). Clinical evidence indicates that rocking in a slow, rhythmical pattern seems to produce a general calming effect. Rhythmical rolling therefore can be an important preliminary input in cases of hypertonia, for example, patients with multiple sclerosis or Parkinsonism. A hyperactive child can be calmed by this repetitive motion, and thus the way can be prepared for higher level postures and activities.

Although a systematic rolling pattern may decrease the output from the reticular activating system, a more irregular, accelerating pattern may be effective in increasing the arousal state of comatosed or severely hypotonic patients.

In summary:

- Because of its multiple connections in the CNS, the vestibular system can exert widespread effects on skeletal muscle tone. The exact nature of these effects and the manner in which they can be elicited are still under investigation.

EXTEROCEPTIVE ELEMENTS

■ Light Touch

Light touch stimuli may be provided either manually or with ice. In both instances, the stroking or sweeping stimulus is lightly applied over the muscle belly for only a few repetitions to avoid receptor adaptation. Fast-adapting skin receptors that connect with the large A fibers rapidly transmit impulses from the periphery. The efferent pathway is uncertain. According to Shahani (personal communication, August 1979), when cutaneous receptors, particularly those in the face, are stimulated, segmental responses are produced. However, the possibility that impulses are transmitted from the periphery to higher centers, where connections are made with descending pathways directly to motoneurons, cannot be excluded. If the muscle is activated, the contraction must be resisted immediately to perpetuate the response. If the response is not resisted, the influences of the GTOs, which are very sensitive to active tension, may predominate and may lead to inhibition to the muscle stimulated and reciprocal facilitation, or a rebound effect in the case of the antagonist (53). Thus, quickly applied stimuli may result in either autogenetic muscle facilitation or inhibition, depending on whether the elicited response is resisted.

Light touch, although not generally considered to be a particularly potent method of stimulation in a mature central nervous system, is often effective in distal musculature because of the abundance of specific encapsulated cutaneous receptors (54). Light touch may also produce a response in the facial muscles, which of course are very responsive to cutaneous inputs. The effectiveness of phasic input to the face may be due to the predominance of fast-twitch fibers in these muscles (55). Patients with Parkinsonism, for example, can benefit from light touch stimuli to facial muscles followed by techniques such as repeated contractions that will enhance and perpetuate the facilitatory response.

Precautions and contraindications:

- The therapist should avoid the use of phasic stimuli with patients with autonomic instability or extraneous movement patterns because general arousal can result (1). Because of the location of sympathetic ganglia, these and all stimuli should be applied to paravertebral musculature with caution.

In summary:

- Light-touch stimuli are generally used to elicit a phasic response. If the response produced is not resisted, inhibition may result. With the exception of the facial and distal musculature, light touch does not appear to be an effective stimulus in the case of adults.

Brushing

The element of brushing, which was introduced by Rood, can be used to:

1. Reduce pain

2. Increase stretch sensitivity of muscle spindles
3. Reduce excessive perspiration

Brushing is applied with a battery-operated brush and differs slightly in its application, depending on which goal is to be accomplished. The optimal effects are thought to occur when brushing is applied to a functional skin area (FSA), that is, wherever the dermatomes and myotomes correspond. When an FSA is lacking, brushing can be applied directly to the skin overlying the muscle to be facilitated (1). It is usually applied distally to proximally in the direction of the hair growth. Although it has been suggested that brushing should be applied against the direction of the hair growth (56), experience indicates that such application is uncomfortable for the patient and may result in an undesirable withdrawal response.

Reduction of Pain. Brushing is applied over the painful site in the manner described for approximately 3–5 minutes. Subjective clinical findings indicate that brushing can effectively decrease pain, but which mechanisms are involved is not clear. The anatomical organization of dorsal root fibers and their multiple connections in the spinal cord are very complex; as a result, although much has been learned about pain in recent years, the pathways through which pain is transmitted and subsequently reduced are difficult to determine at the present time.

Rood's theory, which is based on research by Young and King (57), has been interpreted by Stockmeyer to suggest that the efficacy of brushing on pain is due to primary afferent depolarization (PAD) occurring in the dorsal horn of the spinal cord (1). PAD is defined by Bishop as a decreased release of transmitter substance at a synapse that results in a smaller postsynaptic potential. This phenomenon is called presynaptic inhibition (58). The dorsal horn is divided into different laminae, each composed of nerve cells serving various functions in the relay of impulses to higher centers (59–60). Rood hypothesized that lamina III, which forms part of the substantia gelatinosa of the dorsal horn, provides the key to the suppression of painful stimuli. When lamina III is excited, presynaptic inhibition or PAD is exerted at lamina IV. Rood proposed that impulses may be transmitted from lamina IV to other parts of the neural axis. If lamina III is not excited, or is inhibited, the possibility exists that pain impulses will then be allowed to travel to higher centers. Rood further suggested that unwanted inhibition of lamina III can be brought about in the following manner: Pain impulses traveling over C size fibers may synapse at lamina II. When excited, the cells in lamina II presynaptically inhibit the cells in lamina III [Figure 5–3(a)]. Such lamina III inhibition allows the pain impulses to be transmitted to other areas or, in terms of Melzak and Wall's pain theory, it "opens the gate" (61). Brushing, however, theoretically "closes the gate." Impulses produced by brushing may possibly be transmitted by a separate "nonnoxious" C fiber pathway that synapses, not at lamina II, but directly onto cells in lamina III. As a result of this direct stimulation, lamina III cells may then presynaptically in-

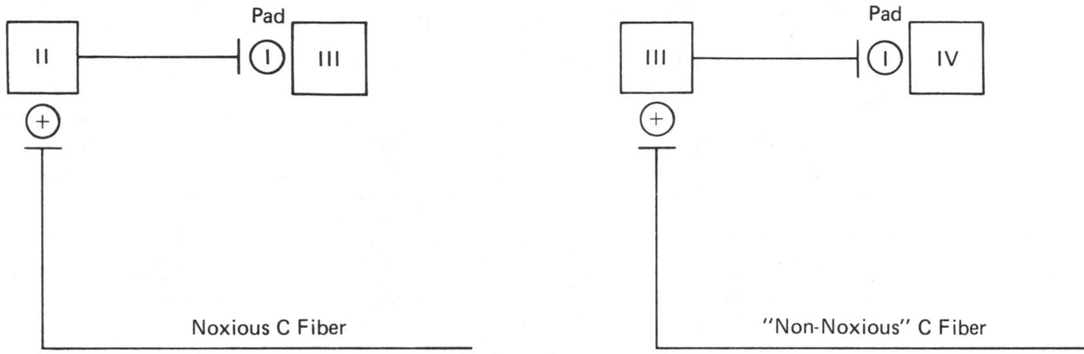

(a) Presynaptic Inhibition at Lamina III

(b) Presynaptic Inhibition at Lamina IV

FIGURE 5–3

hibit or "put a PAD" on other connections in the dorsal horn, primarily those connections at lamina IV [Figure 5–3(b)]. Thus, according to this hypothesis, the PAD produced by brushing can prevent pain stimuli from reaching conscious awareness (1).

Recent studies tend to substantiate Rood's PAD theory, but indicate that the reduction of the dorsal horn connections to the three lamina just described may be an extreme oversimplification and may not adequately reflect the complexity of the mechanisms involved in the decreasing of pain (58).

Increasing Muscle Spindle Stretch Sensitivity. Brushing is applied over the FSA or muscle belly (62). The impulses may travel as high as the thalamus and, as with most ascending and descending tracts, branching is likely to occur in the reticular formation (RF) (1, 62). From the RF it is theorized that descending tracts synapse with static gamma motoneurons in the anterior horn of the spinal cord, which in turn innervate the intrafusal fibers of the muscle spindles (1, 62). Static gamma motoneurons, which are more abundant in tonic than in phasic muscles (63), increase the sensitivity of muscle spindles to stretch. Adequate gamma bias or internal stretch is important in postural muscles, which must constantly respond to external stretches from the environment. Brushing, therefore, would be appropriately applied to a postural muscle prior to its being stretched or resisted, as occurs during tonic holding or in weight-bearing postures. If spindle bias can be enhanced, then the chances of providing motoneuron pools with more facilitatory than inhibitory impulses will be increased. Because there is branching in the RF, which contains many reverberating circuits, a latency period of 30 seconds has been associated with brushing. Rood also suggests that the effects are not optimal until 30–40 minutes after the stimulation (62). Investigations conducted both on normal subjects and on hemiplegic patients suggest, however, that the effects of brushing may be immediate and not long lasting (64–65).

Reduction of Perspiration. Excessive perspiration or hyperhidrosis in the distal areas of the extremities can be a problem for patients who, as a result of trauma or disease, exhibit signs of increased sympathetic functioning. Brushing can be used to effectively decrease hyperhidrosis in the palm of the hand or the sole of the foot when applied to the affected region for approximately 5 minutes two or three times daily (1). Why a decreased sympathetic effect occurs is uncertain. The results could be a consequence of efferent pathway stimulation. Autonomic tracts from the hypothalamus innervate sweat glands and may be affected by impulses from brushing that ascend to the hypothalamic region.

Precautions and contraindications:

- Because brushing, like vibration, produces a rapid artificial volley of impulses and appears to have widespread connections in the CNS, the use of brushing should be avoided or used cautiously in the case of a young child or an adult with neurological dysfunction. Caution must also be taken if brushing is applied to paravertebral musculature because of the presence of sympathetic ganglionic chains.
- Brushing of spastic muscles should be avoided or used with careful monitoring. Because of the rapid maintained input and reverberating circuits, brushing is likely to produce arousal effects in a system that may already be suffering from a deficiency of inhibitory responses.

In summary:

- Brushing produces a tonic volley of impulses into the CNS. Because of brushing's theoretical connections with the reticular system, reverberating effects may be produced which result in a decrease of pain and hyperhidrosis or an increase in muscle spindle stretch sensitivity.

Temperature

Methods incorporating temperature can be divided into three categories: those based on heat, cold, and neutral warmth. Both heat and cold have been extensively used for years in treating injuries to soft tissues, painful musculoskeletal conditions, and hypertonia. Recently, both have been found to be effective in producing a delayed response of muscle strengthening (66–68).

Heat and cold can be applied several ways. Superficial heating can be administered with hot packs or infrared lamps, whereas deeper penetrations require applications of diathermy, microwave, or ultrasound. Depending on the surface to be cooled and the goal of the treatment, cold can be applied in the form of packs, dips, iced towels, massage, sprays, or baths. The effects of heat and cold are a product of many variables: temperature of the stimulus, duration of application, depth of penetration, amount of body surface covered, and the condition of the patient. The physiology underlying the various modes of thermal application are complex and beyond the scope of this text. The reader is referred to other sources for more indepth information (69–70).

Rood advocates the use of *neutral warmth* or retention of body heat to reduce pain and to increase relaxation (62). Patients such as those with rheumatoid arthritis, whom she speculates have an increased sympathetic outflow, seem to respond to neutral warmth (16). Although cold or heat may initially elicit desired responses, a rebound effect is apt to occur with intensification of the original symptoms. More neutral temperatures appear to bring the system into a state of homeostasis (1, 62).

Local neutral warmth can be applied by wrapping a part in a turkish towel or covering it with a down pillow for approximately 20 minutes (1, 62). A warm sweater for upper extremities may also be appropriate. More widespread effects can be produced by a tepid bath or by totally wrapping a patient in a blanket for 20 minutes before other elements such as rhythmical rolling are added to enhance parasympathetic responses.

In summary:

- Various forms of thermal stimuli have been widely used to decrease pain and swelling as well as to alleviate muscle spasm and spasticity. Empirical evidence indicates that neutral warmth provided by the retention of body heat may play an important role in the reduction of pain and enhancement of muscle relaxation without the danger of harmful rebound effects.

Slow Stroking Down Posterior Primary Rami

Slow stroking down the posterior primary rami (PPR) can be used to decrease muscle tone and produce a general calming effect. Indications for use are similar to those discussed under rhythmical rolling. With the patient sidelying or prone, the therapist alternately strokes distally over the paravertebral musculature just lateral to the vertebral column from the cervical area to the buttocks. The stimulus is applied with the flat of the hand by using firm but not heavy pressure. As one hand approaches the coccyx, the other begins stroking in the cervical region. The sensory input continues without interruption for approximately 3 minutes, or until relaxation occurs (1, 62).

Why relaxation occurs as a result of this particular pattern of sensory input applied over sympathetic ganglionic chains is not clear. The exact effects of caudal stroking on the autonomic system need to be documented for both normal subjects and patients with various disorders. Without definitive data, it is difficult to speculate about the neurophysiological mechanisms responsible for the effectiveness of slow stroking down PPR.

COMBINED PROPRIOCEPTIVE AND EXTEROCEPTIVE ELEMENTS

Manual Contacts

Skin receptors are facilitatory to the muscles over which they lie (71–72). Although facilitation can occur on a segmental level (73), studies have demonstrated that input appears to play an important role in the stimulation of the motor cortex (74–75). For this reason, manual contacts are placed on the muscle to be facilitated whenever possible. If the goal is a movement, touch may be light or intermittent while firmer, more maintained contacts may be applied more appropriately to elicit a holding response. If movement or holding in only one direction is desired, as with slow reversal or slow reversal hold, manual contacts should be positioned to facilitate that particular direction of movement. If, on the other hand, cocontraction is the goal, as with rhythmic stabilization, the hand placement should be more diffuse—that is, both sides of the joint should be facilitated simultaneously.

The role of fast and slow nerve fibers in the conduction of various types of impulses from the periphery and the adequate stimuli for their endings have not been clearly delineated (12, 76). Touch stimuli may be conducted by the A size fiber endings if the stimulus is more intermittent or by the C size fiber endings if the stimulus is maintained. If pressure is firm, the muscle spindles may be externally stretched resulting in firing.

In summary:

- The direction of movement and the type of muscle response produced can be influenced by the location, pressure, and time of application of manual contacts.

Pressure on Long Tendons

Firm maintained pressure on long tendons appears to dampen muscle tension and can be incorporated advantageously into the treatment of a patient with hypertonia (1). During treatment this pressure may be applied man-

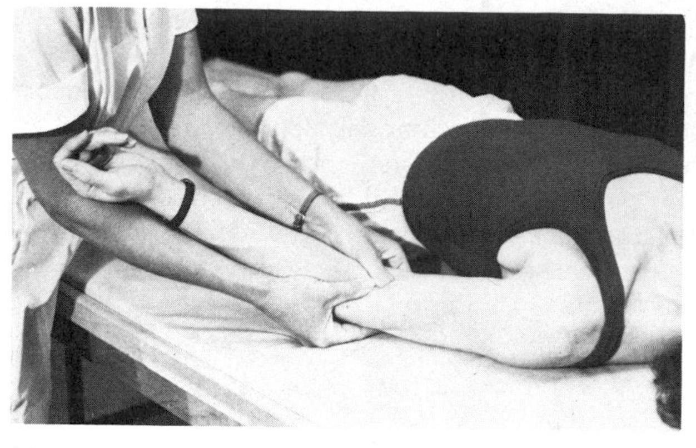

(a)

A. Supine.
E. Manual pressure on biceps tendon.

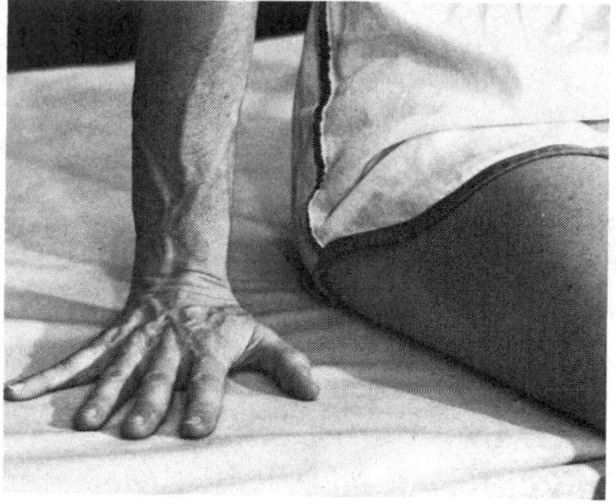

(b)

A. Supported sitting.
E. Prolonged pressure on wrist and finger flexors.

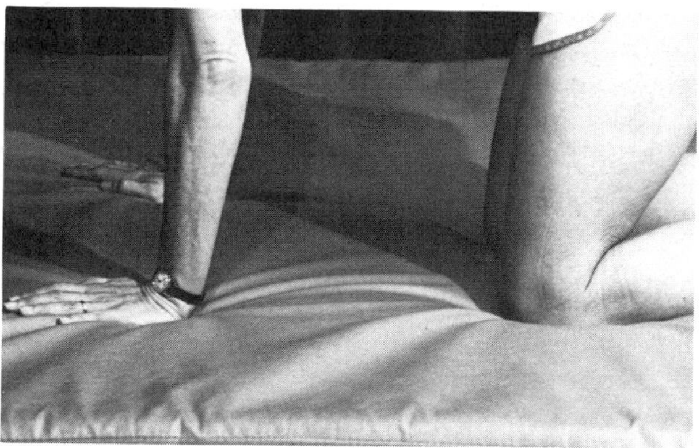

(c)

A. Quadruped.
E. Prolonged pressure on wrist and finger flexors, plus quadriceps tendons.

(d)

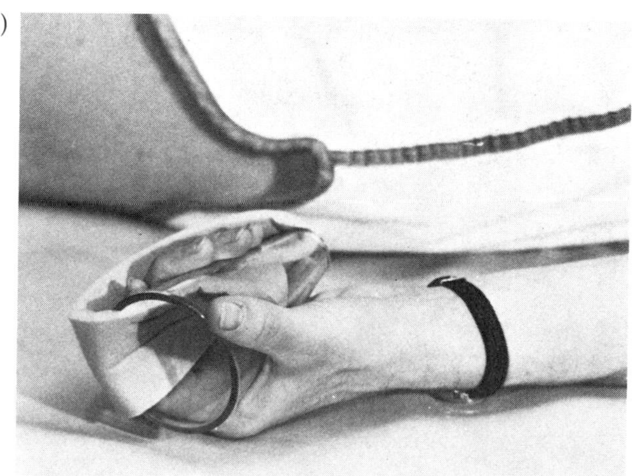

A. Supine.
E. Prolonged pressure on wrist and finger flexors.

FIGURE 5–4

ually [Figure 5–4(a)], or by a supporting surface [Figures 5–4(b) and (c)]. A firm object placed in the hand of a patient with wrist and finger spasticity during nontreatment hours can have the same dampening effect [Figure 5–4(d)]. If the object is soft or spongy, facilitation of stretch reflexes in the already hyperactive musculature can take place and therefore should be avoided.

The dampening of a muscle response by firm pressure on tendons could be partly affected by GTOs, which may be stimulated by the initial passive stretch of the muscle. Spindle afferents and phasic cutaneous receptors also may respond to the initial stretch and touch stimuli. Because the pressure is maintained, however, adaptation of both the spindle afferents and cutaneous receptors could possibly occur and could decrease the facilitatory influences to motoneuron pools.

Precautions and contraindications:

- Caution must be taken during treatment to avoid the use of postures that force weight bearing on long tendons of hypotonic muscles. Such sensory input would be inconsistent with the goal of muscle strengthening.

TELORECEPTIVE ELEMENTS

Teloreceptors refer to the exteroceptors of sight, hearing, and smell and are so named because they make possible perception at a distance (77). Visual input is one of the most important elements a therapist can use in treatment. It can be vital to the initial learning of activities, especially when other feedback systems are not operative. Because visual and vestibular systems are closely associated with each other (45), a patient will be more apt to coordinate an activity when he is directed to watch the movement.

All cranial nerves synapse in the reticular formation. From this formation reticulospinal tracts descend and synapse with both alpha and gamma motoneurons (45). The quality of both verbal and visual stimuli thus play an important role in the magnitude of a cortically elicited response (78–80). Brisk, dynamic verbal commands, bright colors, or moving stimuli can all contribute to arousal while more gentle instruction, soothing music, and a dimly lit, quiet environment can have the opposite effect.

Cranial nerve V, the largest cranial nerve, is a very complex structure with numerous sensory and motor components (45). Sensory endings of the trigeminal nerve, located in the mucous membrane of the nasal passages, can respond to noxious olfactory stimuli. Activation of facial muscles can be promoted through reflex contractions of trigeminal fibers with the motor nuclei of the facial nerve. Such activation is important in establishing protective responses of facial muscles, particularly those of patients with Parkinsonism and may be the first step in the mobilization of neck and trunk musculature (16). The noxious stimulation may be provided by either ammonia or vinegar.

Precautions and contraindications:

- Noxious odors may be facilitatory to the autonomic nervous system. Such stimulation therefore, should be guardedly used for patients who are not in homeostasis.

In summary:

- Because of the connections of the cranial nerves with the reticular system, visual, verbal, and olfactory stimuli can affect the magnitude and quality of a muscle response. Depending on the method or intensity of stimulation, muscle response can be enhanced or dampened.

INTEROCEPTIVE ELEMENT

The carotid sinus is a slight enlargement located at the beginning of the internal carotid artery. The carotid sinus nerve continually exerts a depressor effect on blood pressure. Increased pressure on the carotid sinus will only enhance the frequency of the afferent impulses and magnify the depressor effect upon medullary centers (81).

The carotid sinus reflex can be used in treatment to produce a decrease in muscle tone and is accomplished by lowering the patient's head in relation to his trunk (16, 82). This reflex can be elicited in quadruped, in sitting, or by lying prone over a large ball, depending on both the size and age of the patient and his ability to tolerate the various postures (Figure 5–5).

Precautions and contraindications:

- The head down position should not be maintained for more than a few seconds as prolongation of the posture could result in a marked drop in blood pressure and an increase in intracranial pressure. Close monitoring of pulse and pressure is therefore important. The therapist should also be aware that while general relaxation may be attained initially, prolonged head inversion, aside from being uncomfortable, can result in axial facilitation owing to the stimulation of the otoliths.

In summary:

- When the head is lowered for a few seconds in relation to the trunk, the result is a general decrease in muscle tone. The carotid sinus reflex, repetitive rolling, and neutral warmth, and a slow stroking down PPR may all be used to produce calming effects.

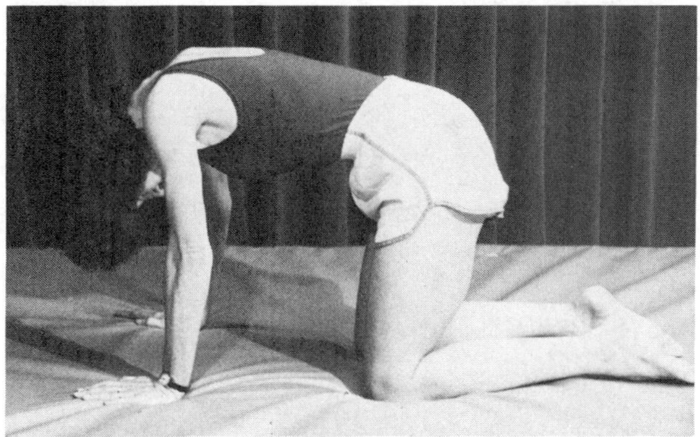

(a)

A. Quadruped.
E. Head down.

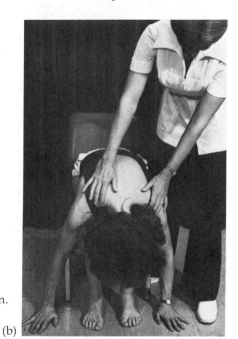

A. Sitting.
E. Head down.

(b)

(c)

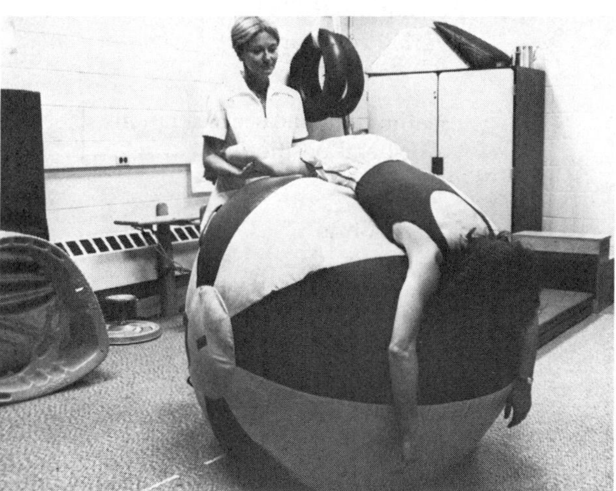

A. Prone over ball.
E. Head down.

FIGURE 5–5

A general guideline of the elements as they relate to patient treatment is included in Table 5–1. When using any type of sensory input, the reader should keep in mind the opening comments of this chapter. Responses to sensory stimulation are often unpredictable. Each patient must be closely observed for excessive or unwanted autonomic and somatic effects. If they occur, treatment must be altered until the desired goals are attained.

TABLE 5–1
Summary of Responses Capable of Being Produced by Elements

Elements	Response
Quick stretch Traction Light touch Visual input Verbal commands	Localized phasic response
Angular or transient linear acceleration Light touch Noxious odors Visual input Verbal commands	Generalized phasic response
Vibration Approximation Brushing Maintained touch Stretch to intrinsics Visual input Verbal commands	Localized tonic response
Maintained linear acceleration or head positioning	Generalized tonic response
Vibration to antagonist Prolonged stretch Pressure on tendons Thermal stimuli Light touch Visual input Verbal commands	Localized decrease in tone
Rhythmical rocking Thermal stimuli Slow stroking down PPR Head down Visual input Verbal commands	Generalized decrease in tone

REFERENCES

1. Stockmeyer SA: Procedures for improvement of motor control. Unpublished notes from Boston University, PT 710, 1978
2. Mathews PBC: Mammalian Muscle Receptors and Their Central Connections. London, Edward Arnold Ltd, 1972
3. Granit R: The Basis of Motor Control. New York, Academic Press, 1970
4. Freeman MAR, Wyke B: Articular contributions to limb muscle reflexes. Brit J Surg 53:61–69, 1966
5. Millar J: Joint afferent fibers responding to muscle stretch, vibration and contraction. Brain Res 63:380–383, 1973
6. Houk J, Henneman E: Responses of Golgi tendon organs to active contractions of the soleus muscle of the cat. J Neurophysiol 30:466–481, 1967
7. Jansen JKS, Rudjord T: On the silent period and Golgi tendon organs of the soleus muscle of the cat. Acta Physiol Scand 62:364–379, 1964
8. Houk J, Singer J, Henneman E: Adequate stimulus for tendon organs with observations on mechanics of ankle joint. J Neurophysiol 34:1051–1065, 1971
9. Henneman E: Peripheral mechanisms involved in the control of muscle. In Mountcastle VB(ed): Medical Physiology, ed 13. St Louis, CV Mosby, 1974, vol 1
10. Stuart DG, Mosher CG, Gerlach RL: Properties and central connections of Golgi tendon organs with special reference to locomotion. In Banker BQ, Przbylski RJ, Vander Meulen JP and Victor M(eds): Research in Muscle Development and Muscle Spindle, part 2. Amsterdam, Exerpta Medica, 1972
11. Urbscheit N: Reflexes evoked by group 11 afferent fibers from muscle spindles. Phys Ther 59:1083–1087, 1979
12. Mendell LM, Henneman E: Input to motoneuron pools and its effects. In Mountcastle VB(ed): Medical Physiology, ed 14. St Louis, CV Mosby, 1980. vol 1
13. Kirkwood PA, Sears TA: Monosynaptic excitation of motoneurons from secondary endings of muscle spindles. Nature 252:242–244, 1974
14. Stauffer EK, Watt DGD, Taylor A, et al: Analysis of muscle receptor connections by spike triggered averaging .2: Spindle group 11 afferents. J Neurophysiol 39:1393–1402, 1976
15. Crutchfield CA, Barnes MR: The Neurophysiological Basis of Patient Treatment, ed 2. Atlanta, GA, Stokesville Publishing Co, 1975, vol 1
16. Stockmeyer SA: An interpretation of the approach of Rood to the treat-

ment of neuromuscular dysfunction. Amer J Phys Med 46:950–956, 1966

17. Ayres, JA: Integration of information. In Henderson A(ed): The Development of Sensory Integrative Theory and Practice. Dubuque, IA, Kendall Hunt, 1974
18. Scholz JP, Campbell SK: Muscle spindles and the regulation of movement. Phys Ther 60:1416–1424, 1980
19. Lawrence MS: Strengthening the quadriceps: Progressively prolonged isometric tension method. Phys Ther Rev 36:658–661, 1956
20. Burg D, Szumski AJ, Struppler A, et al: Influence of a voluntary innervation on human muscle spindle sensitivity. In Shahani M(ed): The Motor System: Neurophysiology and Muscle Mechanisms. New York, Elsevier, Publisher, 1976
21. Cheney PD, Preston JB: Classification of fusimotor fibers in the primate. Neurophysiol 39:9–19, 1976
22. Granit R: The functional role of the muscle spindles—facts and hypotheses. Brain 98:531–556, 1975
23. Kabat H: Central facilitation: The basis of treatment for paralysis. Permanente Foundation Bulletin. August 1952, vol 10
24. Eklund G, Hagbarth KE: Normal variability of tonic vibration reflexes in man. Exp Neurol 16:80–92, 1966
25. Bishop, B: Neurophysiology of motor responses evoked by vibrating stimulation. Phys Ther 54: 1273–1282, 1974
26. Gilles D, Lance JW, Neilson PD, et al: Pre-synaptic inhibition of the monosynaptic reflex by vibration. J Physiol 205:329–339, 1969
27. Shahani BT, Young RR: Effect of vibration on the F response. In Shahani M(ed): The Motor System: Neurophysiology and Muscle Mechanisms. New York, Elsevier, Publisher, 1976
28. Eldred E: Recent advances in the physiology of muscle receptors. In Buerger AA and Tobis JS(eds): Neurophysiologic Aspects of Rehabilitation Medicine, Springfield, IL, Charles C Thomas, 1976
29. Hagbarth KE: The effect of muscle vibration in normal man and in patients with motor disorders. In Desmedt JE(ed): New Developments in Electromyography and Clinical Neurophysiology. Basel, Karger, 1973, vol 3
30. Burke D, Hagbarth KE, Lofstedt L, et al: The responses of human muscle spindle endings to vibration of non-contracting muscles. J Physiol 261:673–693, 1976
31. Burke D, Hagbarth KE, Lofstedt L, et al: The responses of human muscle spindle endings to vibration during isometric contraction. J Physiol 261:695–711, 1976
32. Lance JW, Burke D, Andrews CJ: The reflex effects of muscle vibration.

In Desmedt JE(ed): New Developments in Electromyography and Clinical Neurophysiology. Basel, Karger, 1973, vol 3

33. Goldfinger GH, Schoon CG: Reliability of the tonic vibratory reflex. Phys Ther 58:46–50, 1978

34. Bishop, B: Possible applications of vibration in treatment of motor dysfunctions. Phys Ther 55:139–143, 1975

35. Bishop B: Spasticity: Its physiology and management. Phys Ther 385–395, 1977

36. Shaw, J: The Inter and Intraday Reliability of the TVR. Thesis. Boston, MA, Boston University Sargent College of Allied Health Professions, 1980

37. Smith C: Effects of Twenty Minutes of Heat and Ice on the TVR. Thesis. Boston, MA, Boston University Sargent College of Allied Health Professions, 1980

38. Eastman J, Krosschell K, Larrivee B, et al: The effects of five and ten minutes of ice on the TVR. Unpublished study, Boston, MA, Boston University Sargent College of Allied Health Professions, 1980

39. Knott M, Voss DE: Proprioceptive Neuromuscular Facilitation, ed 2. New York, Harper & Row, 1968

40. Wyke B: Neurology of Joints. Ann Roy Coll Surg Eng L 41:25–49, 1967

41. Dee, R: Structure and function of hip joint innervation. Ann Roy Coll Surg Engl 45:357–374, 1969

42. Cyriax J: Diagnosis of soft tissue lesions. In Textbook of Orthopedic Medicine. London, Balliere Tindall and Cassell, 1969, vol 1

43. Gottlieb G: Behavioral Embryology: Studies on the Development of Behavior and the Nervous System. New York, Academic Press, 1973

44. Wilson VJ, Peterson BW: Peripheral and central substrates of vestibulospinal reflexes. Phys Rev 58: 80–105, 1978

45. Carpenter MB: Human Neuroanatomy. Baltimore, Williams & Wilkins, 1976

46. Fiebert IM, Brown E: Vestibular stimulation to improve ambulation after a cerebral vascular accident. Phys Ther 59:423–426, 1979

47. Chee KW, Kreutzberg JR, Clark DL: Semicircular canal stimulation in cerebral palsied children. Phys Ther 58:1071–1075, 1978

48. Kanter RM, Clark DL, Allen LC, et al: Effects of vestibular stimulation on nystagmus response and motor performance in the developmentally delayed infant. Phys Ther 56:414–421, 1976

49. Montgomery PC, Richter EW: The effect of sensory integrating therapy on the neuromotor development of retarded children. Phys Ther 57:799–806, 1977

50. Montgomery P, Gauger J: Sensory dysfunction in children who toe walk. Phys Ther 58:1195–1204, 1978

51. Pederson DR: The soothing effect of rocking as determined by the direction and frequency of movement. Can J Behav Sci 7:237–243, 1975

52. Ter Vrugt D, Pederson DR: The effects of vertical rocking frequencies on the arousal level of two-month-old infants. Child Dev 44:205–209, 1973

53. Stockmeyer SA: A sensorimotor approach to treatment. In Pearson PH and Williams CE(eds): Physical Therapy Services in the Developmental Disabilities. Springfield, IL, Charles C Thomas, Publisher, 1976

54. Mountcastle VB: Sensory receptors and neural encoding: Introduction to sensory processes. In Mountcastle VB(ed): Medical Physiology, ed 13. St Louis, CV Mosby, 1974, vol 1

55. Shahani B: The human blink reflex. J Neurol Neurosurg Psychiat 33: 792–800, 1970

56. Harris FA: Facilitation techniques in therapeutic exercise. In Basmajian JV(ed): Therapeutic Exercise, ed 3. Baltimore, Williams & Wilkins, 1978

57. Young RF, King RB: Excitability changes in trigeminal primary afferent fibers in response to noxious and nonnoxious stimuli. J Neurophysiol 35:87–95, 1972

58. Bishop, B: Pain: Its physiology and rationale for management. Phys Ther 60:21–23, 1980

59. Rexed B: The cytoarchitectonic organization of the spinal cord in the cat. J Comp Neurol 96:415–495, 1952

60. Rexed B: A cytoarchitectonic atlas of the spinal cord in the cat. J Comp Neurol 100:297–379, 1954

61. Melzack R, Wall PD: Pain mechanisms: A new theory. Science 150:971–979, 1965

62. Rood M: The use of sensory receptors to activate, facilitate, and inhibit motor response, autonomic and somatic, in developmental sequence. In Sattely C(ed): Approaches to the Treatment of Patients with Neuromuscular Dysfunction. DuBuque, IA, WM C Brown, 1962

63. Boyd IA: The response of fast and slow nuclear bag fibers and nuclear chain fibers in isolated cat muscle spindles to fusimotor stimulation and the effect of intrafusal contraction on the sensory endings. Quart J Exp Phys 61:203–254, 1976

64. Spicer SD, Matyas TA: Facilitation of the TVR by cutaneous stimulation. AM J Phys Med 59:223–231, 1980

65. Spicer SD, Matyas TA: Facilitation of the TVR by cutaneous stimulation in hemiplegics. AM J Phys Med 59:280–287, 1981

66. Chastain P: The effect of deep heat on isometric strength. Phys Ther 58:543–546, 1978

67. Oliver RA, Johnson DJ: The effect of cold water on post treatment leg strength. Phys Sports Med, November 1976

68. Oliver RA, Johnson DJ, Wheelhouse WW, et al: Isometric muscle contraction response during recovery from reduced intramuscular temperature. Arch Phys Med Rehabilitation 60:126–129, 1979

69. Licht S: Therapeutic Heat and Cold, ed 2. Baltimore, Waverly Press, 1972

70. Griffen JE, Karselis TC: Physical Agents for Physical Therapists. Springfield, IL, Charles C Thomas, 1978

71. Hagbarth KE: Excitatory and inhibitory skin areas for flexor and extensor motoneurons. ACTA Physiol Scand 26, suppl 94:1–58, 1952

72. Eldred E, Hagbarth KE: Facilitation and inhibition of gamma efferents by stimulation of certain skin areas. J Neurophysiol 17:59–65, 1954

73. Struppler A, Velho F: Single muscle spindle afferent recordings in human flexor reflex. In Shahani M(ed): The Motor System: Neurophysiology and Muscle Mechanisms. New York, Elsevier, Publisher, 1976

74. Asanuma H, Rosen I: Topographical organization of cortical efferent zones projecting to distal forelimb muscles in the monkey. Exp Brain Res 14:243–256, 1972

75. Rosen I, Asanuma H: Peripheral afferent inputs to the forelimb area of the monkey motor cortex: input-output relations. Exp Brain Res 14:257–273, 1972

76. Vallbo AB, Hagbarth KE, Torebjork HE, et al: Somatosensory, proprioceptive, and sympathetic activity in human peripheral nerves. Physiol Rev 59:919–957, 1979

77. Powers, WR: Nervous system control of muscular activity. In Knuttgen HG(ed): Neuromuscular Mechanisms for Therapeutic and Conditioning Exercise, Baltimore, University Park Press, 1976

78. Burg D, Szumski AJ, Struppler A, et al: Afferent and efferent activation of human muscle receptors involved in reflex and voluntary contraction. Exp Neurol 41:754–769, 1973

79. McCandless CA, Rose DE: Evoked cortical response to stimulus change. J Speech Hear Res 13:624–634, 1970

80. Shahani M: Visual input and its influence on motor and sensory systems in man. In Shahani M(ed): The Motor System: Neurophysiology and Muscle Mechanisms. New York, Elsevier, Publisher, 1976

81. DeCoursey RM: The Human Organism. New York, McGraw-Hill, 1955

82. Gellhorn EL: Principles of Autonomic-Somatic Integration. Minneapolis, University of Minnesota Press, 1967

chapter 6

Implementation

INTRODUCTION

The initial treatment procedures are chosen to enhance the patient's existing capabilities before proceeding to higher level functioning. These procedures are also geared toward the attainment of functional goals such as rolling in bed or ADL in the sitting position. During the application of these procedures, the therapist may determine that modifications in the exercises may be needed. Modifications are made if the desired response does not occur or if it occurs too readily and thus indicates the need for a more difficult treatment. Any one or more of the units of a procedure can be changed to meet the needs of the patient. The following examples will illustrate how the procedure can be modified to:

1. Reduce the challenge
2. Maintain the same relative degree of challenge
3. Increase the challenge

1. Dressing in the sitting position over the edge of the bed is a skill level activity and is an appropriate goal for many hemiparetic patients. This functional activity requires both stability and controlled mobility in this posture. If the patient is having difficulty with balance in the posture, the first procedure chosen may be:

A. Sitting, upper trunk movements

T. SRH

E. MC scapulae

If this procedure is too demanding, it can be altered either by using a less stressful posture or by using a less challenging technique:

A. Sitting

T. RS

E. MC scapulae

This alteration in the procedure has decreased the difficulty of the technique from one that promotes controlled mobility to one that enhances the stability level of motor control.

2. This same hemiparetic patient may have difficulty rolling toward prone. The initial procedure chosen may be:

A. Log rolling

T. SRH

E. MC scapula and pelvis

If the goal of rolling is not accomplished by this procedure, the therapist must then determine the cause of failure—for example, the trunk and involved extremity may not have been participating optimally in the movement. The activity therefore may need to be changed to enhance arm function. The procedure might then be modified to:

A. Rolling with a reverse chop

T. SRH

E. MC scapula and wrist

Unlike the first example, this alteration was not introduced to lessen the difficulty of the procedure, but rather to provide the patient with the means of attaining the same level of motor control and the same functional goal.

3. The hemiparetic patient often has difficulty with rotational trunk motions. Sidelying may be the appropriate posture to facilitate these movements. The first procedure chosen may be to promote upper trunk movements:

Stages of Motor Control

Activities	Mobility	Stability	Controlled mobility	Static-dynamic	Skill
Rolling	N	P	O	O	O
Sitting	N	P	O	O	O
Prone on elbows	N	P	O	O	O
Modified plantigrade	N	P	O	O	O
Quadruped	N	P	O	O	O
Standing	N	P	O	O	O

Evaluation of a Patient with a deficit in Stability

FIGURE 6–1

N = Level of control normal
P = Level of control present but quality is poor
O = Level of control absent

Stages of Motor Control

Activities	Mobility	Stability	Controlled mobility	Static-dynamic	Skill
Rolling	N	N	N	N	P
Sitting	N	N	P	P	O
Prone on elbows	N	N	N	P	O
Quadruped	N	N	P	P	O
Modified plantigrade	N	N	P	O	O
Standing	N	P	P	O	O

Evaluation of a Patient with Variations in Motor Ability

FIGURE 6–2

A. Sidelying, upper trunk rotation
T. SRH
E. MC scapula and pelvis

To enhance lower trunk movements the procedure may be:

A. Sidelying, lower trunk motions
T. SRH
E. MC pelvis and scapula

To combine these two motions and to promote the trunk counter-rotation needed during ambulation, a progression of difficulty from these previous two procedures might be:

A. Sidelying, trunk counter-rotation
T. SRH
E. MC scapula and pelvis

This is an example of increasing the difficulty of the entire procedure by increasing the challenge of the activity. If the patient has difficulty with this procedure, an element such as neutral warmth may help to reduce trunk spasticity, should that be the problem.

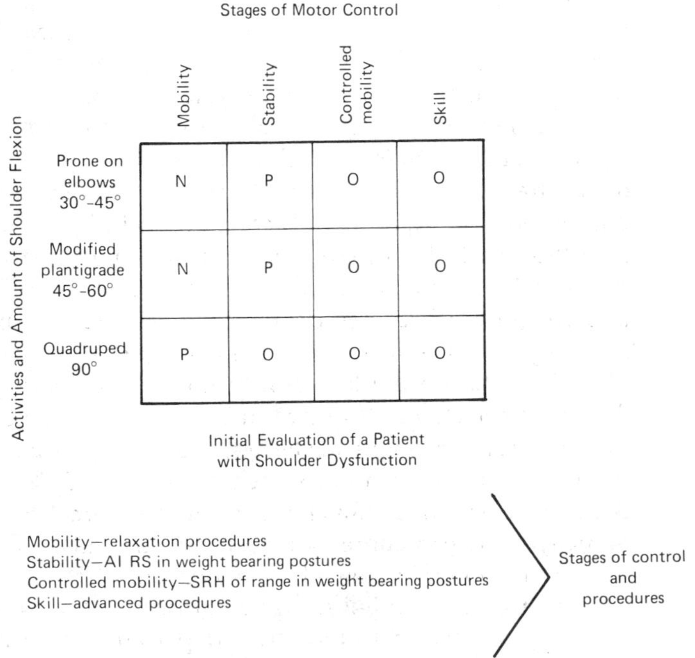

FIGURE 6–3

In general, the progression of procedures is designed to appropriately stress the patient while still providing the reward of goal accomplishment. This requires a logical sequencing of procedures that may differ for each patient. The previous examples have illustrated how procedures can be altered by changing one unit without modifying the posture. The posture can be changed, however, to increase the level of difficulty for the patient.

The therapist may find it difficult to ascertain the postures in which treatment can be initiated and the levels of motor control to be facilitated in each posture. By observing the patient's performance in various developmental postures during evaluative sessions, the therapist should be able to determine the patient's highest level of functioning in each posture. Certain patients may exhibit a lack of stability, for example, in all postures, while others may show a lack of various levels of motor control depending on the difficulty of the posture (Figures 6–1 and 6–2). Treatment of patients who lack one aspect of motor control in every posture should focus on enhancing that particular level of control, while treatment of patients who exhibit variations in motor ability requires more specific planning. The patient with shoulder dysfunction commonly shows a deficit at various levels of motor control as different activities are attempted.

Part of a typical evaluation of a patient with shoulder dysfunction will be given to illustrate how the developmental grid can be used to formulate the initial treatment procedures and provide a mechanism for sequencing. The ROM may show a limitation of shoulder flexion to 80 degrees, abduction to 60 degrees, and external rotation to 20 degrees. Elevation of the arm may only be accomplished by initiating the movement with the scapula. The goals for this patient would include increasing ROM and promoting normal timing by facilitating proximal dynamic stability. Proximal dynamic stability is best achieved in weight-bearing postures by techniques that promote the stability and controlled mobility levels of control. The activities to be used in the treatment of this patient (in order of difficulty) are: sitting, modified plantigrade, and quadruped, with the techniques of RS and SRH. The available ROM will determine the weight-bearing postures that can be used initially in treatment. In transferring the evaluative findings to the developmental grid, it becomes obvious that sitting and modified plantigrade are the only weight-bearing postures the patient can first accomplish (Figure 6–3). To enhance the levels of motor control that are lacking, initial procedures are selected to promote stability in the two postures the patient is able to attain. Once stability has been gained, controlled mobility in these same two postures is enhanced; at the same time, when ROM is sufficient the patient may begin to approach the stability level in the more difficult activity of quadruped. Staticdynamic procedures would follow in the two less stressful postures as controlled mobility is gained in quadruped.

Appropriate selection of procedures makes implementation easier. A task that is familiar to the patient, perhaps one that may be necessary for self-care, will be interpreted by the patient as a meaningful one, and therefore may enhance learning. Following a logical progression of procedures provides no guarantee that the patient will achieve the highest level of motor control in any posture, but it is the most rational way of organizing a treatment plan and of covering all the steps that are needed to reach the goal. In the subsequent chapters the reader is presented with many alternative procedures to accomplish the same goal. By varying the procedures, situation-specific learning can be avoided so that the generalization and transfer of learning from one situation to another may occur.

chapter 7

Clinical Application— An Introduction

The subsequent chapters of this book incorporate the theory presented in the first six chapters into meaningful treatment plans for patients with specific disabilities. Chapters 8 and 9 focus on the evaluation and treatment of patients with cerebral vascular accidents (CVA) and spinal cord injury (SCI). Chapters 10–12 focus on the evaluation and treatment of patients with selected orthopedic disabilities, specifically those with shoulder, knee, and low back problems. These particular disorders were selected not only because they represent a large portion of our patient population, but also because their clinical signs and symptoms are typical of many patients with neurological and musculoskeletal dysfunction.

The chapters dealing with the patients having CNS disorders emphasize the treatment of common problems such as tonal abnormalities, perceptual deficits, and reduced motor control. In the chapters on musculoskeletal dysfunction, treatment is addressed to symptoms such as pain, decreased proximal stability, reduced ROM, decreased strength, and improper timing of movement. Treatment of patients exhibiting any of these symptoms is not discussed in equal depth in each chapter. The reader should be able to transfer the information from one example to another in order to design a comprehensive treatment for patients with one or more of these problems.

The evaluations at the beginning of each chapter draw attention to many of the common assessments that should be performed by the physical therapist. These evaluations are not meant to be all-inclusive nor are the implications of all the possible findings discussed. The purpose is to focus the attention of the therapist on the various methods of determining a patient's problems and assets. Keeping within the scope of this book, only the evaluative findings that respond to therapeutic exercise are emphasized in treatment.

The section on treatment is divided in each chapter into different stages that correspond to the patient's general pattern of recovery. Each section is introduced by the short-range goals that can be achieved by the indicated therapeutic exercise procedures during each phase of recovery. As stated, these goals and treatments do not address every evaluative finding, but rather emphasize the attainment of the various levels of motor control. Many procedures are presented at each phase of recovery to provide the therapist with a wide variety of procedures from which to choose those that will suit the needs of any particular patient. In the chapter on hemiplegia, for example, many of the procedures discussed would promote the goal of crossing the midline. Depending on a specific patient's problems and assets, one or all of these procedures might be appropriate.

The design and sequencing of procedures for each patient follow the principles discussed in the earlier chapters. This format should serve as a guide to the therapist implementing the treatment planning process. For example, procedures generally follow the stages of motor control, progress from proximal to distal, and are performed in increasingly more stressful postures of the developmental sequence.

Although the basic philosophy and treatment concepts of a therapist should be consistent for all patients regardless of age, establishment of goals and specific methods used to reach those goals may have to be altered at times—particularly when treatment involves habilitation rather than rehabilitation. Depending on the patient's age and level of comprehension, certain activities, techniques, and elements may have to be blended in varying combinations by the creative therapist to enhance or dampen muscle tone. Many of the suggested treatments in the subsequent chapters can be modified advantageously to benefit a wide variety of patients with many disabilities. Procedures used to decrease the spasticity of a hemiplegic patient's upper extremity, for example, may be appropriate for a child with cerebral palsy; similarly, many procedures designed for the patient with a traumatic paraplegia can be generalized to patients with lower trunk and extremity problems resulting from multiple sclerosis, spina bifida, or spinal cord tumors. Our structuring of the particular exercise regimens is not in any way intended to provide the reader with a stereotyped recipe for the treatment of all patients with the particular disabilities we have chosen to discuss. Each patient is certainly different and requires an individualized program.

As you read the material in the following sections, recall patients whom you may have encountered with the same or similar problems. How might the described procedures be adapted to meet their needs?

PART II

TREATMENT OF PATIENTS WITH DISORDERS OF THE CENTRAL NERVOUS SYSTEM

chapter 8

Hemiplegia

INTRODUCTION

This chapter focuses on the evaluation and treatment procedures for the hemiplegic patient. Most cerebral vascular accidents (CVAs) affect the middle cerebral artery and have common clinical findings. The upper extremity is usually more affected than the lower extremity and the symptoms—which include diminished sensation and decreased motor control—are usually more evident distally. The extent of language or perceptual deficit is influenced by the hemisphere in which the lesion occurs. When blood vessels other than the middle cerebral artery are involved, problems such as visual deficits, memory impairment, emotional lability, and cranial nerve damage may result (1).

Although many patients exhibit similar deficits, enough variables exist to make the treatment of each hemiplegic patient a unique experience. In addition to the area and extent of the lesion, these variables may include the time lapsed since the insult, the etiology, extent of neurological recovery, and medical complications. The patient's age and amount of family support can also influence the outcome of treatment. Because of these variables, it is difficult to generalize rehabilitation procedures. The evaluation and treatment procedures presented in this chapter focus on alleviating the most commonly found symptoms. Treatment has been divided into initial, middle, and advanced stages to correspond with the typical recovery pattern exhibited by the hemiplegic patient (2). The goals indicated at the beginning of each of the three divisions have been established according to the patient deficits and reflect the desired outcomes at each stage of treatment.

Many unanswered questions exist concerning brain function, particularly in relation to plasticity (3-4), the interdependence of the cortical and brain stem areas that control motor activity (5), the interaction of sensory, perceptual, and motor functioning (6-7), the mechanisms of learning and relearning (8), the effects of the ANS on behavior and hemispheric specialization (9-10). Increased knowledge in these and other areas will undoubtedly improve our treatments in the future.

EVALUATION

The initial evaluation of the hemiplegic patient is performed to assess the current level of functioning. The areas of deficit are transformed into a problem list that is used to establish long- and short-term goals. Equally important, although frequently ignored, is the evaluation of the patient's assets or abilities, which reflect areas of intact neural functioning. To most easily attain the established goals, treatment should be directed toward maximizing the patient's abilities rather than focusing only on the patient's deficits. This concept of working through strength (11) is most applicable to hemiplegic patients for whom relearning of functional movements may have to be organized in other areas of the brain, and executed through different pathways. A patient with poor motor control and decreased sensory feedback, for example, may need other means of sensory input to enhance motor control. Depending on the areas that remain intact, some patients may use added visual cues while others may need detailed auditory commands to supplement sensory input. As the patient's status improves, this additional feedback can be gradually reduced.

Although initially treatment should be centered around the patient's abilities, normal functioning rather than compensatory activities are the goal. In addition, activities that focus solely on compromised functions can frustrate the patient and should be avoided. The evaluation of the hemiplegic patient usually includes but is not limited to the following areas: vital functions; communication ability and mentation; sensory awareness; motor ability and tone; motor control in developmental postures; functional abilities; range of motion; and social, family, and occupational status.

■ Vital Functions

Respiratory. Breathing patterns may be impaired owing to altered tone of intercostal and abdominal muscles (12). Reduced muscular control may result in both a decreased ability to expand the chest walls equally and an ineffective forced expiration. Respiratory evaluation and treatment is essential particularly for the patient remaining on bed rest for an extended period of time because of medical complications.

Chewing and Swallowing. These functions are depressed most commonly in patients with cranial nerve involvement (13). Both decreased sensory awareness and diminished motor control in the facial, tongue, hyoid, laryngeal, and pharyngeal muscle groups may result in reduced function. (Evaluation and treatment of these vital functions are addressed later in this chapter.)

Bowel and Bladder Control. Visceral functions may be affected as a result of either decreased sensory awareness, altered tone, or involvement of the autonomic nervous system (13).

■ Communication Ability and Mentation

Verbal—Receptive and Expressive. Although a complete language evaluation should be performed by a speech therapist, the physical therapist must have an awareness of the patient's ability to understand and express simple or more complex verbal communication. Verbal input during treatment can vary from a one-word command to a series of instructions. If verbal input is to be used effectively, the patient's ability to receive information and then transfer stimuli into a motor response must be assessed. Written and verbal communication may be differentially affected (14).

Nonverbal. Nonverbal communication relies on the patient's ability to accurately process different modes of sensory input, such as visual and perceptual modes. Although communication through these inputs can be assessed in a number of ways, a common method of evaluation is to ask the patient to mimic the therapist's movement patterns. The use of alternative means of communication may be necessary for patients other than those with aphasia.

Mentation. Assessment of the patient's awareness of the disability and orientation with respect to time and place is important. Confusion, depression, and realistic concern for the future should also be noted.

■ Sensory Awareness

Exteroceptive. Exteroceptive sensation is evaluated by means of touch, pressure, and thermal stimuli. The more refined sensory abilities of two-point discrimination and stereognosis also should be noted. Depending on the area of the lesion, the patient may be unable to discriminate between various types of sensory inputs. Localization of sensation on the involved side may be possible, but the sensation may be extinguished when the input is presented bilaterally (13, 15).

Proprioceptive. Proprioceptive sensation is a result of input from the muscle spindle, Golgi tendon organs, and joint receptors. Testing joint position sense, kinesthesia, and the patient's appreciation of tension in a muscle will provide the therapist with general information concerning proprioceptive feedback primarily from the muscle receptors (16). The patient's ability to discern traction and compression applied to a joint may be a means of assessing the feedback from the joint receptors.

The results of the evaluation of both the exteroceptive and proprioceptive sensations are important in the treatment planning process because many sensory inputs can be used either to facilitate or inhibit motor responses. Manual contacts, cold or warmth, vibration, joint traction, or compression may all be included. Even though the patient may not be aware of the sensory input, elicitation of a reflex response may still be possible. If the stimulus response pathway is purely reflexive or is mediated by intact portions of the central nervous system, conscious awareness of the sensation may not be necessary to obtain the desired response. Joint compression, for example, may facilitate activity in postural muscles even though the patient may not sense the stimulation. Perception of sensation may be critical, however, if the response is to be sustained, learned, and made functional. In the standing position, an awareness of weight bearing and position of the joint may be needed before ambulation can become a skilled function. Intact sensory modalities—such as vision, or pressure on the sole of the foot—may be used initially to compensate for a lack of joint sensation.

As discussed in Chapter 5, the effects of many sensory stimuli such as vibration and brushing may differ from the effects of applying these stimuli to people with an intact or normal CNS. Therefore, the initial response and any rebound effects must be carefully monitored.

Body Awareness and Perception. Although body image and perceptual awareness can be assessed by the physical therapist, a more in-depth evaluation is usually performed by the occupational therapist. Many functional abilities such as rolling, dressing, moving in space, locating the brake on the wheelchair, perceiving the distance between the wheelchair and the mat may be impaired by a variety of perceptual deficits (17). The functional severity may be compounded when sensory and visual field deficits are also present.

Visual. Visual field tests help the therapist determine the patient's visual awareness of the environment. The patient's ability to respond to and navigate in the environment may be adversely affected by visual impairment. If a deficit exists, the patient's bed should be properly placed in relation to other objects in the room to ensure optimal sensory input. The therapist's position when treating the patient should also be adjusted.

Vertical orientation may be evaluated by asking the patient to assess the verticality of objects and by observing the patient's posture. A discrepancy may exist between the patient's perception of his vertical orientation and the actual vertical posture. This functional loss is usually related to an imbalance of sensory input from the two sides of the body (18).

■ Motor Ability

Reflexes and Reactions. A reflex assessment can be used to determine the dominance of reflexes that should normally be integrated (19), as well as the presence of postural reactions that will help orient the patient to the environment and assist in normal postural reactions (20). The dominance of lower level reflexes will affect the postures that have the most therapeutic value. When positioned in supine, for example, the patient may demonstrate an increase in extensor tone indicating a dominance of the symmetrical tonic labyrinthine reflex (STLR). Sidelying rather than supine, then, may be the most advantageous position to initiate flexor movements of the lower extremity. An increase in extensor tone may reduce the patient's ability to maintain the knee in flexion in the bridging position, which is an important posture in which to initiate weight bearing. An alternative weight-bearing posture such as kneeling would be indicated with such patients and used in treatment until extensor tone is normalized.

The righting, equilibrium, and protective extension reactions involve higher level motor responses (20). The inability of a patient to respond to a change in the C of G might indicate either a sensory or motor deficit. The sensation of altered position may not be perceived or the patient's motor control may be so impaired that a response is not possible. The disparity between the exteroceptive and proprioceptive feedback from the two sides of the body may also affect the patient's ability to maintain a proper orientation to the environment.

In the clinical setting, few if any objective means of measuring reflexes and reactions exist. Determining the strength of these responses is difficult because they may be affected by many variables, such as medication, positioning, and psychological status. It is important, however, to assess the presence of all these reflexes.

Muscle Tone. Tone can range from flaccidity to hypotonia, to normal tone, to hypertonia. The clinical assessment of muscle tone, like the evaluation of reflexes, is largely subjective. Tone can be measured by testing deep tendon reflexes and resistance to passive stretch (21). A lack of consistency in applying these tests—for example, varying the speed of the passive movement—can reduce objectivity. Furthermore, muscle tone may be affected by environmental and autonomic changes, such as head and body position, medication, and anxiety. In spite of the many variables affecting tone and the lack of objectivity in its assessment, the distribution of altered tone both in specific muscle groups, such as the biceps or finger flexors, and in total movement patterns, such as mass extension of the lower extremity, should be evaluated.

Coordination of the Uninvolved Side. Many hemiplegic patients present symptoms bilaterally, even though one side may be more involved. One cerebral hemisphere influences the other and can affect the functioning of ipsilateral body parts (22). Damage to the hemisphere in which the specialized functions of perception, language, transfer of oral input into motor responses, and modes of learning are located may affect the patient's responses bilaterally. Thus it is not unusual for a patient to demonstrate both hypertonia and a lack of fine coordination on the "intact" side.

Movement Ability of the Trunk and Involved Side. Trunk and extremity movements to be evaluated are: head and neck control, movement patterns, range of control, and threshold of abnormal reactions.

1. *Head and Neck Control.* Head and neck control is a precursor of all trunk and extremity movements and is most commonly affected by brain stem strokes. Although the specific details of motor ability are discussed in the next section, we should note here that the ability to stabilize the head and rotate it across the midline should be evaluated.

2. *Movement Patterns.* The assessment covers various aspects of control. At first, the patient may only be able to initiate voluntary movement in certain muscles. Control usually increases until an entire movement pattern can be performed. This movement may be limited, however, to synergistic primitive patterns (2). The patient may progress to combining movements of the major synergistic patterns before being able to isolate joint movement. Proximal and distal movements should be differentially assessed as control of these segments may vary. Evaluation of the timing and speed of movement and of the ability to perform reversing motions is important and should be included (11, 20).

3. *Range of Control.* The ability to hold in the shortened range, to hold at varied points in the range, and to initiate movement from the lengthened range is noted. The quality of both concentric and eccentric contractions in different parts of the range is also assessed. Exerting control in various ranges can be related to the function and composition of the muscle. It is functionally necessary, for example, for a tonic muscle to hold and move in more shortened ranges, and for a phasic muscle to initiate movement from lengthened ranges (23). The ability of a muscle to contract with good voluntary control and without spasticity needs to be evaluated. The presence of voluntary control means that a muscle contraction can be slowly

increased, maintained at various points in the range, and quickly relaxed; reversing movements can be initiated without difficulty. Hypertonicity prevents these variations in control.

4. *Threshold of Abnormal Reactions.* The therapist should assess the level of exercise that the patient can tolerate without causing an increase in spasticity, lower level reflexes, or associated reactions. Initially, any voluntary or cortical effort, or simply movement of the limb against the resistance of gravity, may increase spasticity. Spasticity or associated movements in the involved upper limb may result if too difficult a procedure is attempted for the lower extremities. As spasticity decreases, these abnormal reactions may be evident only when higher level postures are assumed. Appearance of these reactions at any time usually indicates that the activity is too stressful for the patient. Stress can be produced by any or all units in the procedure: A difficult **activity,** such as quadruped or kneeling; a **technique,** which facilitates movement in a posture before stability has been established; or **elements** that include the application of excessive manual or gravitational resistance. The level of patient effort should not be allowed to reach a point at which it causes or increases abnormal reactions.

■ Motor Control in Developmental Postures

As the patient progresses through the postures in the developmental sequence, the highest level of motor control that can be attained in each posture should be assessed by the therapist. The quality of movement and any bilateral discrepancies should also be noted.

Mobility. Mobility refers to the ability to initiate movement and to the availability of range of motion to assume postures. During the initial stages when the patient is partially flaccid or hypotonic, initiation of movement may be difficult, although range of motion may not be necessarily limited. Initially movements may occur only with reflex support, as in the initiation of wrist extension with the shoulder raised above 90 degrees (Souque's phenomenon) (2). If hypertonia limits movement—for example, in the elbow or hand—the range needed to assume many postures may be limited. If the assisted assumption of a posture causes an increase in spasticity or of associated reactions, the patient does not have free mobility into the posture.

Stability. Tonic holding stability refers to the ability of a muscle to sustain an isometric contraction in the shortened range against resistance. When the triceps or wrist extensors can hold in the shortened range, for example, they have attained this tonic holding level of control. During treatment, this level of stability is usually facilitated by the addition of compression forces. Stability cocontraction refers to the patient's ability to contract muscles on both sides of a joint in a normal manner and is evident when the patient is able to maintain postures such as sitting, sitting with upper extremity support, or quadruped without increasing spasticity or associated reactions. Stability can be further challenged and promoted by the techniques of alternating isometrics (AI) and rhythmic stabilization (RS) and the element of approximation.

Controlled Mobility. The ability to perform trunk rotational movements and to move or rock in weight-bearing postures requires an interaction of the two sides of the body and a reversal of antagonists which seems to be difficult for hemiplegic patients. Rotational movements of the head, neck, and trunk require crossing of the midline, which may be impeded by perceptual deficits. As rocking through increments of range is performed in weight-bearing postures, equilibrium reactions are challenged and promoted, and the ability to assume the posture is developed. Both rocking in a posture or the assumption of the posture may not be performed with equal deftness bilaterally. For example, the patient may have difficulty rocking over the involved limbs in weight-bearing postures or assuming the sitting posture from sidelying on both the right and left sides. Static-dynamic activities, the intermediate step between controlled mobility and skill, emphasizes unilateral weight bearing on the involved limb to further enhance tonic postural control. The increase in body-weight resistance makes unilateral static holding more difficult than the previous stages of motor control, which incorporate bilateral weight bearing.

Skill. In the skill stage of motor control the patient is able to functionally interact with the environment, either by locomotion or manipulation. Skill requires sufficient trunk control for the patient to perform postural adjustments in response to extremity movements. In the extremities, the skill level of control implies proximal dynamic stability to direct the limb movement and the proper sequencing, speed, and timing of movement. Many patients may be able to perform skill level activities such as ambulation or dressing, but not with normal sequencing, timing, or bilateral equality.

During the evaluation of these four major areas of motor control—mobility, stability, controlled mobility, and skill—in developmental postures, the quality of bilateral movement is assessed. Many activities, such as the assumption of sitting may be accomplished with little participation of the involved extremities.

■ Functional Abilities

Functional assessment is a measure of the skill level of motor control. Activities of daily living such as dressing, feeding, hygiene care, and the ability to move either by ambulating or propelling a wheelchair are included. As in the previous evaluations, the quality of movement and bilateral involvement are noted.

■ Range of Motion

Because daily variations in ROM can be caused by hypertonicity, goniometric measurements are not reliable. Limitations in range of motion should become apparent, however, during the application of all the evaluative procedures. Some motions seem to be more critical for function and may frequently become limited because of the usual distribution of spasticity. Mobility of both the noncontractile and contractile tissues is assessed. Particular attention is paid to the mobility of the scapula and shoulder joints. Proximally, the most common pattern of spasticity is in the scapula retractors and downward rotators, which may result in a decrease in the normal movement of the scapula during either passive or active shoulder flexion (20). Elbow extension and forearm supination also frequently become limited because of the typical flexed and pronated resting posture. Prolonged elbow, wrist, and finger flexion will produce a maintained stretch on the antagonistic extensors that may further reduce their ability to contract.

In the lower extremity, ankle dorsiflexion is frequently the most limited movement. Hypertonia of the plantarflexors as well as improper positioning in bed may result in a plantarflexion contracture. The inability to passively dorsiflex the ankle may lead to hyperextension of the knee during the stance phase of gait.

■ Social, Family, and Occupational Status

The status of the patient's personal environment is an integral part of a complete evaluation. A home and occupational assessment will provide the therapist with the information necessary to ensure optimal functioning of the patient when he is discharged from the hospital setting.

■ Goals

The goals for the patient are established following the evaluation. The information gleaned from the evaluation is used to establish both a problem list and an asset list indicating the patient's deficits and abilities, respectively. These lists will help to determine the attainable long-range functional goals. In the remainder of this chapter, short-range goals that would be appropriate at various stages of recovery are listed prior to the procedures selected to reach those goals.

TOTAL TREATMENT PLAN

The total treatment plan is organized to ensure a comprehensive and coordinated treatment. Interaction with other professions including medical, occupational therapy, nursing, speech therapy, social service, and vocational therapy is necessary. The assessment of probable equipment needs—such as orthoses, ambulatory assists, and home equipment—should be included in the total treatment planning process.

Every plan should include a philosophy of treatment to provide a framework in which a progression of procedures can be built. The plan in this chapter was based on the following assumptions:

1. The hemiplegic patient commonly demonstrates deficiencies in many areas of CNS functioning, including sensory, perceptual, and motor integration. The presence and control over higher level reflexes and reactions may be lacking.
2. These problems may be effectively treated by progressing the patient through the stages of motor control and by using the appropriate postures of the developmental sequence.
3. The procedures that are most effective in treatment combine biomechanical, neurophysiological, and developmental principles.

The following discussion will help the reader to understand why certain components of the selected procedures (activity, technique, element) may be particularly important for the hemiplegic patient and thus have been emphasized throughout the entire treatment sequence in this chapter.

Because reflexes and reactions are integrated into and do not dominate normal motor behavior, the sequences of therapeutic procedures is designed to promote an integration of lower level reflexes and to develop normal righting and balance reactions. Trunk rotation in any posture is an effective activity that appears to decrease tonic reflex influences while promoting rotational righting responses (20). Trunk rotation may also be used to: assist the patient in crossing the midline, reduce primitive movement patterns, and enhance segmental motions of the trunk.

Initial control of both the trunk and extremities is gained in postures that provide a great amount of biomechanical support. Trunk control can be promoted independently by means of various activities or can be enhanced in conjunction with extremity control. In the extremities, the procedures are selected to gain first proximal then distal motoric abilities. In keeping with the philosophy of treatment, synergistic patterns are avoided, but the therapist may choose to facilitate these movements if the patient remains flaccid for a prolonged period of time. Normal extremity movement is initially promoted in nonsynergistic, less stressful diagonal 1 (D_1) patterns before progressing to control in diagonal 2 (D_2). To enhance extremity control, trunk combinations precede the use of bilateral and unilateral patterns. Trunk patterns in which the limbs are in contact with each other can be used to capitalize on the sensory input from the uninvolved extremity and provide the CNS with increased feedback. This added information will promote total body awareness when unilateral neglect is present. Experimentation on brain-damaged animals suggests that exercise of the uninvolved extremity may result in decreased functioning of the contralateral involved limb (25). While contralateral inhibition may occur in some experimental conditions, empirical findings indicate that contralateral facilitation, especially in proximal areas, is the predominant response when the unaffected limb is exercised in combination with the affected side.

Developing the ability to accomplish a reversal of antagonists of limb and trunk musculature is an important goal for all patients. The ability to perform a smooth reversal motion with a minimal time delay between the reversal requires a balance of tone between antagonistic muscle groups. Treatment first emphasizes increasing function in the nonspastic or hypotonic muscle groups, which will help to balance tone and subsequently allow a reversal of antagonists to be promoted (20).

In addition to somatic dysfunction, damage to higher centers may influence the autonomic nervous system and affect homeostasis (26). Patients may demonstrate responses that could be considered sympathetic in nature, for example, discrimination among many sensory inputs may be difficult and the patient either may not respond at all or may attempt to respond to all stimuli; movements may frequently lack purpose; and distal circulation may be affected, as evidenced by a lower than normal temperature in the hands and feet. As in normal development, homeostasis of the autonomic nervous system is the goal. Procedures selected to increase parasympathetic control will help to promote a balance between these antagonistic systems.

The program in this chapter was designed in accordance with these general considerations. The specific procedures follow a logical order and are sequenced to reach the short-term goals designated at each stage of treatment. As stated earlier, initial procedures should be selected to enhance the patient's ability and then should gradually be made more difficult. Various modes of sensory input can be used to improve function and then can be withdrawn as motor responses improve.

Treatment Procedures

The sequence of procedures is divided into three stages, which correspond to the initial, middle, and advanced levels of the patient's abilities. Following is a brief description of the patient characteristics at each of these three levels. More specific information will be outlined at the beginning of each stage of treatment.

An evaluation of patients at different levels of recovery may reveal certain general findings as follows.

1. **Initial stage:**
   - Muscle tone—flaccid to beginning hypertonia.
   - Reflexes—increased dominance of spinal and tonic reflexes and decreased higher level balance reactions.
   - Movement ability—no voluntary control progressing to associated reactions and minimal voluntary control in synergistic patterns.

- Motor control—decreased ability to initiate movement and to stabilize within or to assume higher level postures.

2. **Middle stage:**
   - Muscle tone—hypertonia.
   - Reflexes—more normalized integration of lower level reflexes and increased presence of higher level reactions.
   - Movement ability—full movement in synergistic patterns and beginning movement out of synergistic patterns.
   - Motor control—improved ability to initiate movement and to stabilize and move in more difficult postures.

3. **Advanced stage:**
   - Muscle tone—reduced hypertonia to more normalized tone.
   - Reflexes—ability to perform most higher level reactions.
   - Movement ability—isolation of movement more evident with improved ability to combine all patterns of movement.
   - Motor control—a skill level of motor control emerging, but normal timing and speed of movement lacking.

Recovery of other functions, such as sensation and communication, may follow a similar pattern, like the one described for the somatic motor system. The extent and location of the lesion and the amount of neural recovery will influence the speed and progression through the stages of recovery and can determine whether the different stages will be attained.

Initial Stage of Treatment

Patient Characteristics or Problem List. The evaluation at this stage may show flaccidity to minimal amount of hypertonia. The patient may be able to initiate synergistic movement but not be able to isolate movement out of synergistic patterns. Predominance of lower level reflexes, including spinal and tonic reflexes, may interfere with normal movement patterns. Decreased control of the trunk and proximal areas will reduce the patient's ability to maintain or move in many postures. Perceptual deficits combined with the increase in lower level reflexes may diminish the patient's ability to rotate the trunk and cross the midline. Vital functions including respiratory, swallowing, and feeding abilities, may be impaired.

The possible short-range goals are:

- Improve respiratory, swallowing, and feeding functions
- Increase body awareness
- Improve trunk and proximal control

- Increase ability to cross the midline
- Maintain mobility of the scapula, shoulder, elbow, wrist, hand, and ankle joints
- Normalize tone
- Begin reversal of antagonists
- Improve functional abilities

General Considerations. An important consideration during the initial aspect of treatment is the bed positioning of the patient. At this stage the patient is still hypotonic, and synergistic patterns may be just emerging. As the overall goal of treatment is to normalize tone and to promote normal movement patterns, bed positioning should be directed toward the accomplishment of these objectives. In the most comfortable postures for the patient, supine and sidelying, appropriate pillow or towel supports are used to position the trunk and involved limbs out of the most common synergistic patterns. The position of the muscles or movements that most frequently become spastic are those emphasized in proper positioning. Because the finger and wrist flexors are usually hypertonic, either a firm object is placed in the hand (27), or the fingers are maintained in abduction (28). Both, or a combination of these methods, are designed to reduce tone in the flexors.

Passive ROM should be normal during the initial stage and should not become limited until later stages if hypertonia or prolonged immobilization occur. Initially range of motion exercises may not be needed to maintain range, but may be appropriate to provide the patient with some sensation of movement and an awareness of some of the treatment procedures (29). As we have noted, the most critical ranges for function in the upper extremity include the shoulder and hand, and in the lower extremity the ankle. Because so many patients complain of shoulder pain, range of that joint should be performed carefully. Shoulder range is most frequently performed in supine. The scapula elevation and upward rotation that normally accompany shoulder motion should always be incorporated into ROM shoulder exercises. Glenohumeral motion without scapulothoracic movement may overstretch capsular structures and impinge the supraspinatus tendon, and subsequently result in shoulder pain.

Specific Procedures. The *activities* at the initial stage should afford the patient a large B of S and low C of G to decrease the need for balance responses. These postures include sidelying, supine, and sitting. Movements in these postures should emphasize trunk control, interaction of antagonists, trunk rotation, and integration of the two sides of the body. Trunk and proximal control is most easily initiated in the sidelying position, where the effects of gravity and tonic reflexes are diminished. In supine, the use of trunk and bilateral extremity patterns can be used to further develop this control. Because the patient frequently is positioned in sitting, this posture is included in the initial stage of treatment. *Techniques* applied to these pos-

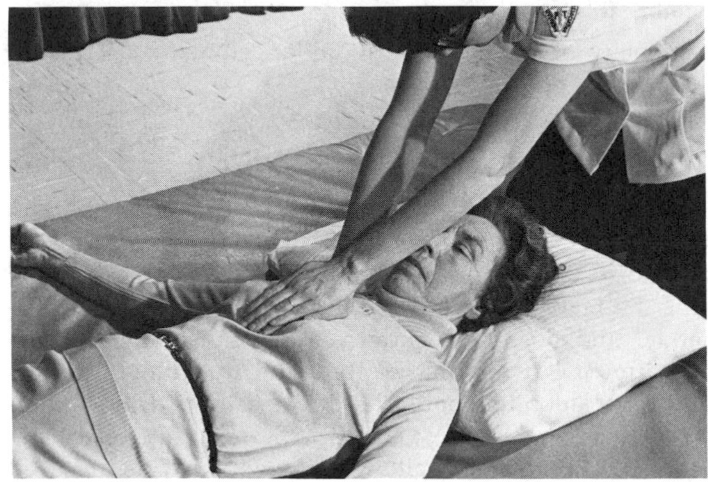

A. Supine: apical breathing.
E. MC sternum.

FIGURE 8–1

tures at this stage are used to emphasize the learning of movement patterns, and the mobility and stability levels of motor control.

The choice of *elements* will depend on the goal of the procedure. Verbal commands should be simple and direct. If the patient is confused or aphasic, verbal communication must be carefully selected. Manual contacts will be most effective if placed on areas that are sensitive to touch and pressure. At this initial stage, the neurological status of the patient may not have completely stabilized. Ice, vibration, and brushing should therefore be used judiciously. As previously mentioned, these stimuli, when applied to a nervous system that is still in flux, may not produce the desired responses and a detrimental effect may result.

Vital Functions. Respiratory function can be promoted in all three postures emphasized during the initial stage of treatment. Breathing exercises are especially important if the patient remains bedridden for a prolonged period of time, or if the intercostal and other trunk muscles are affected. In supine, apical and lateral expansion can be promoted with manual contacts on the sternum and lateral chest walls, respectively (Figures 8–1 and 8–2). In sidelying, with the involved side uppermost, lateral and posterior expansion can be increased. By varying the placement of manual contacts, all areas of segmental expansion can be emphasized in sitting (12).

Mastication and Deglutition. Evaluation of a patient who has suffered a massive CVA or brain stem stroke often reveals deficits in the area of vital functions, including difficulty with both chewing (mastication) and swallowing (deglutition). Attention in treatment should initially be directed at facilitating these important functions, which may be impaired as a result of either sensory or motor dysfunction. Because the physical therapist does not receive extensive training in the facilitation of chewing and swallowing

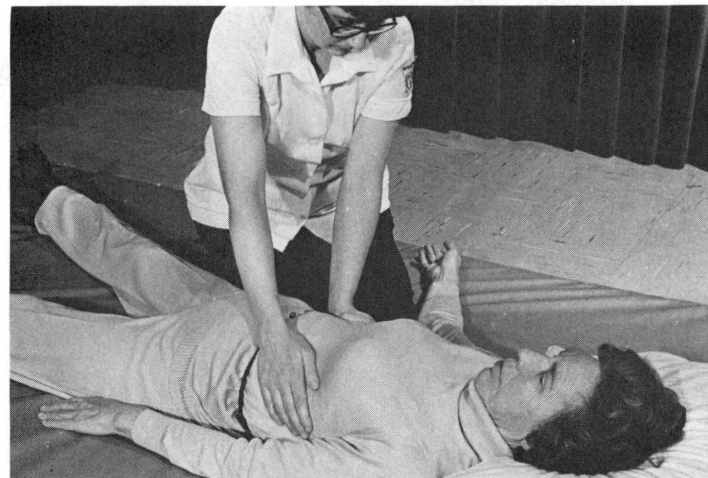

A. Supine: lateral expansion.
E. MC lateral chest wall.

FIGURE 8–2

mechanisms, this important aspect of treatment is often ignored. The purpose of the following paragraphs is to acquaint the reader with the prerequisites of deglutition and to offer suggestions for the facilitation and activation of this complex activity. The procedures to be discussed may be initiated a few days post insult, when the patient is still confined to his bed, and should be continued until the patient can swallow without danger of aspiration. Whenever possible, all the procedures should be performed with the back of the patient's bed elevated approximately 80 to 90 degrees and his head ventrally flexed with a pillow. This position makes swallowing easier and reduces the risk of aspiration (30).

The first and most important treatment goal is head and trunk control. Without proximal control, normal swallowing patterns and intelligible speech are difficult, if not impossible, to attain. Therefore the focus during initial treatment sessions should be on the reestablishment of axial control. When beginning stability is evident, attention can then be directed to the facilitation of the musculature of mouth and jaw, tongue, soft palate, pharynx, and larynx.

In order to chew properly, the patient must first be able to perform fundamental jaw opening and closing and must be able to close his lips around the feeding utensil. Unresisted jaw opening is the function of the pterygoideus externus and suprahyoid muscles, while jaw closing is accomplished by the other muscles of mastication: the pterygoideus internus, masseter, and temporalis. Resistance to jaw opening strengthens the suprahyoid musculature, which plays an important role in the movement of the hyoid bone and the base of the tongue during deglutition as the bolus of food is driven from the mouth into the posterior pharynx (31). Quick ice can be used effectively to stimulate the obicularis oris, hyoid muscles and the muscles of mastication (Figure 8–3). Ice application can be followed by quick stretch and resistance to further facilitate movement and to strengthen

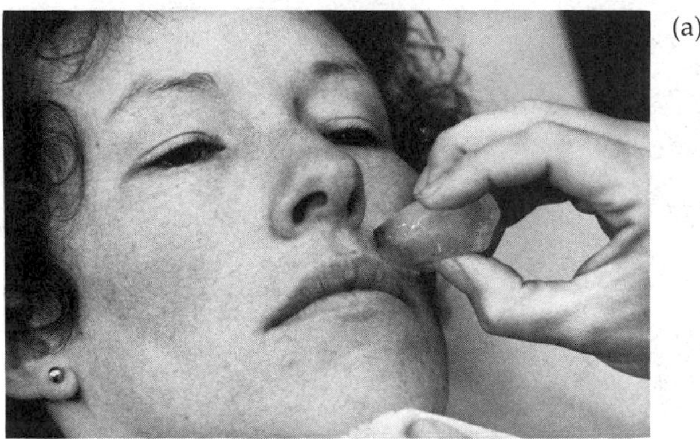

(a)

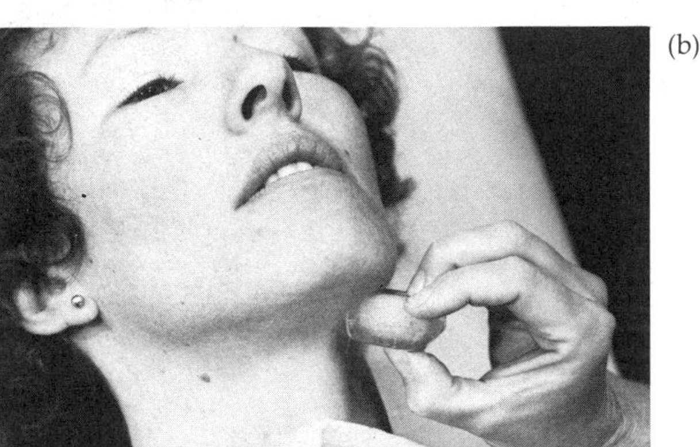

(b)

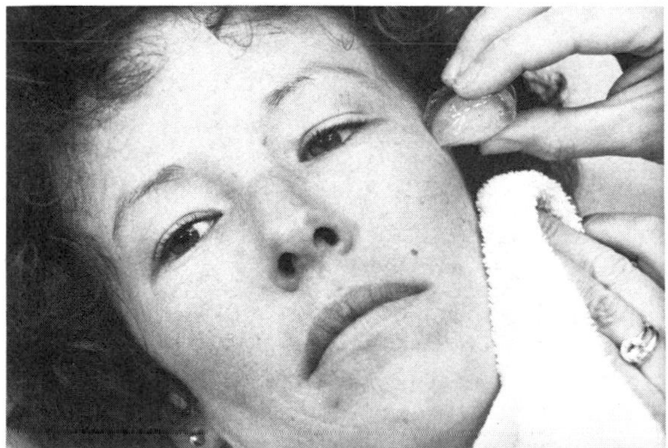

(c)

A. Semireclined.
E. Quick ice to (a) obicularis oris; (b) hyoid; (c) temperalis; (d) masseter; and (e) pterygoideus externus

FIGURE 8–3

the responses of lip closure and jaw opening and closing (Figures 8–4 and 8–5). As we noted in Chapter 5, facial muscles are composed primarily of fast-twitch or phasic muscle fibers and appear to respond well to phasic exteroceptive input. According to some authorities, facial muscles are devoid of muscle spindles (32–33). Because of the lack of the Ia fiber, quick stretch would not appear to be a viable treatment option for facial muscles. Clinical observations indicate, however, that stretch does effectively elicit lip closure and other facial movements. Whether it is the actual stretch or the cutaneous stimulation that is responsible for the positive effects is open to speculation.

The tongue is an intricate and complex structure that is vital for speech, taste, mastication, and deglutition. It is composed of both extrinsic and intrinsic muscles that contain muscle spindles that are dissimilar to those found in the extremity and trunk musculature (34). Multifibrous and tendinous interconnections exist between the tongue and the mandible, soft palate, pharynx, epiglottis, and hyoid bone. To perform all of its varied functions, the tongue must be able to achieve the four levels of motor control: mobility, defined as phasic or random movements in all directions; stability, defined as holding a groove for sucking; controlled mobility, defined as fix-

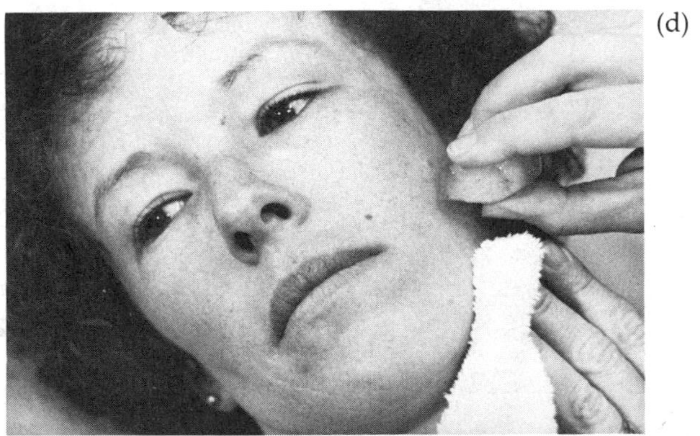

(d)

(e)

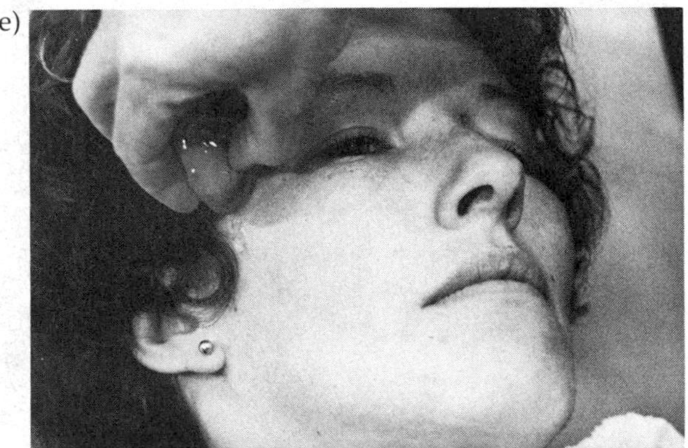

FIGURE 8–3 (Cont'd.)

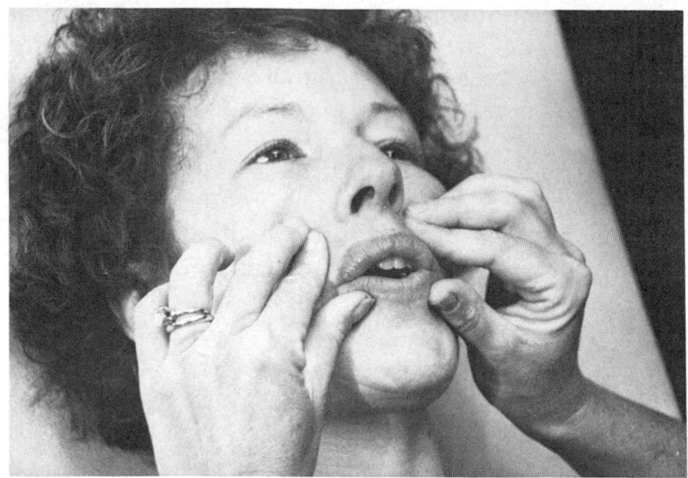

A. Lip closure.
T. Resisted movement.
E. MC around lips, stretch.

FIGURE 8–4

ating the tip on the teeth while the proximal portion elevates during swallowing; and skill, defined as holding proximally in a dynamic manner while the distal portion is used for speech (23).

Treatment of the tongue is aimed at the facilitation of the first three levels of motor control. For mobility, a moist tongue depressor can be used to

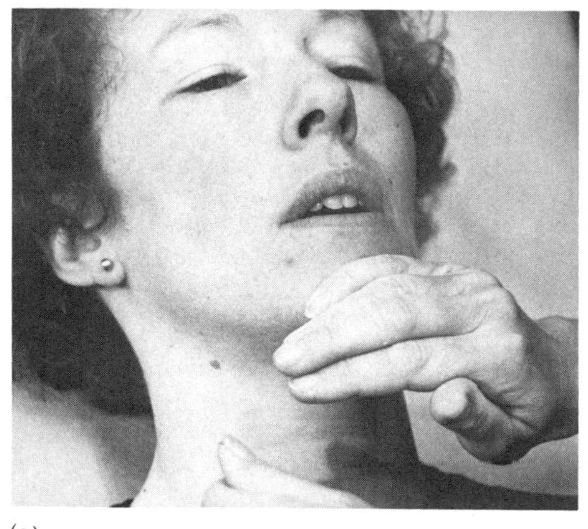

(a)

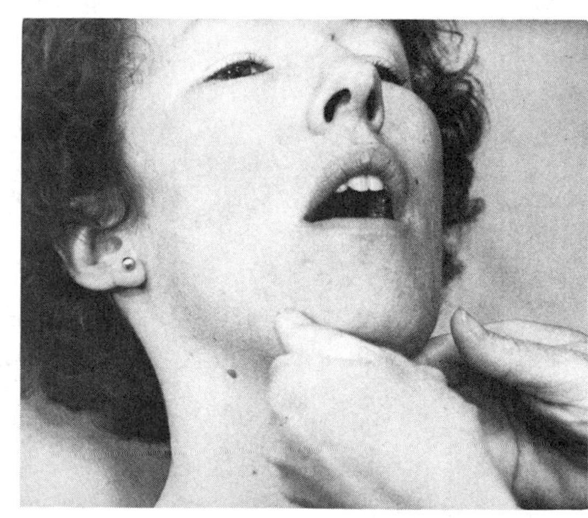

(b)

A. Jaw closure and opening.
T. Resisted movement.
E. MC jaw.

FIGURE 8–5

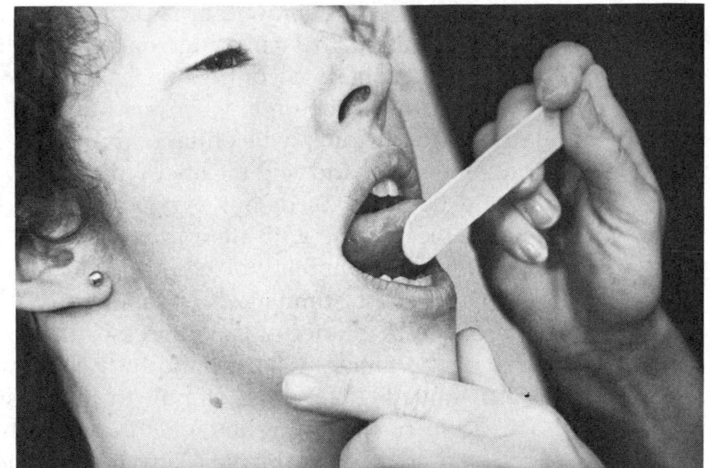

A. Tongue mobility.
T. Resisted movement.
E. Tongue depressor.

FIGURE 8–6

stimulate a combination of forward, lateral, and rotatory tongue movements by quickly stretching, then guiding or resisting these movements with the tongue blade (Figure 8–6). As with the facial muscles, tongue mobility may be preceded by quick icing applied to the different areas of the tongue. If the tongue depressor method does not produce results, the therapist can grasp the tongue with a moistened sterile gauze pad or gloves and can stretch and resist the movements (11) (Figure 8–7). Such stimulation may not be pleasant for either the patient or the therapist, but it is an effective means of eliciting tongue movement.

Stability of the tongue can be facilitated by having the patient suck

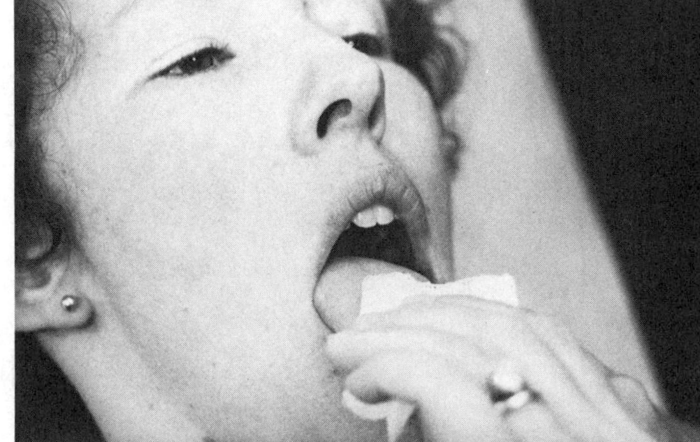

A. Tongue mobility.
T. Resisted movement.
E. MC tongue gauze.

FIGURE 8–7

through an empty straw that is placed against any object such as his finger tip. In addition to facilitating tongue stability, resisted sucking through a straw can facilitate cocontraction or stability of the neck musculature in sitting, or in a prone-on-elbows posture (24). Sucking on a lollipop, particularly a chewy one, will enhance both the mobility and stability levels of tongue control and will facilitate lip and jaw musculature (30). This exercise should be supervised, however, and should be discontinued if the patient is not able to cope with the increased saliva production.

Controlled mobility or elevation of the posterior tongue to the soft palate may also be stimulated with a dampened tongue depressor. If the direction of the resistance of the depressor is downward and backward, then the base of the tongue will respond to the stimulation with an upward and forward movement. Stretch stimuli to the posterior tongue may result in the activation of the gag reflex which, although uncomfortable for the patient, can be a goal of treatment. Many hemiplegic patients lack the protection of the gag reflex and can easily aspirate liquids or solid foods. Controlled mobility tongue exercises are important, therefore, to facilitate a tongue movement that is an integral component of swallowing, to facilitate a hypoactive gag reflex, and lastly, because of fibrous interconnections, to indirectly stimulate contraction of the soft palate and pharyngeal muscles.

During swallowing, the muscles of the soft palate, interact with those of the pharynx and larynx. The larynx elevates anteriorly and the soft palate ascends to prevent passage of food into the nasopharynx (35). The pharynx is simultaneously drawn upward and dilates to receive the bolus of food from the mouth. Subsequently, the vocal cords adduct and the entrance to the larynx closes, thus preventing aspiration into the trachea (36); the pharyngeal elevator muscles relax, and the pharyngeal constrictors contract to move the food into the esophagus. Once the food is in the esophagus, the soft palate and the larynx return to their resting positions.

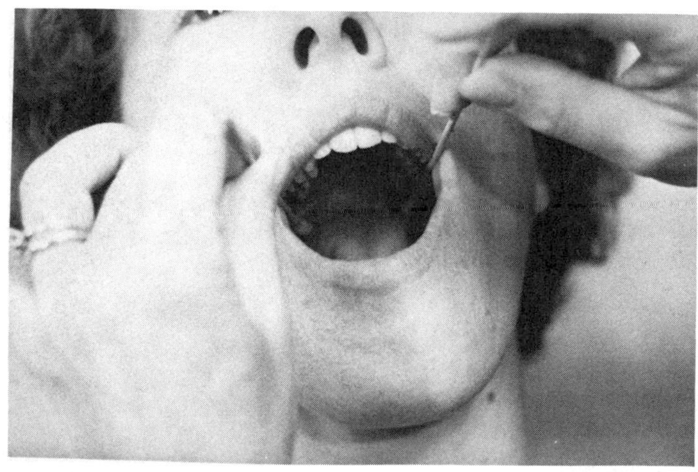

A. Soft palate movements.
E. Quick stretch, cotton swab sticks.

FIGURE 8–8

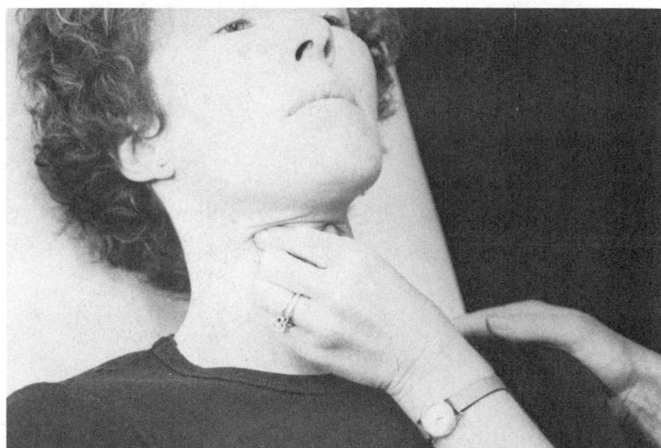

A. Laryngeal elevation.
E. MC larynx.

FIGURE 8–9

Elevation of the soft palate may be directly achieved by bilateral stretching of the folds of the soft palate with moistened cotton swab sticks (Figure 8–8). While the stimulus is applied, the patient should be instructed to phonate with a series of staccato "ahs" performed at both low and high pitches (11, 35, 37). This repeated stretching and phonating sequence should result in contraction of the soft palate and pharyngeal musculature, upward mobility of the larynx, and abduction and adduction of the vocal cords.

Vocal cord adduction can also be stimulated by having the patient hum (36). Performance of the Valsalva maneuver is yet another means of achieving laryngeal adduction, but obviously should be used with caution or even avoided in many cases. Manual elevation of the larynx can assist the patient with swallowing and give him the appropriate sensory feedback (35) (Figure 8–9).

As stated, pharyngeal muscles may be also stimulated indirectly by contractions of the tongue. They also may be stimulated by contractions of the obicularis oris and buccinator muscles. Like the tongue, both of these muscles interconnect with the pharyngeal muscle group. Contractions of either the obicularis oris or buccinator will therefore result in stretch and facilitation of the muscles of the posterior pharynx (24).

The buccinator is an accessory muscle of mastication. Aside from reflexly affecting the pharyngeal muscles, stimulation of the buccinator is important because of the role it plays in holding food within the oral cavity. Facilitation of this muscle can be easily achieved by means of a quick icing application followed by repeated contractions that are bilaterally resisted with tongue depressors (37) (Figure 8–10).

Although the techniques and procedures discussed in this section have focused on the treatment of the patient with hemiplegia, the reader is reminded that this series of exercises may be adapted to the treatment of any patient who has hypotonia and dysphagia as a result of either CNS deficit

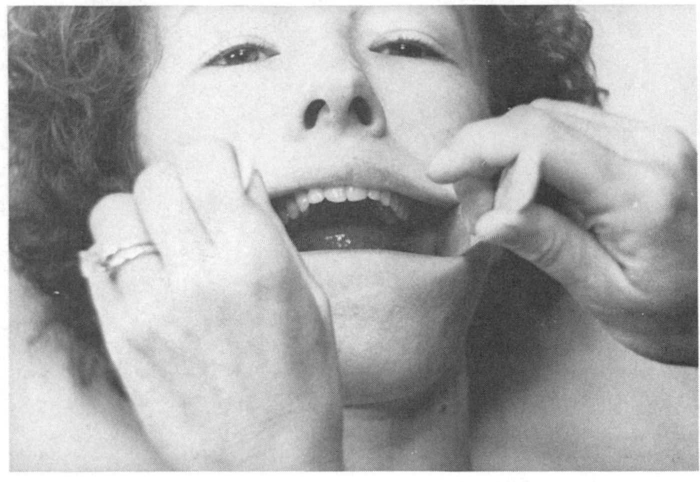

A. Cheek compression (buccinator).
E. Tongue depressor inside mouth, stretch, quick ice.

FIGURE 8–10

or surgical complications. Intraoral exercises are also indicated for patients who exhibit a hyperactive gag reflex and tongue thrust. The eventual goals for these patients are similar to those for patients with hypotonia, but the methods used to accomplish the goals differ (38).

Selected Procedures for Trunk Control. The development of trunk control begins with the activity of rolling. Rolling can be performed by means of total body movement or by segmental movement. Patients with reduced tone in the trunk muscles or with motor learning problems may have less difficulty with rolling when the segmental movement precedes the total body rotation. Segmental trunk movement performed prior to the total body pattern is not the usual developmental sequence of movement, but because of the special needs of some hemiplegic patients this sequence of activities may be easier to perform. The technique of rhythmic initiation (RI) can be applied to either of these activities (Figure 8–11). The rolling movement begins in sidelying and progresses through larger excursions of range. The technique begins with passive movement; then the patient is asked to assist in the movement before finally participating in a more active fashion. The goal of this procedure is the initiation of movement in both directions. Both upper trunk and lower trunk protraction and retraction may be promoted during this initial stage. If spasticity is marked, however, the forward protraction motion of both trunk segments may be emphasized later in treatment to counteract the hyperactivity commonly seen in the retractors. Forward rotation of the lower trunk in this sidelying posture and in other, more advanced activities will help to promote the lower trunk control needed for gait. Once movement can be initiated, stability can be emphasized. Although the techniques may differ, the sequence of the activities is similar to the progression during the mobility stage just described. Alternating isometrics (AI) applied in sidelying can be used to enhance isometric control of the extensors and flexors of the total trunk. When performed separately to the upper and lower trunk segments, AI will help to promote isolated control of the trunk musculature. The application of rhythmic stabilization (RS), which facilitates the cocontraction level of stability, results in counter-rotational isometric control. Although this technique may be attempted during early treatment stages, the patient may not be capable of responding in the desired manner. Many patients have difficulty performing RS during the initial stage because they lack rotational control and are unable to contract the muscles on both sides of the trunk simultaneously. Trunk stability is necessary, however, to maintain all higher level postures and should be a goal of treatment during all stages of recovery. Thus even though the patient may have difficulty responding to the demands of RS, attempts at cocontraction in the initial phase of treatment are important.

(a)

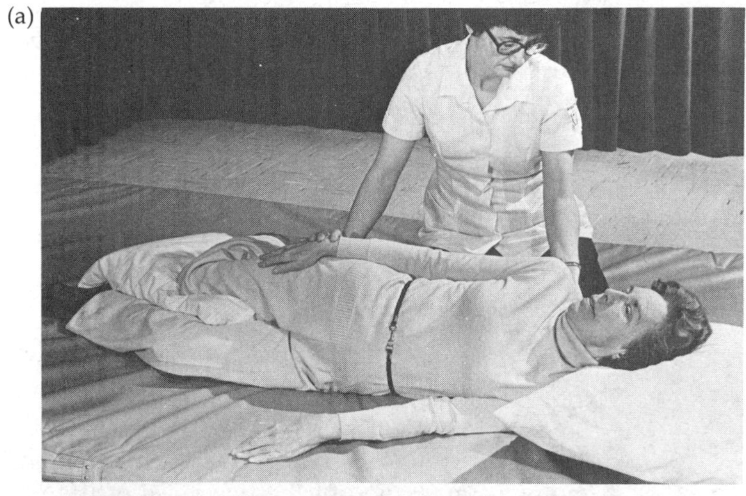

(b)

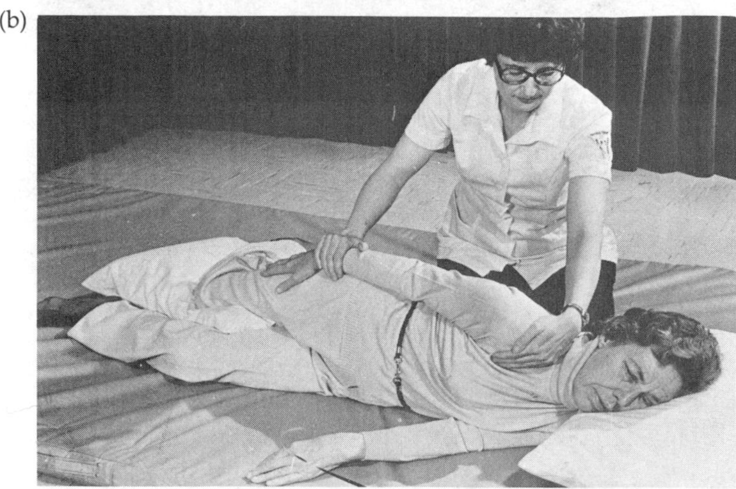

A. Sidelying: upper trunk motions.
T. RI.
E. MC scapula and pelvis.

FIGURE 8–11

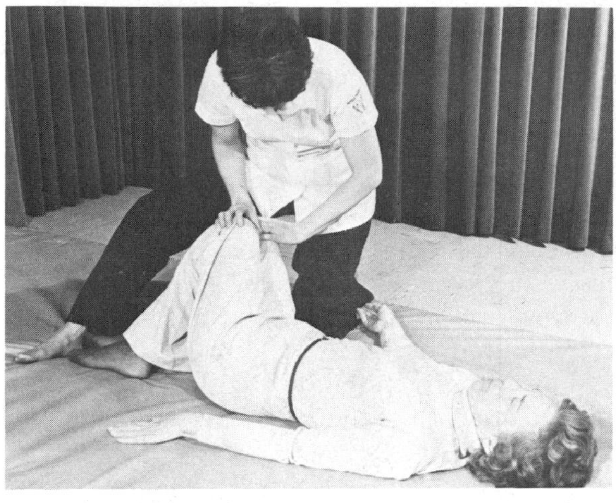

(a)

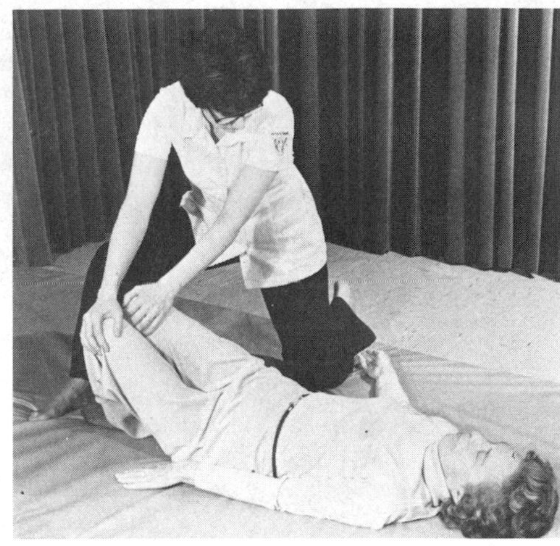

(b)

A. LTR.
T. RI increments of range.
E. MC knees.

FIGURE 8–12

In supine, segmental trunk motions that incorporate lower extremity movement can be performed. The activity of lower trunk rotation (LTR) can be used to achieve many goals that are important for the hemiplegic patient. The extremities cross the midline; muscles are bilaterally activated to promote an integration of the two sides of the body; and lastly, because there is a flexor and extensor phase of the movement, an interaction of antagonists occurs (11, 39). The lower trunk rotational motion may help to reduce hypertonia and, as in sidelying, will promote the pelvic forward rotational movement necessary for ambulation. If the entire trunk moves as a unit, the technique of RI performed through increments of range will help to ensure the isolation of motion to the lower trunk (Figure 8–12). The upper extremity may be positioned at the patient's side out of synergistic patterns, with the shoulder slightly abducted, the forearm supinated, and the hand extended. The feet may need to be supported by the therapist during this activity because of the decreased proximal control. Extensor spasticity, a dominance of the STLR, or an extensor thrust may all reduce the patient's ability to maintain the hip and knee in flexion.

Selected Procedures for Lower Extremity Control. Lower trunk flexor and extensor patterns can also be performed in supine. As with the LTR

(c)

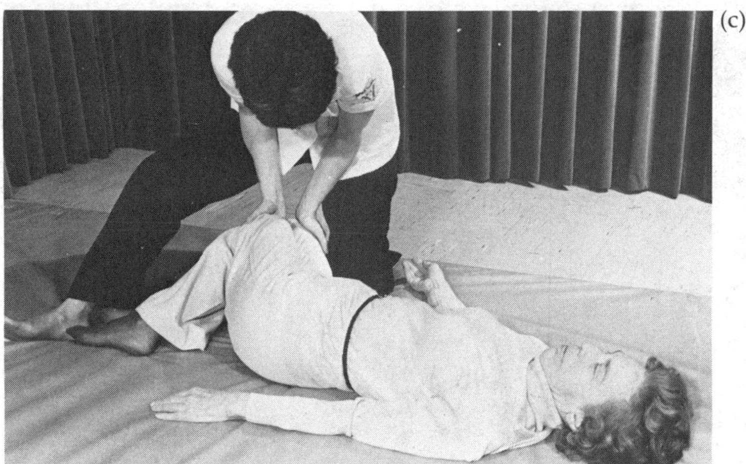

(d)

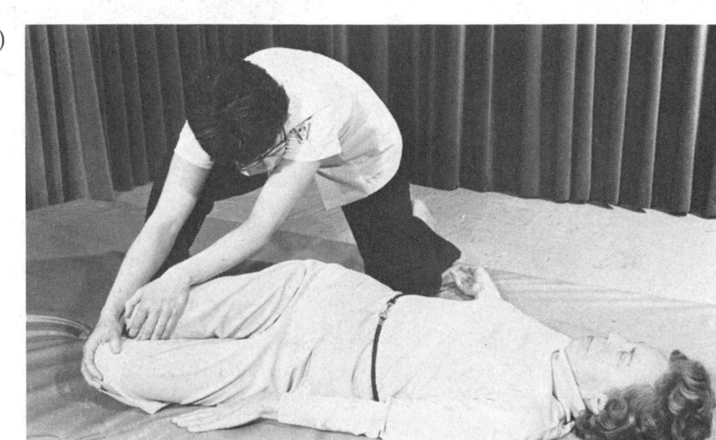

FIGURE 8–12 (Cont'd.)

activity, contact between the lower extremities will improve sensory feedback and provide a "tracking" response in the involved lower extremity (40). The lower trunk patterns incorporate a rotational component, but the emphasis at this time is on the mass flexor and extensor movements of the extremities. To avoid movement into the synergistic pattern, the involved leg should perform a D_1 pattern that incorporates hip adduction with flexion and abduction with extension (40). If extensor tone is dominant, emphasis on the flexor phase of the lower trunk patterns will promote a balance of tone. The lower extremities first may be positioned in the shortened range of flexion to facilitate flexor tone. As flexor control increases, movement can be initiated from more lengthened ranges, in which the effects of gravity and the length of the lever arm are increased. For patients who have a generalized decrease in tone or a predominant flexor withdrawal response, the

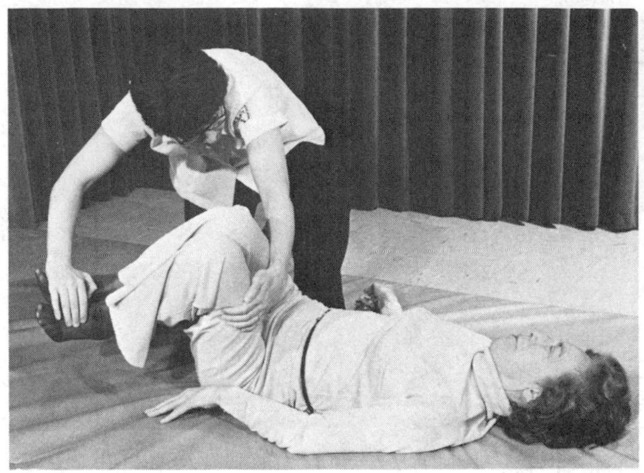

(a)

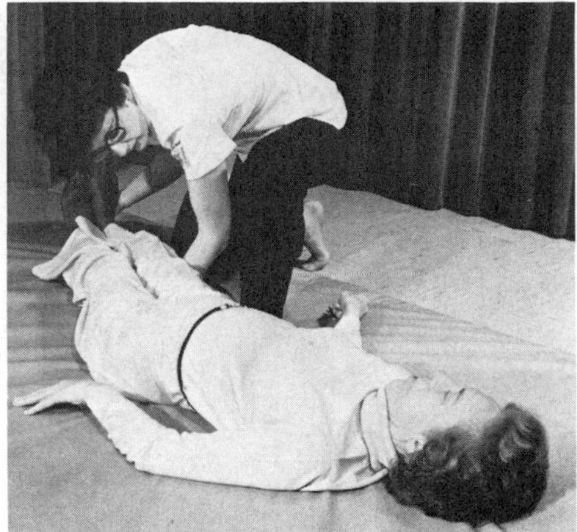

(b)

A. Lower trunk: flexion and extension.
T. Holding in shortened range.
E. MC thigh and foot.

FIGURE 8–13

extensor rather than the flexor phase should be emphasized (Figure 8–13). For all hemiplegic patients, the combination of hip extension with abduction is important for the stance phase of gait (2) and can be enhanced by facilitation of isometric contractions in the shortened range of the trunk extensor pattern.

Selected Procedures for Upper Extremity Control. Activities to enhance upper extremity control are the next focus of treatment. As described, control of the upper trunk can begin with sidelying. To incorporate both upper extremities into the movement and to promote proximal scapula and shoulder control, the trunk pattern of a reverse chop is performed as a segmental upper trunk rotational movement in the supine position (Figure 8–14). The reverse chop also may be incorporated into the activity of rolling from supine toward prone to assist the upper extremity in participating in this functional movement (40) (Figure 8–15). The involved extremity during this activity is in a D_1 flexor pattern, which facilitates scapula protraction and shoulder flexion with adduction. These movements are an important step in the promotion of proximal control out of synergistic patterns.

The patient is frequently positioned in the sitting posture. Many patients may have difficulty maintaining this posture because of decreased muscle tone, reduced balance reactions, or imbalance in sensory feedback from the two sides of the body. Emphasizing holding in an anterior, posterior, or lateral direction may help to prevent the patient from falling backward or forward or to either side. Thus, AI can be performed in any direction that may be beneficial and usually is followed by RS to further enhance cocontraction control (Figures 8–16 and 8–17). By altering the placement of manual contacts, these techniques can be used to emphasize head, neck, and trunk control (37, 40). Sitting balance can be further enhanced by movement in the directions of flexion and/or extension with rotation, depending on the patient's needs (Figure 8–18). Like RI, the techniques of slow reversal (SR) or slow reversal hold (SRH) may need to be initiated by guided movement through range to teach the patient the pattern before resistance through range can be added. When sitting balance is extremely poor, trunk control should first be gained in the lower level postures of sidelying and supine, as already indicated. Once control in these less stressful postures is

(a)

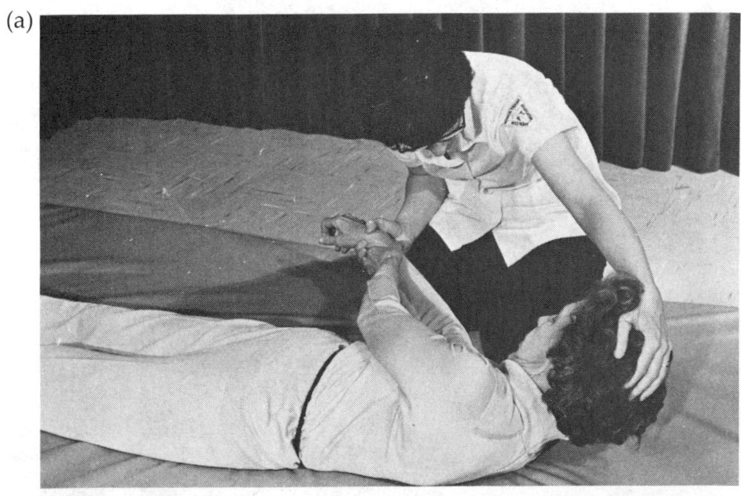

(b)

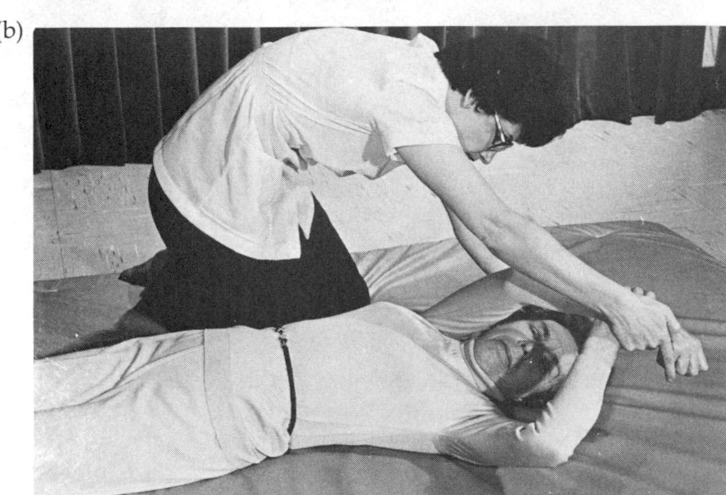

A. Supine: reverse chop.
T. RI.
E. MC head and wrist.

FIGURE 8–14

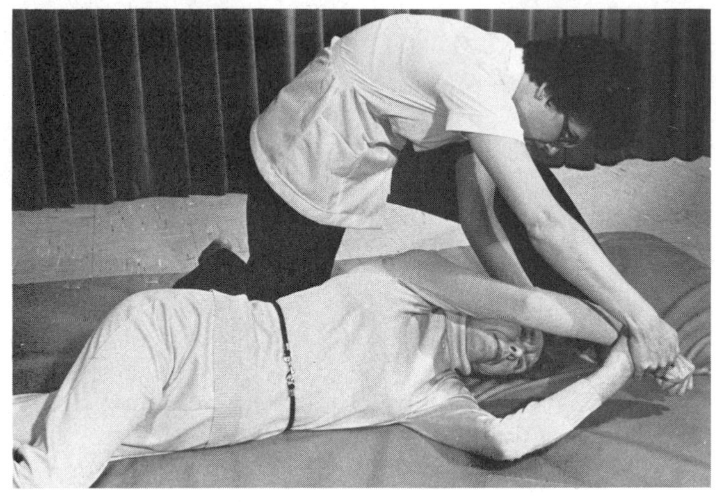

A. Rolling: reverse chop and D_1 of LE.
T. RI.
E. MC head and wrist.

FIGURE 8–15

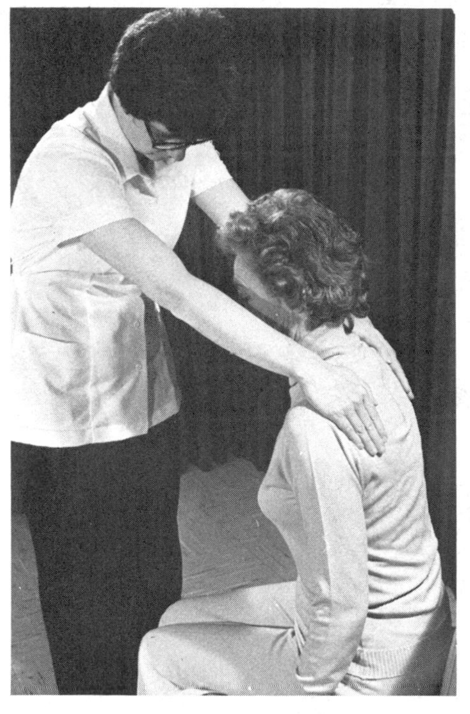

A. Sitting.
T. AI.
E. MC scapulae (extension indicated).

FIGURE 8–16

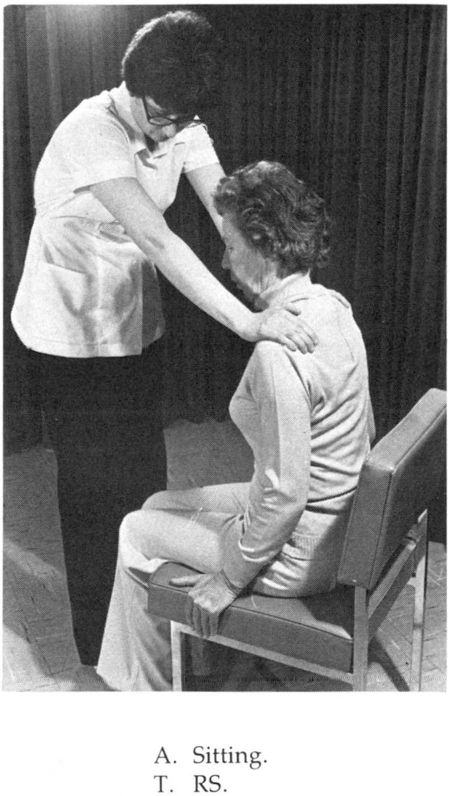

A. Sitting.
T. RS.
E. MC scapulae.

FIGURE 8–17

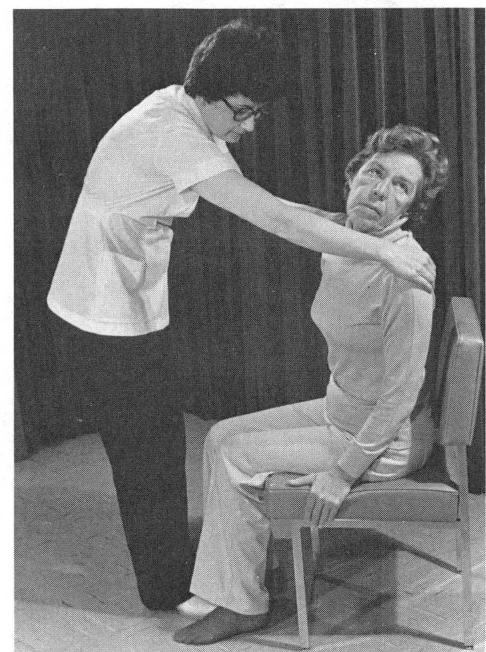

A. Sitting: upper trunk extension with rotation.
T. SRH.
E. MC scapulae.

FIGURE 8–18

evident, trunk balance can be emphasized in the sitting posture in which the patient is having difficulty.

In summary, the procedures in the initial stage of treatment for the hemiplegic patient should emphasize facilitation of vital functions and the development of the mobility and stability levels of trunk control in the sidelying, supine, and sitting postures. Mobility of the extremities is promoted during the performance of trunk patterns that also may be used to gain proximal control.

■ Middle Stage of Treatment

Patient Characteristics. The middle stage of treatment is appropriate for patients in the third and fourth stages of recovery, as described by Brunnstrom (2). During the beginning of this middle stage, only the strongest components of each of the synergistic patterns may be activated by the patient; toward the end of the stage, complete synergistic movement patterns may be evident and some movement out of synergy may occasionally be performed. Spasticity may range from moderate to marked and may interfere with the initiation of movements antagonistic to the spastic patterns. Controlled movement of the spastic musculature is extremely difficult. An increase of flexor tone often prevails in the upper extremity while extensor tone is common in the lower trunk and leg. Compared to the initial stage of recovery, the dominance of tonic reflexes is reduced and the righting and balance reactions are more prominent.

In the initial stage of treatment, trunk and proximal control were promoted as well as movement out of synergy. These goals may be further stressed in the middle stage. Treatment goals appropriate to this middle stage of recovery include:

1. Promote a balance of antagonists.
   - Inhibition of spastic musculature.
   - Facilitation of antagonistic movements.
2. Promote advanced patterns.
3. Enhance control of proximal musculature during the performance of higher level activities.
4. Promote initial stages of control in the intermediate joints (elbow, knee).

General Considerations. Because extensor tone is commonly dominant in the lower extremity, the flexor motions that were promoted during the initial stage of treatment with activity of the lower trunk flexion should be further facilitated in this stage. Advanced functional movement patterns can only be performed when a balance of tone has been established. Care must be taken, however, when an attempt is made to decrease extensor tone and increase flexion. Because of the location of the lesion, the patient may not regain volitional control. In such instances extensor spasticity can be used functionally during transfer and gait activities. Although a balance of tone is always a desired goal, if a choice has to be made, extensor spasticity in the lower extremity is more useful to the patient than a predominance of flexor tone.

In gait, the common problems that can be alleviated most easily are those reflecting a lack of trunk, pelvis, and hip control. Emphasis on proximal control in the low-level postures of sidelying, supine, lower trunk rotation, and bridging during both the initial and middle progressions may prevent the development of these problems.

Procedures. *Activities* are chosen in relation to the stage of motor control that is being promoted. In sidelying and supine, for example, the mobility stage can be easily enhanced. Trunk or unilateral patterns in these postures may facilitate the desired movement patterns. The hooklying posture is used to improve trunk, hip, and knee control, which is further challenged in bridging where the lower extremities are weight bearing. Stability functions in the upper extremity are gained first in sitting with the arm supporting and next in the modified plantigrade posture. In modified plantigrade, weight bearing also occurs through the lower extremities. The position of the trunk and lower extremity is similar to the position during the most advanced functional activity of the middle stage of treatment, that is, standing.

The choice of *techniques* for these various postures depends on the goal of the procedure. To promote mobility, the techniques of RI and a modified hold relax active movement (HRAM) may be used. Because hypertonia may be evident in this middle stage, quick movement is avoided to prevent an increase in spasticity. The technique of HRAM is thus adapted to the needs of the patient, and the fairly rapid movement appropriate for other patients is performed at a much slower pace for patients with hypertonia. The goal of this technique is to have the patient contract the muscles antagonistic to the spastic movement, first isometrically in the shortened range, then isotonically from a more lengthened to shortened range. This modified HRAM helps to improve control in the nonspastic muscles before reversal activity is attempted. During stability procedures, the techniques of AI and RS are most appropriate. Because an imbalance of tone may still be problematic, a gradual gradation in the amount of resistive force is indicated. Spasticity may increase if too much resistance is given. Controlled mobility is best achieved by SRH through increments of range. This technique is used to increase weight-bearing resistance and to develop balance control.

Elements may be used to balance homeostasis in the autonomic nervous system and also to enhance the various stages of motor control. Extremes of thermal stimuli may be used to decrease spasticity. A rebound effect, however, may actually increase spasticity (24, 41). If this occurs, a more neutral temperature may be appropriate. Brushing and vibration may be effective in improving motor ability.

These units of the procedure are sequenced to improve proximal control, then to promote control of the intermediate joints, the knee, and the elbow. As mentioned earlier, the mobility, stability, and controlled mobility levels of control are enhanced in the trunk, and upper and lower extremity. Although the skill level is gained as ambulation is initiated at this stage, the patient should not be expected to walk with normal control.

Selected Procedures—Trunk and Lower Extremity Control. In sidelying, forward pelvic rotation can be coupled with hip flexion to promote the proximal control needed to initiate the swing phase of gait and to increase flexor tone in the lower extremity (20). Isometric contractions of pelvic protraction and hip flexion in the shortened range are followed by controlled isometric contractions of these movements in more lengthened ranges. Unidirectional isotonic control is initiated with movement from the more shortened range; then movement progresses from more lengthened ranges into the shortened range, ending with movement from the fully lengthened to the shortened range of pelvic protraction and hip flexion. This forward movement is performed in a mass pattern that will help to initiate and strengthen the flexor motion (Figure 8–19). When tone in the flexor pattern has been increased and a balance of tone has developed, emphasis can be placed on reversal movements. As already noted, the patient frequently has developed or can be expected to develop a pattern of mass extension. Therefore, when resis-

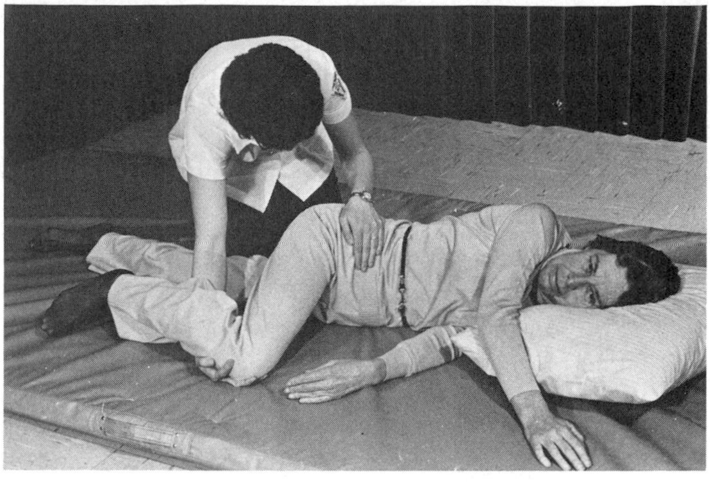

A. Sidelying: pelvic protraction and mass flexion of LE.
T. Holding in shortened range: initiation from lengthened range, modified HRAM.
E. MC pelvis and thigh.

FIGURE 8–19

tance is applied to the reversal motion, hip extension is coupled with knee flexion in an advanced combination of movement (11, 20) (Figure 8–20).

Flexion can also be initiated in *supine*. Because body-on-body contact is lacking, the performance of unilateral D_1 patterns in this middle stage of treatment may be more difficult than the trunk or bilateral combinations that were performed in the initial stage. Both hip and knee flexion and ankle dorsiflexion are most easily facilitated during this mass flexor motion (2). Because a reversal of antagonistic movement patterns may be difficult for the patient to control, a lower trunk pattern is chosen before a unilateral motion is attempted so that the uninvolved extremity can assist the involved limb with the difficult reversal activity.

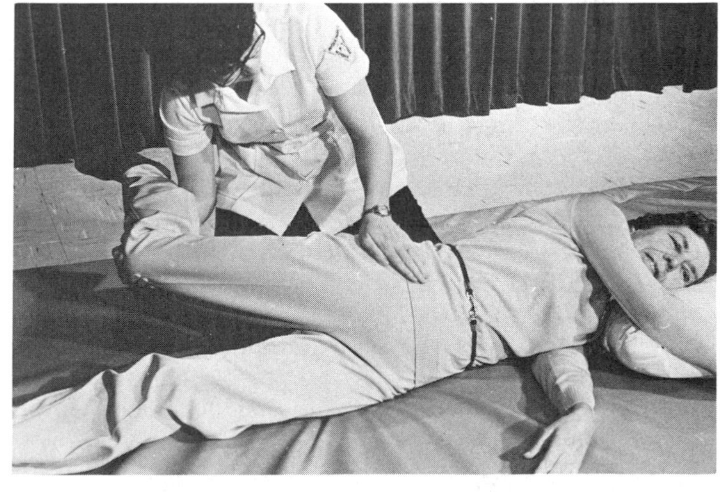

A. Sidelying: hip extension with knee flexion.
T. Modified HRAM.
E. MC pelvis and thigh.

FIGURE 8–20

The balance between flexor and extensor tone can be enhanced in the hooklying position. When the hips and knees are initially positioned near full flexion, the quadriceps are placed on a prolonged stretch to reduce the tendency toward a mass extensor motion. The techniques of AI and RS can be performed with manual contacts positioned on the knees (Figure 8–21). When the patient can cope with resistance in this flexed range, the hips and knees are positioned in more extension and the techniques are repeated. As full knee extension is approached, greater control is required to prevent a phasic contraction of the quadriceps from occurring. To further promote normal control and also to enhance cocontraction, resistance can be applied more directly to the knee musculature by placing the manual contacts on the ankles and by repeating the techniques of AI and RS (Figure 8–22). In summary, in hooklying: (1) the activity can be altered by beginning with the hips and knees flexed and by progressing toward hip and knee extension; (2) the techniques can progress from AI to RS; and (3) the elements (placement of manual contacts) can progress from the knees to the ankles. The overall goal of these procedures is for the patient to cocontract the musculature around the hip and knee when knees approach full extension. The patient may respond to these activities with an extensor thrust or increased extensor tone. If so, modification of the foot position so that only the heel is in contact with the mat may reduce the tendency for this uncontrolled extensor movement (42).

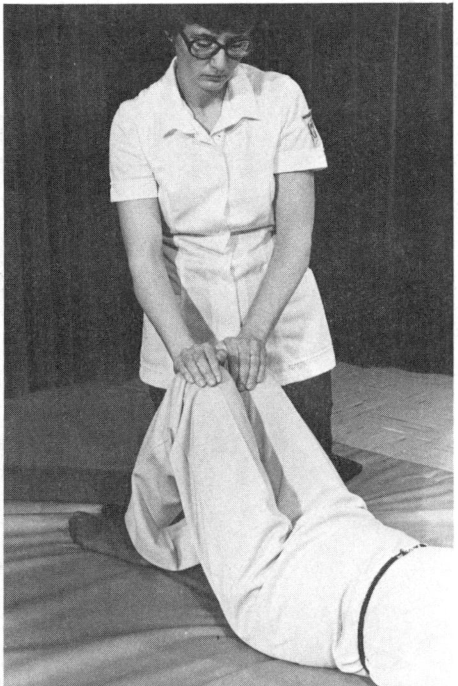

A. Hooklying.
T. AI, RS.
E. MC knees.

FIGURE 8–21

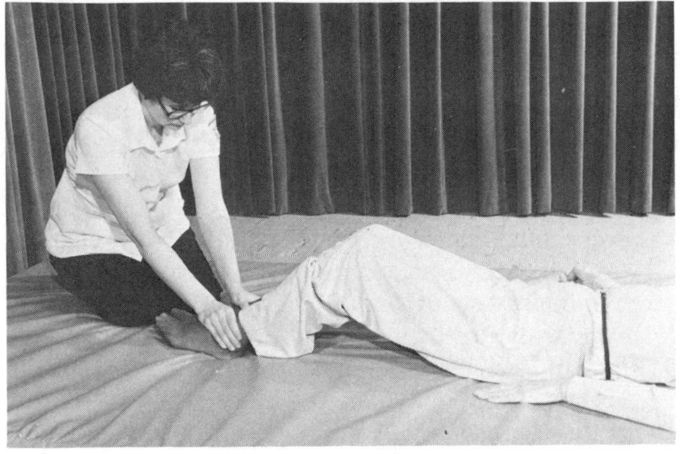

A. Hooklying: knees near full extension.
T. AI, RS.
E. MC ankles.

FIGURE 8–22

Lower trunk rotation in hooklying was used in the initial stage with RI to initiate movement. This activity is now coupled with the techniques of SR or SRH to improve control through range and to further enhance a reversal of antagonists. Two aspects of this activity should be emphasized: forward rotation of the pelvis on the involved side in preparation for the control needed during the swing phase of gait; and holding in the shortened range of the extensor phase where the hip extensors and abductors simultaneously contract in a pattern needed for the stance phase of gait (43) (Figure 8–23).

The bridging activity can be attempted once some control in the hip and knee has been gained with the previous procedures. The patient may need assistance in assuming the posture, but once bridging is attained, the patient should be able to maintain bridging independently. The knees should

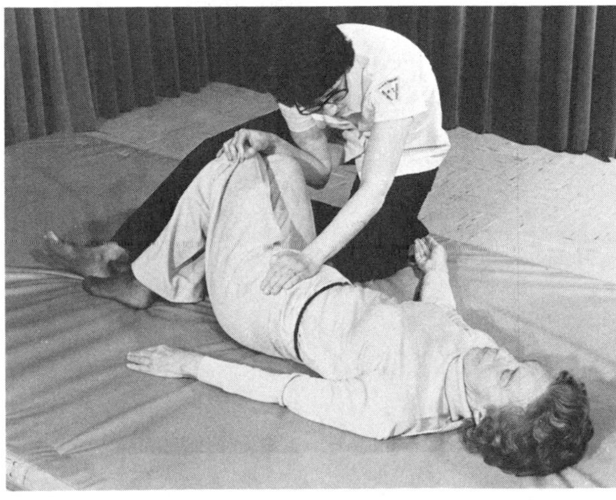

A. LTR.
T. SRH with emphasis on pelvis forward rotation.
E. MC pelvis and knees.

FIGURE 8–23

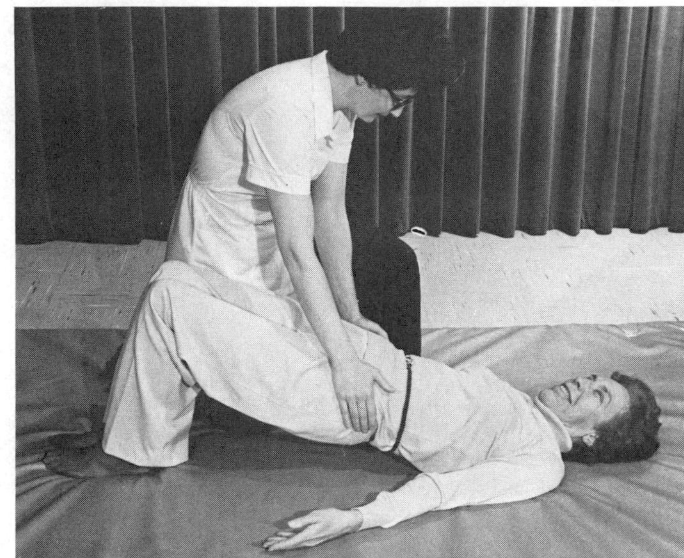

A. Bridging.
T. AI, RS.
E. MC pelvis.

FIGURE 8–24

again be positioned initially in full flexion to reduce the tendency for mass extension (Figure 8–24). In this posture, the low back and hip extensors contract in their shortened range; this contraction should help to promote the lower trunk control needed in upright postures. The activities and techniques performed in bridging can specifically emphasize many of the determinants of gait, such as lateral shifting and rotation of the pelvis (43) (Figure 8–25). To proceed through the stages of motor control, the stability techniques of AI and RS can progress to the controlled mobility techniques of SRH or SR. If weakness is found in certain parts of the movement, repeated

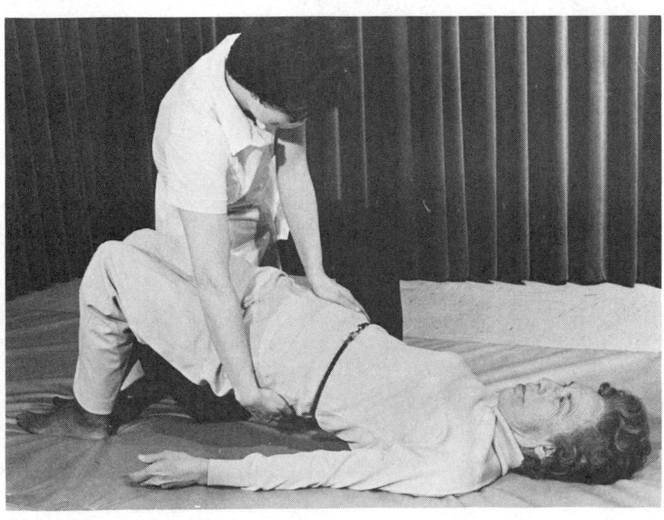

A. Bridging: pelvic rotation.
T. SRH.
E. MC pelvis.

FIGURE 8–25

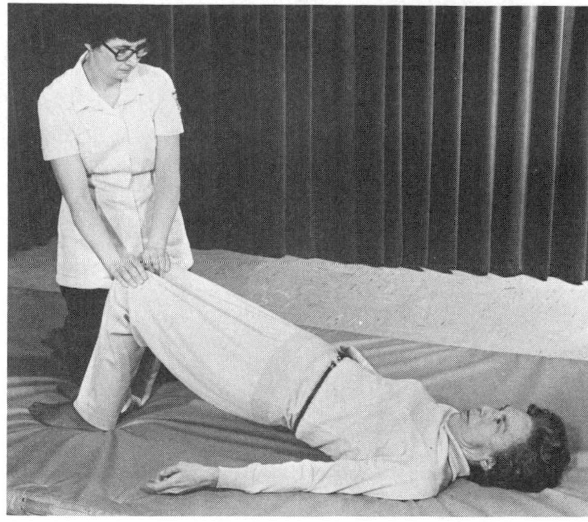

A. Bridging.
T. AI, RS.
E. MC knees.

FIGURE 8–26

contractions (RC) or timing for emphasis (TE) may be appropriate. The manual contacts are first positioned on the pelvis when facilitating proximal control; then they are moved to the knees and ankles to increase the control required both proximally and distally (Figures 8–26 and 8–27). Static-dynamic activities can simulate the unilateral weight bearing of the stance phase of gait. The amount of patient effort is carefully monitored during all of these bridging procedures. The therapist should be aware of the presence of any associated reactions in the upper extremity or of an increase in spasticity in the lower extremity. These abnormal responses may indicate to the therapist that the procedure is too stressful and that the difficulty of the activity or the amount of resistance should be decreased (20).

To summarize, the procedures in bridging can be used to increase control of the lower trunk and lower extremities and to enhance the control needed for ambulation. Procedures can be made more difficult by: 1) altering the activity with increased knee extension and decreasing the B of S with unilateral weight bearing; 2) varying the techniques so that isometric

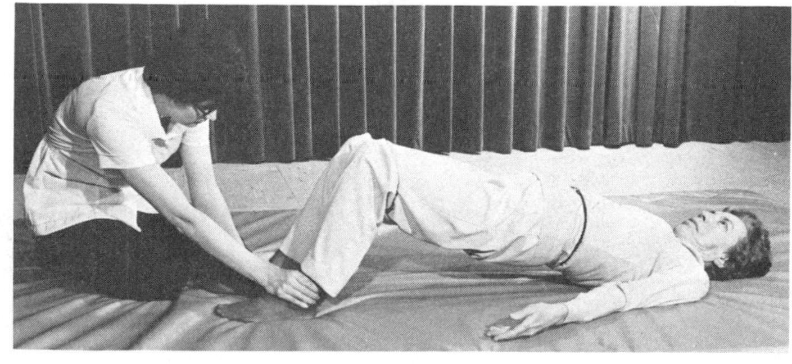

A. Bridging.
T. AI, RS.
E. MC ankles.

FIGURE 8–27

then isotonic control is enhanced; and 3) altering the placement of manual contacts from proximal to distal segments.

Selected Procedures—Upper Extremity Control. Upper extremity control begins with mobility and progresses to stability in weight-bearing postures. During the initial phase of treatment, mobility of the upper trunk and proximal areas was promoted by trunk patterns in supine and in combination with rolling. In this middle stage, mobility of the upper extremity is promoted first in the sidelying posture by means of unilateral patterns, then in the supine position. The following guidelines indicate appropriate sequences by which the difficulty of the activity can be increased: 1) activity in the proximal scapula and shoulder should be promoted before control in the more distal elbow and hand; 2) isometric contractions of muscles antagonistic to spastic muscles should be initiated in the shortened range before movement from the lengthened range; 3) unidirectional control of antagonistic muscles should be enhanced before reversing movements; 4) both gravity and tonal influences should assist the motion, or be eliminated before positions in which these factors resist the movement are attempted; 5) specific movements should be initiated before combining movement into a functional pattern; and 6) manual resistance should be gradually increased (20). In sidelying, for example, movement begins with protraction of the scapula followed by protraction of the scapula combined with shoulder flexion, adduction, and elbow extension (Figure 8–28). This combination of movements is antagonistic to the synergistic pattern and is sequenced in a proximal to distal progression. Movement is first facilitated in the shortened range before unidirectional movement through range is attempted. If reversing movements can be accomplished without triggering spasticity, then a balance of tone has been achieved. This same sequence can be applied in

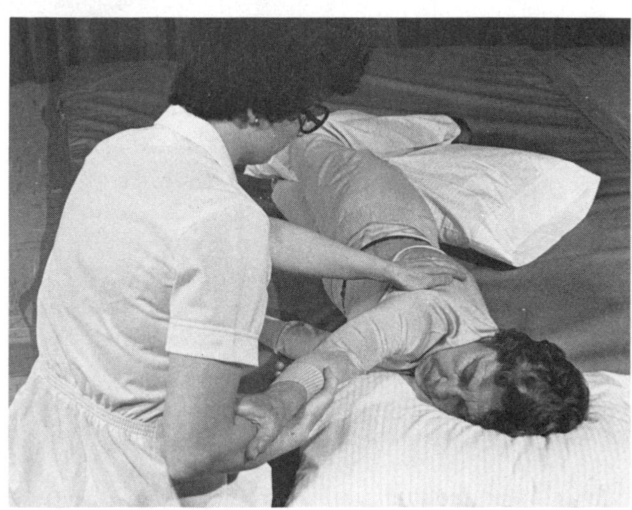

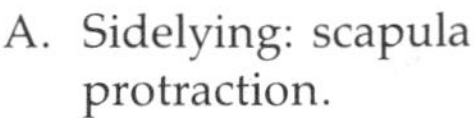

A. Sidelying: scapula protraction.
T. Modified HRAM.
E. MC scapula and arm.

FIGURE 8–28

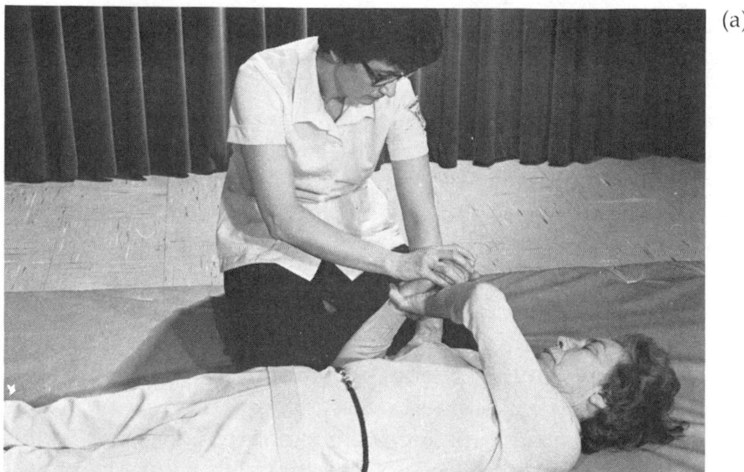

(a)

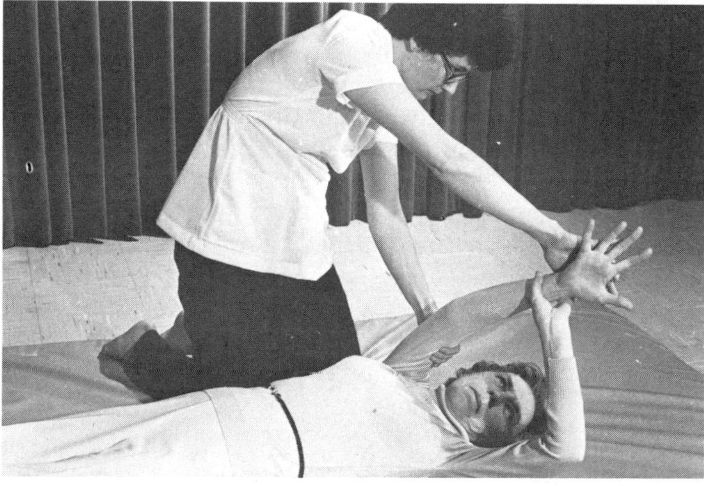

(b)

A. Supine: D_1 thrust assisted.
T. RI.
E. MC wrist and arm.

FIGURE 8–29

supine, where gravity will resist most of the upper extremity movements. An assisted D_1 thrust in the supine position will incorporate all of the desired proximal movements as well as facilitate hand opening (2, 40) (Figure 8–29). These guidelines can be applied to the selection of procedures for the lower extremity.

Stability control in the upper extremity follows the mobility stage and is first promoted in sidelying, then in sitting with upper extremity weight bearing. In sitting, the arm is positioned posteriorly with the shoulder slightly abducted and externally rotated, the elbow extended, forearm supinated, and the hand opened in order to disassociate the strongest synergistic patterns. Approximation through the arm should facilitate holding in this position (11, 20). Weight-bearing resistance is increased by rocking over the involved limb. Positioning the arm from the side to the front of the patient increases the stretch on the proximal muscles. Lateral rocking over the extended elbow with the shoulder in the three positions—posterior, lateral, and anterior—increases the weight-bearing resistance with the triceps maintained in the shortened range. Gradually flexing of the elbow puts the triceps on a prolonged stretch. If the tone of the triceps is sufficient, the inhibitory influences caused by the increase in weight-bearing resistance will not predominate. A balance of muscular tone around the elbow should result. If, however, increasing range into elbow flexion reduces the ability of the triceps to hold, tonic holding in the shortened range of elbow extension is again facilitated to further develop the gamma bias of the triceps.

The modified plantigrade position can be used to increase control in the upper extremity (Figure 8–30). More weight bearing occurs through the upper extremity than in sitting and the proximal muscles are further challenged by the increase in shoulder flexion range. As in sitting, the hand is opened and in prolonged contact with the supporting surface, which may lead to inhibition of spasticity in the finger flexors (23). Stability techniques in the posture are followed by weight shifting—controlled mobility—which will promote more range in the proximal joints and increase the amount of weight bearing.

The quadruped position is the most difficult weight-bearing posture in which upper extremity control can be gained because of the amount of weight borne through the limb and the range in which the proximal muscles

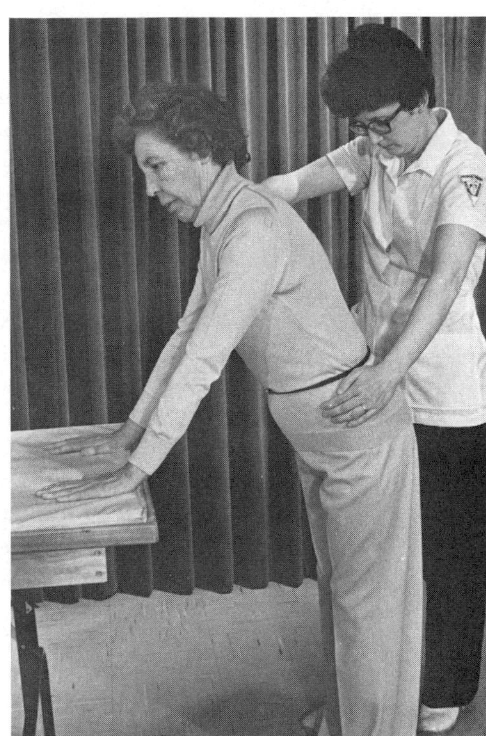

A. Modified plantigrade.
T. RS.
E. MC scapula and pelvis.

FIGURE 8–30

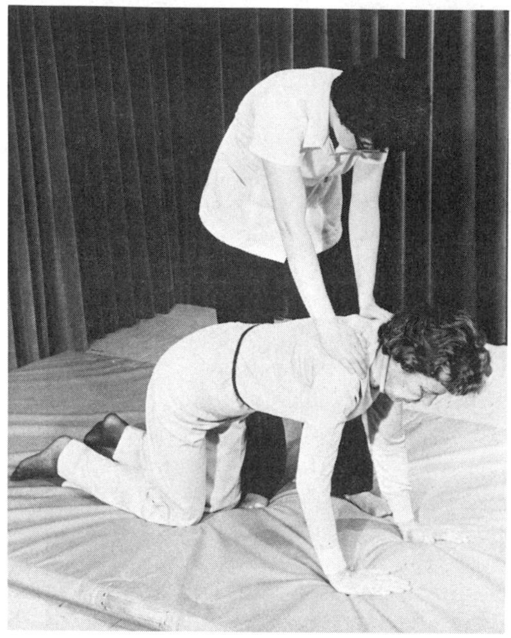

A. Quadruped.
T. RS.
E. MC scapulae.

FIGURE 8–31

are functioning (Figure 8–31). In quadruped, as in modified plantigrade and sitting, triceps control can be enhanced by weight shifting onto the extended elbow then by gradually allowing the elbow to flex. Static-dynamic activities will enhance even further the weight bearing on the involved limb. Many patients, however, may have difficulty with the amount of wrist and finger extension required to maintain this posture. For this and other reasons, such as inadequate balance reactions, the response to quadruped may be an increase in spasticity. Patients for whom the position is too stressful may find that other previously mentioned postures may be more appropriate.

Lower extremity control also can be promoted in these modified plantigrade and quadruped postures. In quadruped, the lower extremity position is mass flexion. The hip extensors and quadriceps are on a prolonged stretch and there is weight bearing on the quadriceps tendon. If extensor spasticity totally dominates movement, the inhibition of quadriceps activity occurring in quadruped may be necessary to balance tone. If, however, a balance in tone has already been achieved by prior procedures or if flexor tone predominates, the quadruped position may not be appropriate.

Modified plantigrade promotes control in the lower extremity with less weight-bearing resistance than occurs in standing (43). The position of the lower extremity is advanced with the hip minimally flexed, the knee extended, and the ankle dorsiflexed. The range at the knee should be carefully monitored so that extension, not hyperextension, occurs. Hyperextension during gait may be caused by a variety of reasons, including: 1) spasticity in the triceps surae leading to limited dorsiflexion at the ankle, 2) spasticity or weakness of the quadriceps; and 3) decreased tone in the hamstrings (2). Rocking over the involved lower extremity simulates the knee and ankle control needed during the stance phase of gait (Figure 8–32).

The lower extremity position in modified plantigrade can be varied. The feet may be symmetrical or in stride and the involved leg in the anterior or posterior position. In the symmetrical position, proximal stability is followed by controlled mobility movements in anterior-posterior, lateral, and rotational directions. Anterior weight shifting causes the tibia to ride over the talus and thus increases the range of dorsiflexion and the amount of stretch on the gastroc-soleus. If posterior tightness exists or if the stretch results in an increase in spasticity, the knee will tend to hyperextend. Rocking in the anterior direction in such instances should be performed through increments of range while maintaining the proper knee alignment to enhance the control needed for the mid to late stance phase of gait (43). Lateral shifting over the involved limb will increase the resistance of body weight on that limb, which can be increased further by static-dynamic activities performed in this posture. During rotation of the lower trunk, emphasis is on forward rotation of the involved side in preparing the patient for the rotation needed during the swing phase of gait. Motion during these procedures should be restricted to the lower trunk. The stabilization of the upper trunk by weight bearing will help to prevent total trunk movement during these preparatory gait activities.

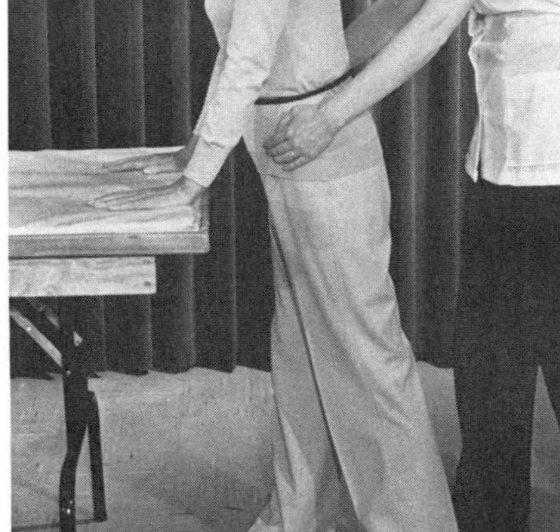

A. Modified plantigrade: LE in stride, weight shifting.
T. SRH.
E. MC pelvis.

FIGURE 8–32

The involved lower extremity can be positioned forward in stride. Weight shifting over that limb simulates the ability to accept weight during the stance phase of gait. The three pelvic motions that were performed as separate activities with the feet symmetrical can now be combined into one smooth diagonal rocking motion which incorporates forward and lateral movement over the stance limb with forward rotation of the contralateral pelvis. The position of the extremities can be changed with the involved leg in the posterior position to simulate the beginning of the swing phase of gait. Emphasis in this case would be on forward pelvic rotation, initiation of hip flexion, and controlled heel rise.

Standing erect has a small B of S and a high C of G and requires the greatest control over balance reactions. As often occurs throughout the sequence of procedures, the patient may be capable of maintaining the position and weight shifting within small ranges. Very often, however, the patient may need assistance with the assumption of the posture (Figure 8–33). The sequence of procedures in standing is similar to the order described in the modified plantigrade posture. Stability techniques can be performed

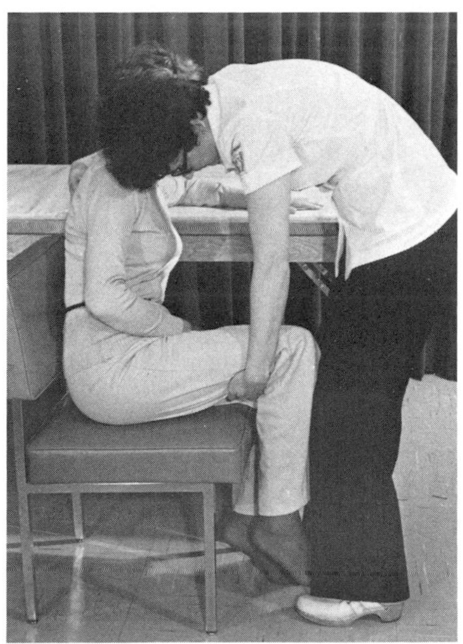

(a)

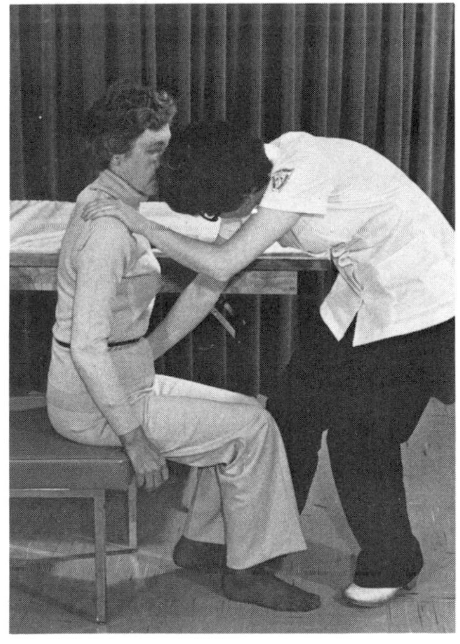

(b)

A. Sitting to standing.
T. Assist to position.
E. MC as needed.

FIGURE 8–33

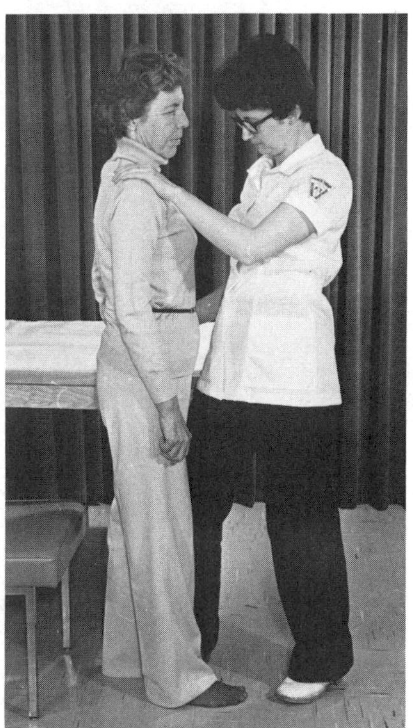

A. Standing.
T. RS.
E. MC scapula and pelvis.

FIGURE 8–34

with manual contacts on the pelvis, scapula, or on both scapula and pelvis to alter areas of emphasis (Figure 8–34). To specifically enhance cocontraction around the knee and to reduce the tendency toward hyperextension, AI and RS with manual contacts placed both proximally and distally to the knee may be performed. Controlled mobility with the lower extremities in a symmetrical position includes anterior-posterior, lateral, and rotational movements of the lower trunk. Manual contacts on the pelvis can be used to emphasize movement in this area. Isolated rotation of the lower trunk is preliminary to the counter-rotation needed during a normal gait pattern. Rotational movements of the trunk in this posture may be particularly difficult to perform and may need to be further improved in less stressful postures and activities such as sidelying, LTR, bridging, and modified plantigrade. Weight acceptance can be promoted by standing in stride (Figure 8–35). As in modified plantigrade, the three pelvic motions that were previously performed separately are now combined to assist the patient in weight shifting forward and laterally over the involved limb and in rotating the contralateral side of the pelvis forward to begin the swing phase on that side. When the involved lower extremity is positioned posteriorly, the end of stance and the initiation of swing can be emphasized, particularly pelvic rotation and hip flexion.

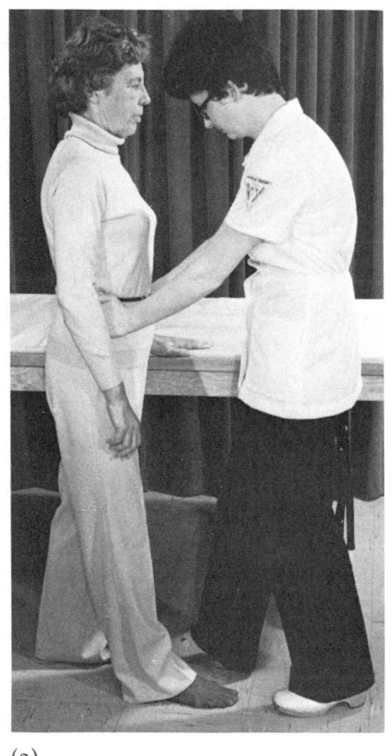

(a)

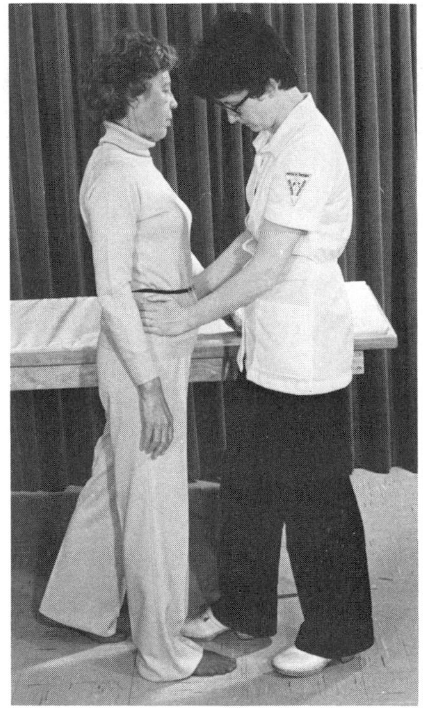

(b)

A. Standing in stride.
T. SRH.
E. MC pelvis.

FIGURE 8–35

The patient should not practice movements that are not part of normal gait, such as exaggerated knee flexion on the stance limb. Although slight knee flexion at heel strike is normal, the exaggerated motion should be avoided. If too much knee flexion at heel strike is encouraged, a more forceful hyperextension movement may occur during the later stance phase. This exaggerated recurvatum may be caused by the quadriceps responding to the increased stretch or the limited dorsiflexion that occurs when the tibia cannot roll over the talus. If a balance of tone around all the lower extremity joints was achieved during the activities of LTR, bridging, and modified plantigrade, more normal movements during ambulation should occur.

Slow deliberate walking can be used to emphasize each phase of gait (Figure 8–36). The manual contacts usually are positioned on the pelvis to guide the proximal movement. By constant evaluation during all phases of gait training, the therapist will be able to determine areas of deficit and

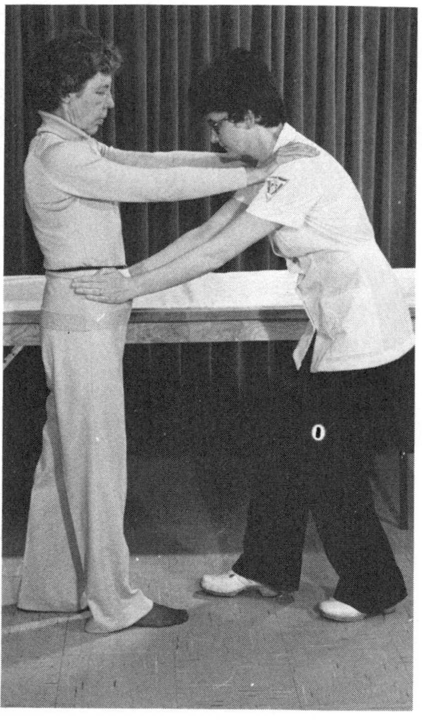

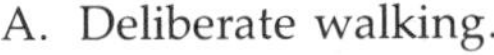

A. Deliberate walking.
T. Resisted progression (RP).
E. MC pelvis.

FIGURE 8–36

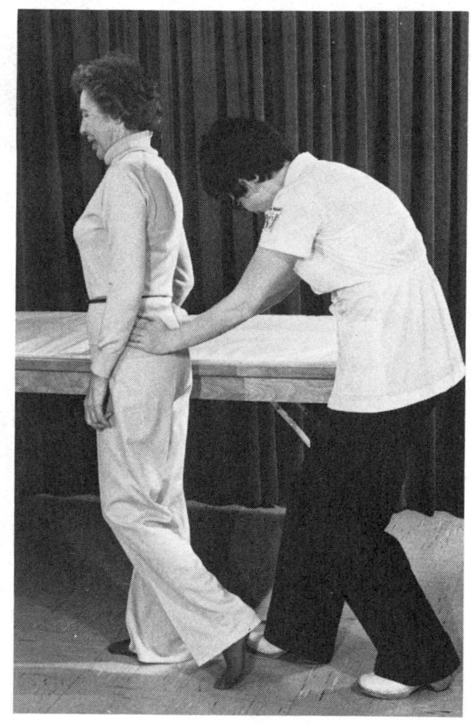

A. Walking backward.
T. RP.
E. MC pelvis.

FIGURE 8–37

therefore the activities and levels of motor control that may need to be stressed during the mat exercise segment of treatment.

Walking in all directions is the next sequence of procedures. Walking backward requires the advanced movement combination of hip extension and knee flexion (20) (Figure 8–37). Circumduction and mass extensor movements that reinforce synergistic patterns are discouraged. Sidewalking should be performed in both directions (2) (Figure 8–38). Walking away from the involved limb requires stabilization of the pelvis and trunk by the abductors on the involved side. Movement toward the involved side requires dynamic proximal control of the hemiplegic leg. Because isolated abduction is a difficult movement, the patient frequently may substitute hiphiking or lateral trunk flexion. Patients may also attempt to turn their trunk and flex and abduct with the tensor fascia lata, rather than abduct with the gluteus medius. Braiding is considered the most difficult activity in

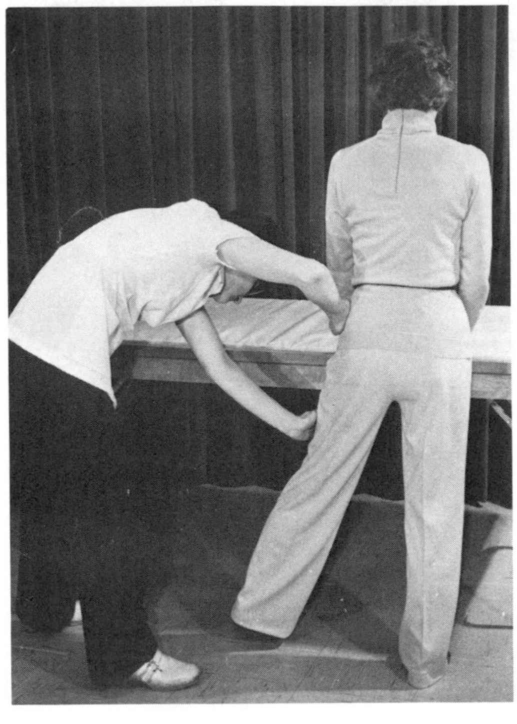

A. Sidewalking.
T. RP.
E. MC pelvis and thigh.

FIGURE 8–38

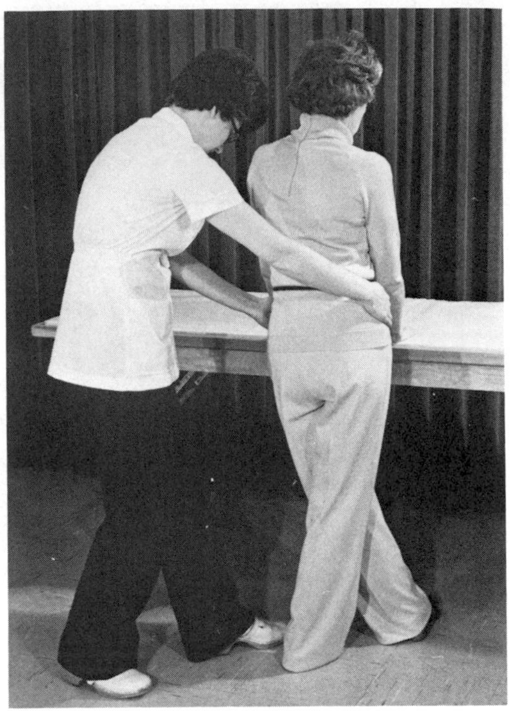

A. Braiding.
T. RP.
E. MC pelvis.

FIGURE 8–39

this sequence of walking procedures because it combines lower trunk rotation while the lower extremities are crossing the midline both anteriorly and posteriorly (43) (Figure 8–39). The four diagonal movement patterns incorporated into braiding can be promoted individually in standing before the entire progression is performed.

Standing activities require good motor control and balance reactions. For most patients, standing early in the treatment progression is necessary psychologically, even though an adequate foundation for this posture has not been established. Unsuccessful attempts at ambulation will demonstrate to the patient the need to develop control in less stressful, lower level postures. While short periods of standing and stepping may be important for psychological support, emphasis on ambulation, a skill activity, with maximal assistance and many external supports will only tend to frustrate the patient and the therapist, and will promote poor gait patterns.

In summary, the procedures of the middle stage have been chosen to promote stability and controlled mobility of the trunk, as well as mobility, stability, and controlled mobility of the upper and lower extremities. The activities in which these levels of control have been enhanced include side-lying, sitting, LTR, bridging, modified plantigrade, quadruped, and standing. Although a skill level activity is the long-range goal, the gait pattern performed by the patient at this time may not be of normal quality (see the next section).

■ Advanced Stage

Patient Characteristics. This stage is characterized by the ability of the patient to move out of synergistic patterns with good proximal control. Spasticity is decreasing and imbalances of tone are not as prevalent. Difficulty with distal movements, the normal timing of activity, eccentric control, and reciprocating movement may still be evident. Abnormalities in the gait pattern may persist as a result of any or all of these factors.

Because of the location and extent of the lesion, many patients may not be able to perform the procedures suggested for this stage of recovery. Volitional distal control, particularly fractionalization of movement, is primarily a cortical function and may be permanently lost owing to damage in the motor or sensory strip or the internal capsule (44).

Goals. The goals during the advanced stage are to promote the skill level of motor control, to improve the gait pattern, and to improve the ability to perform ADL. Skill may be accomplished by: 1) improving function of the distal segments, 2) improving eccentric control, 3) improving reciprocating movements, 4) increasing the speed of movement, and 5) facilitating the normal timing of movement.

General Considerations. By this stage, ambulation is usually a functional activity but the pattern of gait may not be normal. Because of decreased trunk counterrotation, the upper extremity may show a decrease in arm swing and the lower extremity step length may not be equal. Delayed timing of muscular contraction and relaxation can affect the speed and quality of the gait pattern. During the various stages of normal gait, eccentric control of most of the lower extremity muscles is required. Many hemiplegic patients find it difficult to achieve this eccentric ability. Finally, a proper sequencing and timing of advanced movement combinations, an integral part of skilled gait, may be lacking.

Skilled movement incorporates both proximal dynamic stability and distal mobility. Proximal control is needed to guide the limb in space and to provide the balance reactions to maintain the upright posture. Therefore in this advanced stage the focus is on both improved proximal and distal control.

Procedures. Many of the procedures already described during the initial and middle stages of treatment can be made more difficult to promote the goals of this advanced stage. The *activities* may be altered both to emphasize advanced combinations of movement and to improve distal function; the *techniques* are selected to enhance the control of the existing movements and to initiate movements that still may be difficult; the *elements* may be varied by altering the position of manual contacts, by increasing the gravitational or manual resistance, or by decreasing the amount of external stimuli that may have been necessary in earlier procedures.

Specific Procedures—Trunk. To improve the trunk counter-rotation needed during normal gait, adversive trunk movements or counter-rotation may be performed in sidelying. This activity can be initiated with the technique of RI and continued until a smooth reversal of antagonists is accomplished. The activity may begin with slow deliberate movements, and speed can be gradually increased to facilitate a quick reversal of antagonistic muscle groups. During the initial and middle stages of treatment segmental trunk motions were performed first by using the upper trunk pattern of a reverse chop followed by the LTR activity. At this advanced stage, these two patterns can be combined in the supine position to promote trunk counterrotation (Figure 8–40). The participation of the upper extremities in the performance of this activity may improve the coordination of arm swing during gait.

As already mentioned, LTR was initially incorporated into treatment to enhance various goals. Now that spasticity has decreased this activity can be used to specifically emphasize pelvic forward rotation. With one manual contact positioned on the pelvis and the other on the knees, the technique of timing for emphasis (TE) can be performed (Figure 8–41).

Specific Procedures—Lower Extremity. The bridging activity may be repeated in the advanced stage to further enhance the hip, knee, and ankle control needed during gait. The difficulty of bridging may be increased by positioning the knees near full extension and by providing resistance with manual contacts on the ankles. The technique of RS will improve cocontraction around the knee (Figure 8–42). The altered direction of the resistive forces will promote a reciprocal contraction between the lower extremity muscles; for example, the hamstrings on one limb will contract isometrically along with the contralateral quadriceps. The speed of the altering resistive forces is gradually increased to improve the relationship between the timing of the contraction and relaxation of the lower extremity muscles. This alternating control is first gained isometrically before isotonic reciprocal activities are attempted. Lateral weight shifting is followed by reciprocal unilateral weight bearing in bridging to improve the ability to accept weight on the stance limb in standing. The speed of this activity should eventually match the cadence of gait. Bridging is also an effective posture in which eccentric control of the hip and knee extensors can be promoted. The technique of agonistic reversals (AR) promotes a reversal of concentric and eccentric contractions of these muscle groups as the pelvis is raised and lowered to the

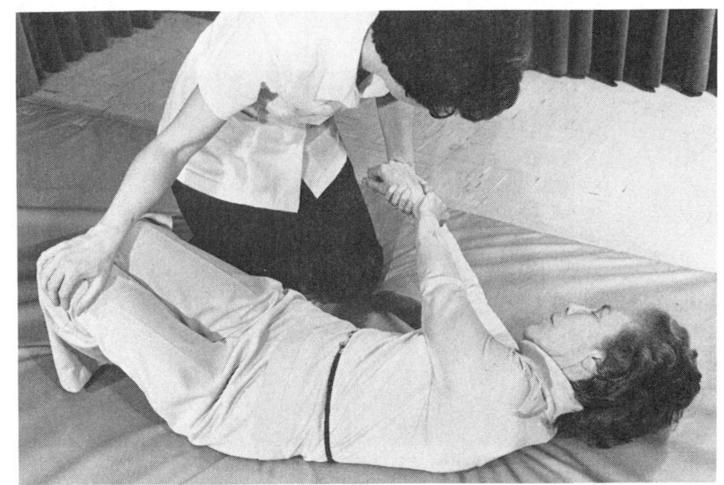

A. LTR with reverse chop and chop.
T. RI.
E. MC knee and wrist.

FIGURE 8–40

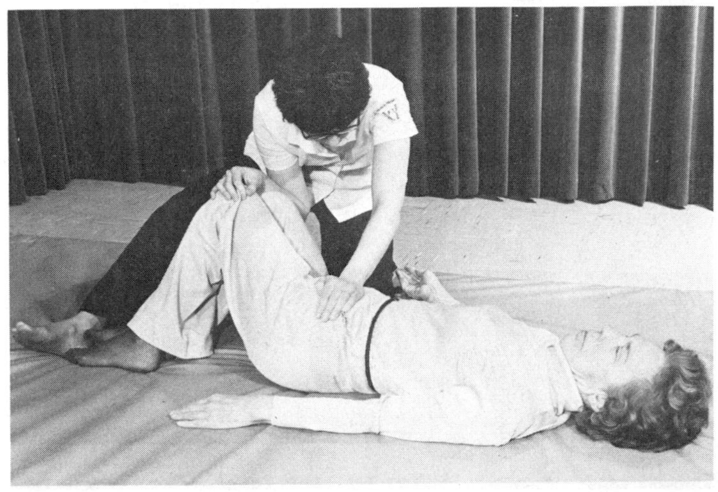

A. LTR.
T. TE on pelvic forward rotation.
E. MC pelvis and knees.

FIGURE 8–41

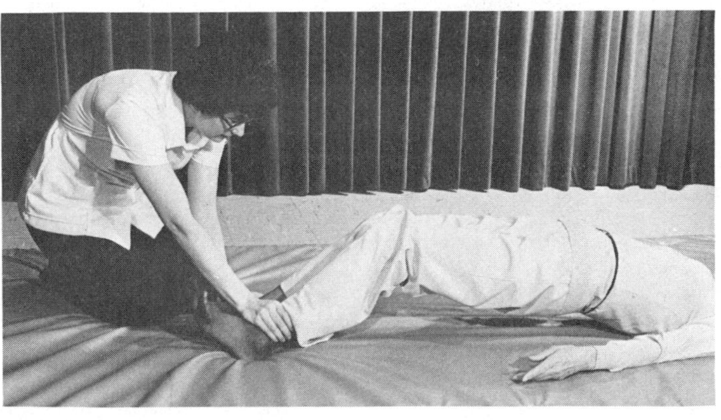

A. Bridging: knees near full extension.
T. AI, RS.
E. MC ankles.

FIGURE 8–42

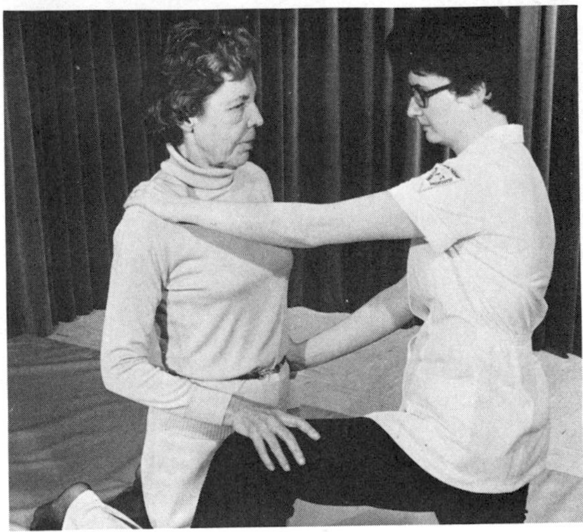

A. Kneeling.
T. RS.
E. MC shoulder and pelvis.

FIGURE 8–43

supporting surface. To add more weight-bearing resistance to this activity, the procedure may be performed with unilateral weight bearing.

A normal gait pattern requires eccentric control of the hamstrings from the mid to lengthened range during the swing phase of gait. Control of these lengthening contractions can be gained in the prone posture by combining the activity of bilateral knee flexion with the technique of AR. Be-

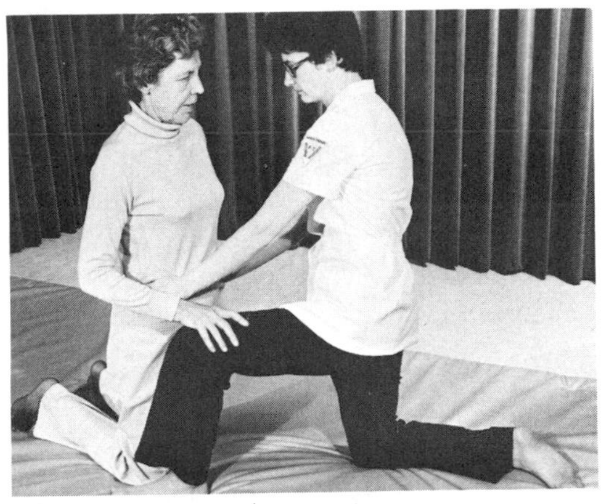

(a)

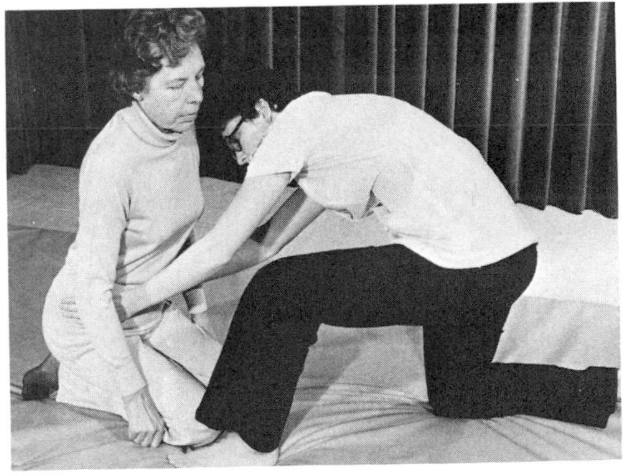

(b)

A. Kneeling (a); Heelsitting (b).
T. SRH, AR.
E. MC pelvis.

FIGURE 8–44

cause visual input is eliminated or reduced in prone, sensory input from the uninvolved limb may be necessary. For this reason, AR in this posture is most easily performed initially in a bilateral pattern. Eccentric control of the hamstring can also be enhanced in supine with unilateral patterns. Hamstring control can be improved concentrically in the advanced combination pattern of hip extension with knee flexion (11). This concentric shortening simultaneously over both joints will enhance the control needed during backward walking.

As mentioned, eccentric control in the shortened to midranges of the hip and knee extensors is an integral component of gait. Eccentric contractions in these ranges can be best promoted in the modified plantigrade and bridging postures and with unilateral lower extremity patterns. Sitting or descending stairs requires eccentric control of the quadriceps and hip extensors in more lengthened ranges. Control in this range can be enhanced with the technique of AR in the kneeling to heelsitting activity. Kneeling is incorporated late in the sequence of treatment procedures because of the amount of balance that is needed to maintain or move within the posture. Unlike other postures, kneeling has the B of S under and posterior to the C of G, so that balance control is needed primarily in the muscles on one side of the joint: the extensors of the trunk, hip, and knee flexors. The hamstrings are in a position of active insufficiency, which contributes to the difficulty of controlling balance in this posture. Although the development of eccentric control of the quadriceps is the major goal of kneeling for the hemiplegic patient, stability and other controlled mobility procedures to improve pelvic control may precede the eccentric activity (Figures 8–43 and 8–44). As in other postures, flexion-extension, and lateral and rotational pelvic movements can be enhanced individually before they are combined into the single movement pattern needed for gait. Because the upper trunk is not stabilized in kneeling, the patient may substitute total trunk motion for the desired isolated lower trunk and pelvic movement. Stabilizing the upper trunk by positioning the patient's arms on the therapist's shoulders or by placing one hand on the therapist's knee, may discourage this total body substitution. If isolated movement is difficult to achieve even though upper trunk stability is provided, then less stressful postures would be appropriate.

Half-kneeling is an intermediate position in the assumption of standing from lower level postures and is probably the most difficult mat activity for hemiplegic patients. The involved limb can be positioned either posteriorly or anteriorly to enhance different aspects of control of different muscle groups. When the involved limb is positioned posteriorly in an advanced combination of hip extension with knee flexion, for example, the amount of weight bearing through the hip is similar to that occurring during the stance phase of gait. Rocking through increments of range will greatly challenge this proximal control. When the involved limb is placed anteriorly, flexion of the hip, knee, and ankle occurs in extremely shortened ranges. Although the patient may be able to initiate these flexor movements in other postures, these motions may be difficult to perform in this stressful half-kneeling posture. Rocking with the involved limb in the anterior position is beneficial, however, in that it can increase the controlled dorsiflexion of the involved limb while the gastrocnemius is on slack. Because the position of the involved limb is one of mass flexion, this position should be avoided among patients who are still demonstrating an increase in flexor tone.

Improved distal control is a major goal in this advanced stage of treatment. As we have noted, both ankle stability and controlled mobility can be promoted in the bridging, modified plantigrade, standing, and half-kneeling activities. Once these are accomplished, the patient can progress to the skill level of motor control. In the lower extremity, skilled activities are those in which the distal segment is no longer weight bearing but is free to move. Balanced dorsiflexion combined with normal timing is necessary for a skilled gait pattern. Balanced dorsiflexion can be defined as a normal synergistic action of the inverters and everters that allows flexion of the ankle to occur without an imbalance between these two movements (45). In the case of the hemiplegic patient, inversion is incorporated into both the flexor and extensor pathological synergistic patterns. Eversion is a very difficult movement to facilitate and therefore must be emphasized during this advanced stage of treatment.

Because facilitation and strengthening of dorsiflexion with eversion is the goal, a mass flexor pattern of the lower extremity is initially the most appropriate. Once eversion is initiated, the flexion of the proximal components can be gradually reduced until the distal movements can be performed with the hip and knee in extension (2). The progression is to an advanced pattern, which is the movement required for gait. This applied sequence of patterns from easiest to most difficult can be used to initiate and strengthen distal movement both concentrically and eccentrically.

Eversion with dorsiflexion is specifically facilitated in the D_2F pattern (11). The pattern, as we have noted, would first be performed in a mass flexor combination progressing to the point at which eversion can be facilitated with the hip and knee in extension. Balanced dorsiflexion while the hip is flexing and the knee is extending is the most skilled activity for the ankle, both in supine and in upright postures. Strengthening techniques such as RC or TE may be effective in improving the ability to sustain the concentric contraction through full range of ankle motion. The technique of NT in combination with an advanced pattern would be appropriate to further enhance the ankle control and the sequencing of segments needed at both toe off and during the swing phase of gait. The eccentric control of the dorsiflexors that normally occurs at heelstrike to foot flat can be improved with the technique of AR. Balanced medial lateral ankle control between posterior tibialis and peroneal muscles is also required during the stance phase of gait and may be enhanced most effectively in weight-bearing postures, such as modified plantigrade, with techniques to promote stability and controlled mobility. Other important functions of the ankle, including eccentric control of the gastro-soleus, can be promoted with other techniques. This control was promoted first in the modified plantigrade posture and may need to be further enhanced at this advanced stage.

Selected Procedures—Upper Extremity. The most advanced level of control for the upper extremity is required for the performance of ADL skills. During these skilled movements, the distal hand is free while the proximal shoulder and scapula muscles provide the dynamic stability needed to guide the limb in space (24).

If during early stages procedures were successful in weight-bearing postures, the patient now should be able to:

1. Initiate movement
2. Stabilize in various points in the range
3. Move with control through range
4. Unilaterally bear weight on an extended hand

(a)

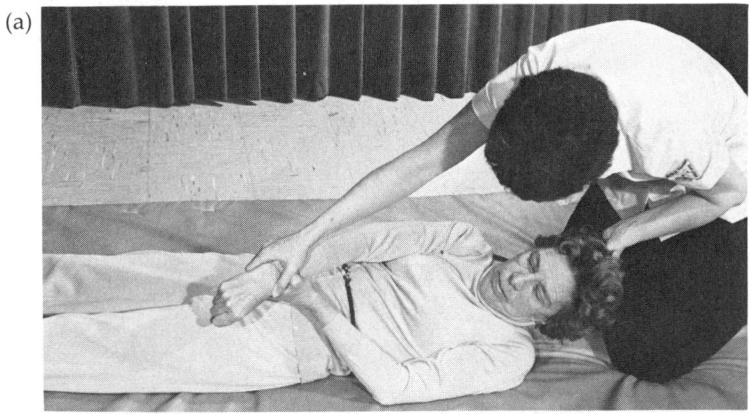

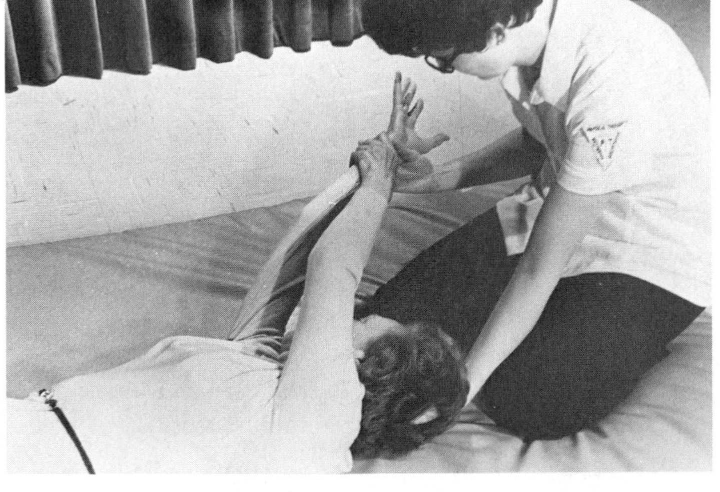

(b)

A. Supine: lifting.
T. SRH.
E. MC head and wrist.

FIGURE 8–45

Once the proximal control of the upper extremity has been achieved in weight bearing, control of the entire limb with nonweight-bearing activities is the goal.

Before the more difficult unilateral patterns are attempted, control at this stage can first be promoted by trunk patterns, followed by bilateral combinations. This sequence of combinations may be necessary now that the facilitating approximation force that occurred in weight bearing has been eliminated. The trunk and bilateral patterns may provide additional sensory input that will enhance the desired proximal control. The sensory input is reduced during the performance of unilateral patterns and the demand on the proximal shoulder muscles is increased. As mentioned in the discussion of the previous stages, initially movement should be enhanced in the D_1 pattern. Because the dominance of spasticity and synergistic patterns is reduced at this advanced stage, movement in the D_2 pattern should also be encouraged. The sequencing of patterns may therefore progress from the trunk combinations of a reverse chop or an assisted D_1 thrust to a lifting pattern, during which the involved limb performs D_1 and D_2 movements, respectively (Figures 8–45 and 8–46). Bilateral combinations that enhance the D_1 pattern before D_2 may also be selected (Figure 8–47).

The techniques applied to these patterns can be used to facilitate many aspects of control that may still be lacking. A smooth reversal of antagonists can be enhanced by the SRH or SR techniques. A faster reversal of antago-

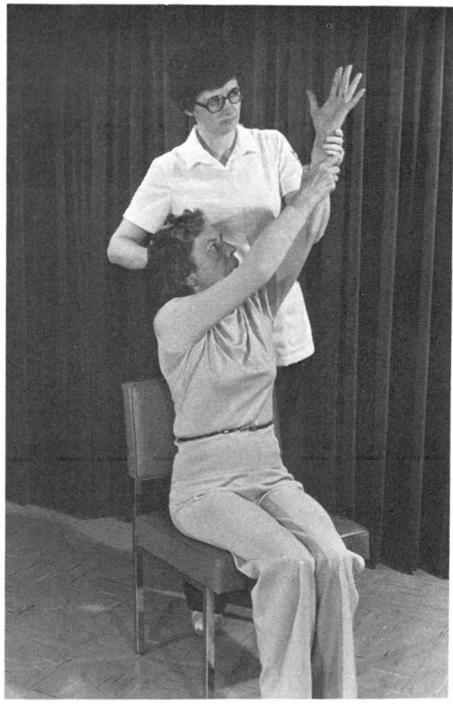

A. Sitting: lifting.
T. SRH.
E. MC head and wrist.

FIGURE 8–46

(a)

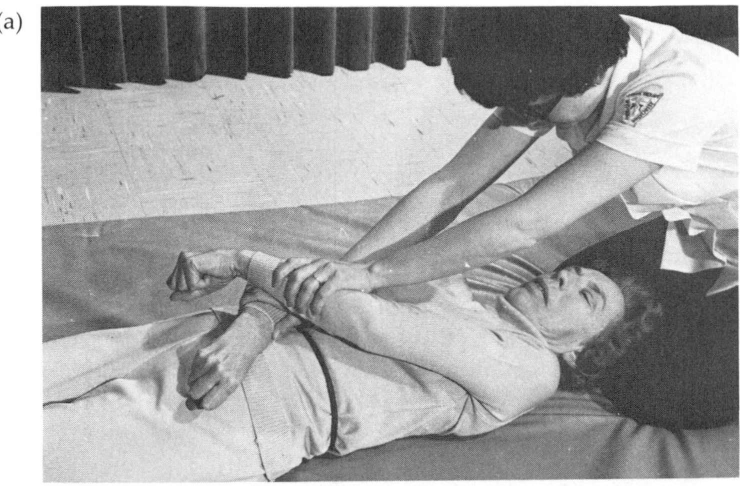

(b)

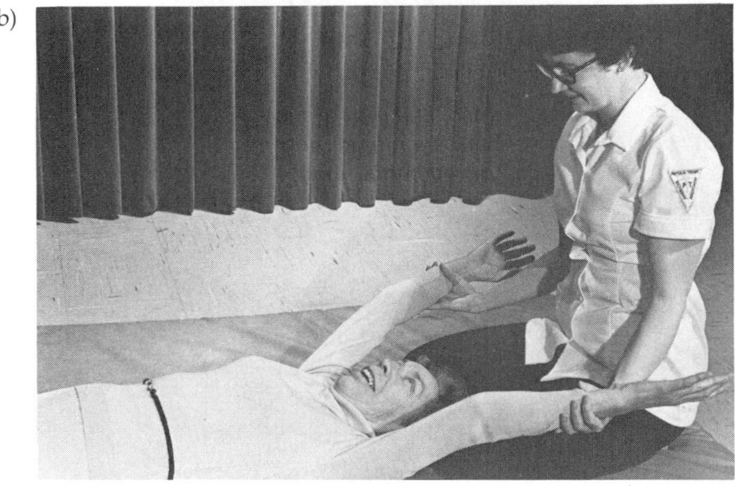

A. BS D_2F.
T. SRH.
E. MC wrists.

FIGURE 8–47

nists can be encouraged if the speed of the SR technique is increased. Strengthening may be best accomplished with the techniques of RC or TE.

All combinations of unilateral movements with the normal distal to proximal timing is the ultimate goal. The four patterns of D_1 and D_2 flexion and extension can be performed with the elbow remaining straight, flexing, or extending. By choosing from these twelve combinations, the therapist can combine all of the normal movement combinations. The D_1 thrusting pattern, which combines shoulder flexion and adduction with finger wrist and elbow extension, is appropriate for the hemiplegic patient and is easily facilitated. The finer aspects of proximal and distal control can best be promoted with unilateral patterns primarily because the therapist has both manual contacts on the involved limb.

The techniques applied to the unilateral patterns will depend on the specific aspects of skill that are to be improved. To reiterate, a smooth reversal can be gained by SR; initiation of movement by the distal segment is enhanced with the technique of NT; and eccentric control through range occurs with AR. First, fine coordinated distal movement may be gained in different patterns by means of these various techniques before being made functional by practicing activities of daily living.

In summary, the goals of all of the procedures in this advanced stage of treatment are: (1) controlled contraction and relaxation of hypertonic muscles; (2) initiation and control of movement in all ranges by muscles antagonistic to the spastic muscles; (3) movement of distal segments with a normal timing of activity; (4) control of balance reactions in all postures; and (5) alteration in the speed of movement.

The examples of procedures that have been presented in this chapter for the initial, middle, and advanced stages of treatment for the hemiplegic patient were developed within the following conceptual framework:

1. The reestablishment of motor control may be enhanced by ordering procedures to follow the original sequencing of control as it occurs in normal development.
2. Because central control mechanisms of movement are altered with hemispheric lesions, peripheral mechanisms may need to be enhanced until the balance between the two systems can be achieved.
3. Before movement can be automatic and therefore functional, the motor control that is the foundation of automatic movement needs to be improved.

REFERENCES

1. Pryse-Phillips W, Murray TJ: Essential Neurology. Garden City, NY, Medical Examination Publishing Co, 1978
2. Brunnstrom S: Movement Therapy in Hemiplegia. New York, Harper & Row, 1970
3. Teuber HL, Rudel RG: Behavior after cerebral lesions in children and adults. Devel Med Child Neurol 4:3–20, 1962
4. Goldman PS: Developmental determinants of cortical plasticity. Acta Neurobiol Exp 32:495–511, 1972
5. Buchwald JS: A functional concept of motor control. Am J Phys Med 46:121–128, 1966

6. Siev E, Freishtat B: Perceptual Dysfunction in the Adult Stroke Patient. Thorofare, NJ, Charles B Slack, 1976
7. Teuber HL: Space perception and its disturbances after brain injury in man. Neuropsychologia 1:47–57, 1963
8. Evarts EV: Feedback and corollary discharge: A merging of the concepts. In Evarts EV, et al (eds): Central Control of Movement. Neurosciences Res Prog Bull, 9:86–112, 1971
9. Kimura D: Acquisition of a motor skill after left hemisphere damage. Brain 100:527–542, 1977
10. Cremonini W, Derenzi E, Faglioni P: Contrasting performance of right and left hemisphere patients on short-term and long-term sequential visual memory. Neuropsychologia 18:1–9, 1980
11. Knott M, Voss DE: Proprioceptive Neuromuscular Facilitation, ed 2. New York, Harper & Row, 1968
12. Rusk HA: Rehabilitation Medicine, ed 3. St Louis, CV Mosby Co, 1971
13. Chusid JG, McDonald JJ: Correlative Neuroanatomy and Functional Neurology, ed 17. Los Altos, CA, Lange Medical, 1979
14. Brown JW: Aphasia, Arpaxia and Agnosia: Clinical and Theoretical Aspects. Springfield, IL, Charles C Thomas, 1972
15. De Jong RN: The Neurological Examination, ed 3. New York, Harper & Row, 1970
16. McCloskey DI: Kinesthetic Stability. Physiol Rev 58:763–820, 1978
17. Trombly C, Scott AD: Occupational Therapy for Physical Dysfunction. Baltimore, Williams & Wilkins, 1977
18. Bruell JH, Peszczynski M: Perception of verticality in hemiplegic patients in relation to rehabilitation. Clinical Orthopaedics 12:124, 1958
19. Fiorentino, M: Reflex Testing Methods for Evaluating CNS Development, ed 2. Charles C Thomas Co, Springfield IL, 1973
20. Bobath, B: Adult Hemiplegia. London, William Heinemann Medical Books, Ltd, 1970
21. Bishop B: Neurophysiology of spasticity: Classical concepts. Phys Ther. 57:371–376, 1977
22. Carpenter MB: Human Neuroanatomy. Baltimore, Williams & Wilkins, 1976
23. Stockmeyer SA: Procedures for improvement of motor control. Unpublished notes from Boston University, PT 710, 1979
24. Stockmeyer SA: An interpretation of the Approach of Rood to the treatment of neuromuscular dysfunction. Am J Phys Med 46:950–956, 1966
25. Taub E, Berman AJ: Movement and learning in the absence of sensory feedback. In Freedman SJ(ed): The Neuropsychology of Spatially Oriented Behavior. Homewood, IL, Dorsey Press, 1968

26. Clark C: Essentials of Clinical Neuroanatomy and Neurophysiology, ed 5. Philadelphia, FA Davis Co, 1975
27. Farber S, Huss J: Sensorimotor Evaluation and Treatment Procedures for Allied Health Personnel, ed 2. Indianapolis, Indiana University Foundation, 1974
28. Doubilet L, Polkow LS: Theory and design of a finger abduction splint for the spastic hand. Am J Occup Ther 31:320–322, 1977
29. Brodal A: Self-observations and neuro-anatomical considerations after a stroke. Brain 96:675–694, 1973
30. Zimmerman JE, Oder, LA: Swallowing Dysfunction in the Acutely Ill Patient. Read at the Midwinter Section Meeting of the American Physical Therapy Association, New Orleans, 1980
31. Gray's Anatomy, ed 27. Philadelphia, Lea and Febiger, 1959
32. Shahani B: The human blink reflex. J Neurol Neurosurg Psychiat 33:792–800, 1970
33. Young RR: The clinical significance of exteroceptive reflexes. In Desmedt JE(ed): New Developments in Electromyography and Clinical Neurophysiology, Basel, Kargel, 1973, vol 3
34. Bowman JP: The Muscle Spindle and Neural Control of the Tongue. Springfield, IL, Charles C Thomas, 1971
35. Adkins HV, Winstein C: Swallowing Dysfunction: Assessment and Management. Read at The Annual Conference of the American Physical Therapy Association, Phoenix, 1980
36. Schultz AR, Niemtzow P, Jacobs, SR, et al: Dysphagia associated with criocophalyngeal dysfunction. Arch Phys Med Rehabil 60:381–382, 1979
37. Knott, M: Unpublished class notes, Vallejo, CA, Proprioceptive Neuromuscular Facilitation, 1966
38. Mueller HA: Facilitating feeding and prespeech. In Pearson PH, Williams CE(eds): Physical Therapy Services in the Developmental Disabilities. Springfield, IL, Charles C Thomas, 1972.
39. Konecky C: An EMG Study of Abdominals and Back Extensors during Lower Trunk Rotation. Thesis. Boston MA, Boston University Sargent College of Allied Health Professions, 1980
40. Voss DE: Proprioceptive neuromuscular facilitation. Amer J Phys Med 46:838–898, 1966
41. Rood M: The use of sensory receptors to activate, facilitate, and inhibit motor response, automatic and somatic, in developmental sequence. In Sattely C(ed): Approaches to the Treatment of Patients with Neuromuscular Dysfunction. DuBuque, IA, WM C Brown Co, 1962
42. Heiniger M, Randolph SL: Conceptual Model for the Practical Appreciation of Neurophysiologic Approaches to Treatment. Read at the

Third Annual Forum of the Society for Behavioral Kinesiology, Houston, TX, 1976

43. Voss DE: Therapeutic exercise. Unpublished class notes from Northwestern University, 1975

44. Lawrence D: Anatomical Localization of the Descending Pathways and Their Contributions to Motor Control. Read at conference on Motor Control sponsored by Harvard Medical School, Boston, 1980

45. Rood M: Treatment of Neuromuscular Dysfunction: Rood Approach. Read at conference sponsored by Massachusetts Chapter American Physical Therapy Association, Boston, 1976

chapter 9

Spinal Cord Injury

INTRODUCTION

Spinal cord injuries (SCI) are most commonly a result of vehicular or sporting accidents and inflicted injuries such as gunshot wounds. Such trauma affects primarily young people ranging in age from the late teens to the early twenties. SCI can occur with congenital deficits such as spina bifida, or may be caused by circulatory insufficiency, which usually occurs in an older age group (1).

Physical therapy is a vital component of the rehabilitation process that includes the other health professions of medicine, occupational therapy, social work, nursing, vocational training, and psychiatry. The level and completeness of the lesion will largely determine the functional capabilities of the patient. However, many other factors exclusive of the level of lesion are important determinants of the success of treatment. These variables include age, height and weight, the amount and pattern of spasticity, body image, motivation, family support, and prior occupational experience. Psychological acceptance of the injury may be the most difficult aspect of rehabilitation as the patient is continually confronted with the reality of functional incapabilities and compromises in life-style. The cooperation of health professionals is essential to assist the patient in dealing with the many changes and adaptations that must occur.

Improved emergency care and medical treatment have increased the likelihood of spinal nerve recovery and have permitted the earlier initiation of restorative procedures. Future advances in all aspects of treatment will lead to further improvement of patient care and enhancement of patient capabilities.

EVALUATION

Assessment of sensory and motor function and the status of the anal reflex provide early indication of the level and completeness of the lesion. As spinal shock subsides, innervation of sensory and motor segments below the level of the vertebral involvement may become evident (2). Serial evaluations are a means of documenting the recovery pattern and of providing the therapist with the information necessary to plan an effective treatment. Although important, the initial evaluations are usually limited by bed positioning and external supportive devices used to immobilize the areas of lesion.

■ Specific Evaluations

Vital Functions. The respiratory functions of breathing and coughing may be severely impaired if the innervation to abdominal and intercostal muscles has been interrupted. Diaphragmatic involvement necessitates initial if not long-term mechanical intervention for respiratory support. Decreased forced expiration occurring as a result of impairment to the accessory muscles of respiration will require respiratory training and pulmonary care (3). Since impairment of bowel and bladder control may greatly influence the patient's ability to function in society, a program to regulate these functions is an integral part of the rehabilitation process and is usually established by the nursing and medical staff.

Sensation. The results of the sensory evaluation are important both in treatment planning and patient education. Sensory testing is usually performed according to nerve root levels and may indicate the level of the spinal recovery. Exteroceptive superficial sensation is differentially evaluated from deep proprioceptive and visceral sensations. Because these sensations travel over different ascending pathways to higher centers of the CNS, they may be affected differently by injury (4). The patient may be able to detect deep joint movement, for example, but not superficial touch. The patient may also be able to sense muscle spasm in areas where exteroceptive sensation is not present. Visceral sensations are monitored both through the autonomic nervous system and cranial nerves and may be partially intact. Autonomic signs including an increase in perspiration or headaches may be indicative of a full bladder or a need to defecate (5).

The sensory level of innervation does not always correspond to the level of motor function. Most fracture dislocations of the vertebral column cause damage to the adjacent anterior tracts in the spinal cord. If the posterior tracts are intact, as can occur with an incomplete lesion, then the sensory functions may be partially spared (2).

Learning a movement is always easier if the patient has sensation in that area. An intact body image, which depends partly on sensory feedback, may enhance the patient's functional ability.

When a lack of sensation around bony prominences—such as the pelvic spines, greater trochanters, heels, and scapula spines—exists, special care must be taken to prevent pressure sores. Particularly important are the ischial areas where skin breakdown may easily result from the pressure of prolonged sitting. Frequent relief of pressure by elevating the pelvis in sitting and turning in bed should become a habit. In addition, the use of special cushions or mattresses will help to decrease the occurrence of decubiti. If sensation in the lower extremities, especially the feet, is impaired, trauma or extremes of temperature must be avoided.

Strength. A specific muscle evaluation following myotomal levels will provide the therapist with an indication of the level of innervation. It is not uncommon to find asymmetries of motor innervation between limbs. Sparing of sacral motor tracts is a frequent finding evidenced by minimal motoric ability in the feet. All muscles that are attached to the involved vertebrae should be tested carefully with minimal resistance. In most instances, testing of those muscles around the injured site is postponed until joint stabilization has been gained.

An incomplete lesion may result in a diffuse and spotty motor and sensory return; the condition of the patient may not stabilize for a long period of time. At the time of injury a peripheral nerve root lesion may have occurred, especially if the direction of force was lateral or rotational. Regeneration along that nerve root may lead to motor return one level below the expected innervation.

To a large extent, the results of the manual muscle test will determine the projected functional capacity. Many patients will not attain their potential while others may greatly exceed expectations. Even if the level of innervation is similar, variations in function may occur between patients owing to many other factors (see Introduction).

Range of Motion. Joint range of motion and muscle extendability should be normal initially, unless other trauma has occurred. Limitations in range may eventually develop because of prolonged immobilization or imbalances of muscle tone. Limited passive movement is often found in the following ranges: shoulder hyperextension, elbow, wrist and finger extension, SLR or the ability to toe-touch in long sitting, and ankle dorsiflexion. Although a certain amount of mobility is necessary, adaptive shortening in some muscles can be used functionally and is actually encouraged. Tightness of the finger flexors, for example, will improve the "strength" of a tenodesis grasp. The combined length of low back extensors and hamstrings should be such to allow the patient to balance anteriorly in the long-sitting position without upper extremity support. Overstretching can result in too much mobility and may decrease the support usually provided by the posterior structures. During early stages of treatment of a patient with a low thoracic or lumbar lesion, passive leg or lower trunk movements are usually contraindicated.

Muscle Tone. Deep tendon reflexes and resistance to passive stretch are used as a subjective means of assessing variations in tone (6). Severe hypertonia may greatly affect treatment. The ability to independently assume long sitting can be severely limited when spasticity in the pectoralis major or biceps prevents the patient from positioning his arms posteriorly. A patient with minimal spasticity in the quadriceps may be able to use his spasticity advantageously during transfers, although excessive spasticity may interfere with mobility and dressing.

Trophic Changes and Skin Condition. Trophic changes occur when autonomic innervation is decreased (7). Pressure sores may affect the patient's long-term sitting tolerance and as a result can severely limit and delay rehabilitation. Skin integrity is extremely important and can be enhanced with good nutrition (8).

Social and Psychological Support. Essential to the patient's acceptance of the present and future is the support given by family, friends, and professionals (9). The SCI patient frequently passes through the stages of grief similar to that experienced by patients with other catastrophic illnesses. The achievement of functional potential is usually delayed until some level of acceptance is reached. Many patients maintain belief in full recovery but accept the fact that for the present they must learn how to overcome the limitations of their disability.

Occupational Therapy. Coordination of evaluation and treatment between physical and occupational therapies is always important, but especially so when one is dealing with quadriplegic patients. Hand splints for positioning may be indicated initially, and later functional splints can be designed to assist with upper extremity activities. The ADL abilities of feeding, dressing, and hygiene are usually emphasized by occupational therapists (10). Depending on the availability of other personnel, the occupational therapist may be involved in vocational testing.

Vocational. Vocational counseling will probably be indicated as rehabilitation progresses. The vocational and educational history will affect long-term planning. The accessibility and feasibility of returning to previous positions must be evaluated and viable alternatives suggested.

Home Accessibility. Architectural barriers should be assessed early in the program and changes implemented before the patient is ready to return home temporarily or permanently. Home adaptations and equipment needs such as a wheelchair and orthotic devices should be anticipated early in the rehabilitation process, especially if financial problems exist.

Goals

The information gleaned from these assessments will help to determine the feasible long-range goals. The goals may include: (1) locomotion, which may be limited to wheelchair mobility or ambulation with crutches and orthoses, and (2) performance of ADL skills such as feeding, dressing, personal hygiene, and vocationally directed activities. The short-range goals are adjusted periodically and are geared to improving the patient's internal motivation.

THE TOTAL TREATMENT PLAN

The treatment planning process requires the interaction of the rehabilitation team. Continual communication between all the health care services is essential to provide the necessary continuity of treatment.

Specific Treatment Procedures

The treatment progression in this chapter begins with procedures appropriate for the treatment of a quadriplegic patient and then progresses to procedures applicable to paraplegic patients. The level of lesion and the extent of muscular innervation will determine the procedures appropriate for each patient.

The first sequence of procedures is designed for quadriplegic patients who have minimal or no triceps control. Patients with greater triceps strength should be able to progress through this sequence more quickly and may not need to perform all the intermediate steps.

Treatment begins with procedures to strengthen the innervated muscles. Strengthening procedures are based on the concept that the activity of the weak muscles can be enhanced by promoting overflow from stronger musculature. Procedures are sequenced to progress in a proximal to distal direction (11). Overflow from one group of muscles to another can occur within a limb or from one extremity to the other (12). The findings of a manual muscle test (MMT) will inform the therapist of the patient's particular strengths. The activity of the strongest muscles is first maximized, and then is used to enhance the weaker musculature through the effects of overflow. Following are typical examples of muscle grades obtained during an evaluation of a quadriplegic patient. Included in the subsequent discussion are the optimal patterns of movement for these muscles and suggestions for combining the activities and techniques to enhance function.

Muscle Grades:

- **Scapula**
  - trapezius: G to N
  - rhomboids: G
  - serratus anterior: F+
  - lower trapezius and latissimus dorsi (LD): P to F
- **Shoulder**
  - middle deltoid: G+
  - posterior deltoid: G−
  - anterior deltoid: F+
  - pectoralis major—clavicular portion: F+
  - pectoralis major—sternal portion: T to P−
- **Elbow**
  - biceps brachii: G to N
  - triceps brachii: O to P
- **Wrist**
  - radial wrist extensors (RWE): G to N
  - flexors: O

The following indicates the patterns in which the muscles listed above can be facilitated optimally.

D_2F:

trapezius: G to N
middle deltoid: G+
radial wrist extensors: G to N

D_1F:

serratus anterior: F+
anterior deltoid: F+
pectoralis major—
(clavicular): F+
wrist flexors: O

(Continued on following page)

D_1E:

rhomboids: G
posterior deltoid: G –
latissimus dorsi: F
radial wrist extensors: G to N*

D_2E:

pectoralis major (sternal): P –
wrist flexors: O

These four diagonal patterns can be performed with the elbow remaining straight, flexing, or extending during the movement (11). On normal subjects, the biceps have been shown to be active in all elbow-flexing patterns, particularly during D_1F. As expected, the triceps are active in all elbow-extending patterns, but especially in D_1E. The triceps are also highly active during D_1E and D_2F with the elbow straight (13). The following paragraphs discuss how this knowledge can be specifically applied to activate weakened musculature.

The analysis of the MMT evaluation shows that D_2F with elbow flexion is the strongest pattern for this patient. The muscles involved in this pattern, from proximal to distal, are the trapezius, middle deltoid, biceps and the radial wrist extensors, all of which range from G to N. Because the strength of all of these muscles is almost equal, the strengthening technique of RC is indicated. The first procedure therefore is the activity of D_2F with elbow F combined with the technique of RC. This procedure will further strengthen the muscles as well as teach the patient how to move against resistance (Figure 9–1).

The second strongest group of proximal muscles (G –) are the rhomboids and the posterior deltoid, which are most active in the D_1E pattern. By performing this pattern with the elbow flexing, overflow from the even stronger biceps is obtained. Because the biceps and wrist extensors are stronger than the proximal muscles, the technique of TE is indicated (Figure 9–2). These stronger, more distal muscles are "locked in"; that is they are isometrically resisted in that part of the range where the therapist feels that they can hold the best. For the biceps, that range is usually around 90 degrees; for the wrist extensors it is the shortened range. While the isometric contraction of these stronger muscles is sustained, the weaker proximal muscles—the rhomboids, posterior deltoid, and latissimus dorsi—perform an isotonic contraction against manual resistance with quick stretches superimposed (see Chapter 4). D_1E is the pattern in which the ulnar and not the radial wrist extensors contract optimally in the normal condition (11). When the cord lesion is in the midcervical region, however, the ulnar wrist extensors are not innervated (14). Therefore, patients, will usually extend their wrist with the innervated radial wrist extensor regardless of the pattern. If the radial wrist extensors are strong, which is usually the case, they can be used in either D_2F or D_1E to elicit overflow effects into the weaker

*The ulnar wrist extensors are usually considered prime movers in this pattern.

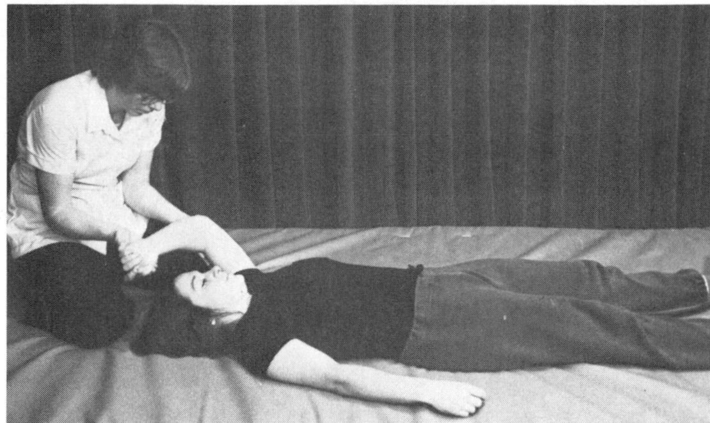

A. D_2 F elbow flexing.
T. RC.
E. MC arm and wrist.

FIGURE 9–1

musculature. Strengthening into the range of shoulder hyperextension, which can be specifically emphasized during this procedure, is preliminary to independent assumption of the postures of supine on elbows and long sitting.

The next group of muscles to be strengthened are the serratus anterior and the anterior deltoid (F+), which are most active in D_1F (11). To promote overflow from the biceps, the pattern is performed with elbow flexion and with the technique of TE. The stronger biceps is locked in and the weaker proximal muscles pivoted into their shortened range. Because the shoulder abductors are stronger than the adductors, the patient may have difficulty flexing in a D_1 pattern, which requires movement toward the midline (Figure 9–3). Although always important, verbal cues and appropriate manual contacts are especially necessary in this instance to enhance the desired movement into D_1F. Functionally, strengthening of the serratus anterior and the anterior deltoid is needed for the assumption of prone on elbows and for lifting the pelvis from the mat in long sitting.

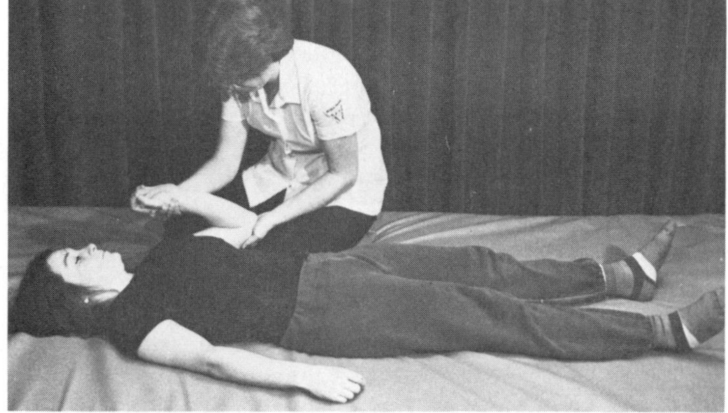

A. D_1 E elbow flexing.
T. TE: emphasis on shoulder extension.
E. MC arm and wrist.

FIGURE 9–2

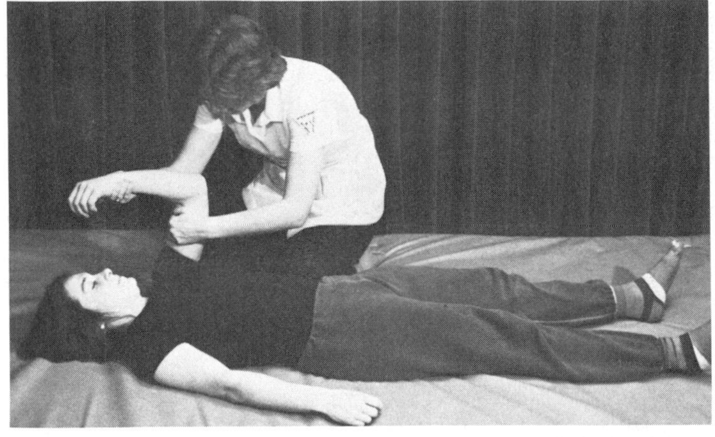

A. D_1 F elbow flexing.
T. TE: emphasis on shoulder flexion.
E. MC arm and wrist.

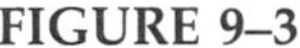

FIGURE 9–3

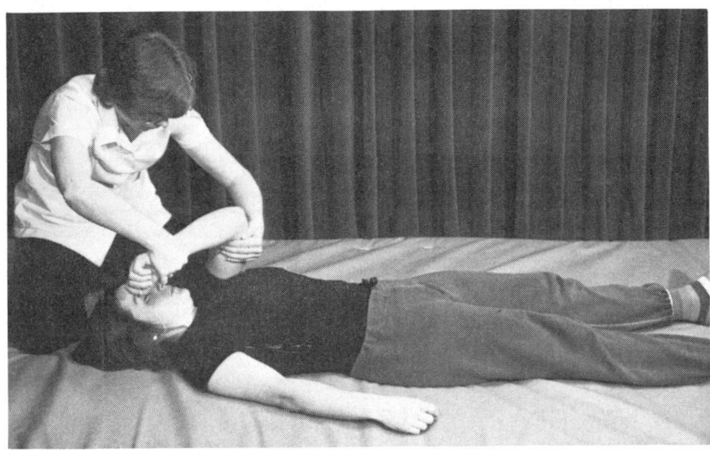

A. D_2 E: elbow flexing.
T. TE: emphasis on shoulder extension.
E. MC arm and forearm.

FIGURE 9–4

The sternal portion of the pectoralis major, usually only partially innervated in a midcervical lesion (14), is most active in D_2E (11). Because of the decreased strength of the proximal muscles, this pattern is the most difficult one for the quadriplegic patient. The technique of TE remains the most appropriate for increasing proximal activity through overflow from the stronger biceps (Figure 9–4). As with the D_1F pattern, additional sensory input may be needed to promote the adduction component of the D_2E pattern. Functionally, activity of the pectoralis major is important for shoulder stability during transfers and for movement of the upper extremities during dressing and other ADL.

Progressing one joint more distally, focus in treatment is directed to strengthening of the triceps. Overflow into the triceps from the strongest shoulder musculature is obtained by performing the D_2F pattern. The elbow is maintained in extension during the pattern and approximation added by the therapist to enhance tonic holding. When triceps strength is sufficient to

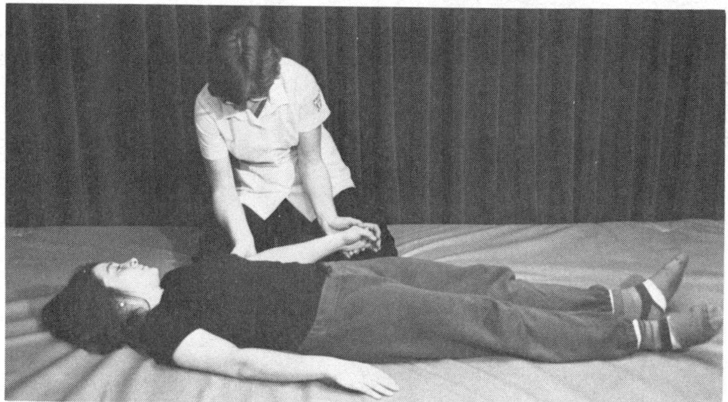

A. D_1 E elbow straight.
T. Holding in shortened range.
E. MC arm and wrist.

FIGURE 9–5

isotonically contract through at least part of the range, the technique of TE is appropriate. The stronger proximal muscles are resisted to the point in the range at which an isometric contraction can best be sustained. For the shoulder, this range appears to be just beyond 90 degrees of flexion. The proximal muscles are locked in and the triceps pivoted. Additional sensory input such as brushing, icing, or vibration may prove effective in increasing the triceps response.

Not only is D_1E another optimal pattern in which triceps activity can be facilitated, but it is also a movement required during many functional mat activities. As with D_2F, the D_1E pattern can be performed with the elbow maintained in extension or extending through range, depending on the strength of the triceps. Emphasis can be placed on holding in the extremely shortened range of the pattern to improve the ability to depress the scapula (Figure 9–5).

Bilateral patterns also may be used to promote overflow if one upper extremity has more innervation. If the right arm is stronger, for example, isometric resistance would be applied to the D_2F pattern in approximately 90 degrees of range to maximize overflow to the weaker left arm. While the right arm is locked in, the weaker extremity isotonically moves against manual resistance with repeated stretches superimposed to facilitate the contraction. The sequence of patterns performed by the left limb would follow that already described for unilateral exercises. The following bilateral combinations would be appropriate with the technique of TE:

1. Bilateral symmetrical D_2F: D_2F on both right and left (Figure 9–6)
2. Cross-diagonal: D_2F on right and D_1E on the left (Figure 9–7)
3. Asymmetrical flexion: D_2F on right and D_1F on left (Figure 9–8)
4. Reciprocal D_2: D_2F on right and D_2E on left (Figure 9–9)

The preceding examples of unilateral and bilateral patterns may be used by the therapist to strengthen the weakened muscles of the quadriplegic patient. These strengthening procedures are designed to complement those in-

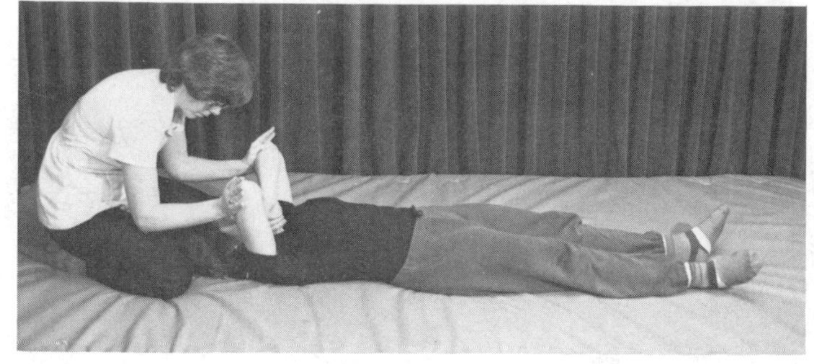

A. BS D_2 F.
T. TE.
E. MC elbows.

FIGURE 9–6

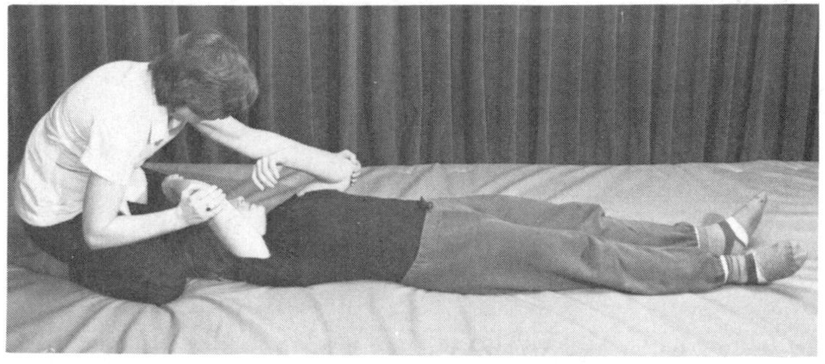

A. Cross-diagonal: D_2F (R) D_1E (L).
T. TE.
E. MC elbows.

FIGURE 9–7

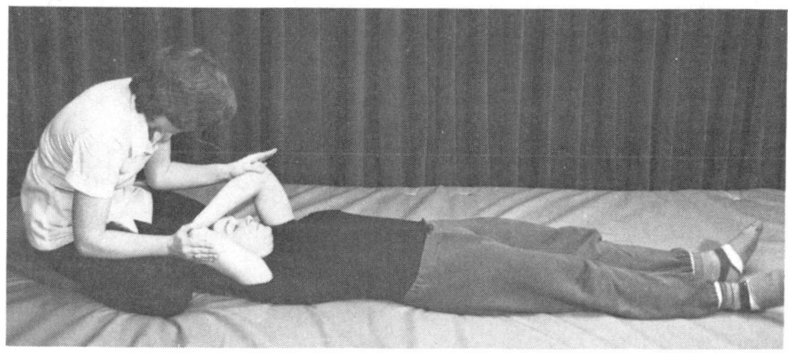

A. Asymmetrical flexion to the right.
T. TE.
E. MC elbows.

FIGURE 9–8

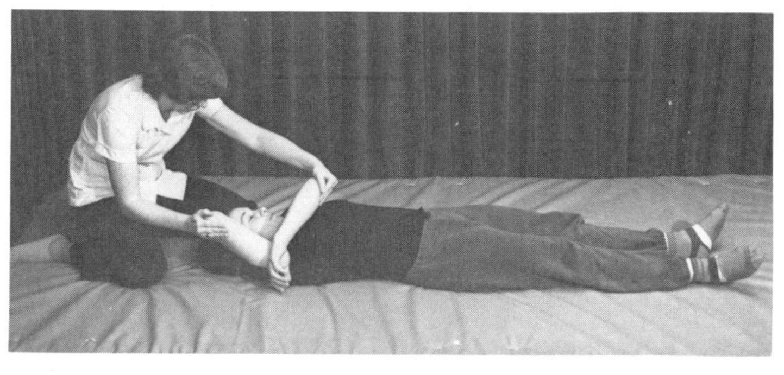

A. BR D_2: D_2F (R) D_2E (L).
T. TE.
E. MC elbows.

FIGURE 9–9

corporated into the mat program. If the patient has difficulty assuming supine on elbows, for example, strengthening of the scapula adductors and shoulder extensors in D_1E is indicated.

MAT PROCEDURES FOR THE QUADRIPLEGIC PATIENT

The mat program is divided into procedures that would be appropriate for patients with three levels of spinal cord injury: cervical, thoracic, and lumbar. The treatment procedures in all cases are geared toward accomplishing the functional goals of wheelchair transfers and bed mobility. To reach this long-range functional stage, the levels of motor control in various postures must first be attained. Procedures for patients with paraplegia are designed to reach more advanced goals, including increased mobility in and out of the wheelchair and, when appropriate, ambulation.

This program is applicable for patients with a C_{5-6} lesion or below. The amount of innervated musculature will obviously affect the speed of progression and ability to accomplish all the procedures of the sequence.

These procedures are divided into three stages: procedures performed in the initial stage emphasize strengthening in functional patterns and stability and controlled mobility in the various postures; middle-stage procedures further enhance controlled mobility; advanced procedures promote skill.

■ Initial Progression

Supine. Manual resistance is applied to bilateral shoulder extension and scapula adduction in preparation for stability in and the assumption of supine on elbows. The elbows are positioned close to the trunk with the forearms supinated and the hands near the shoulders. The patient pushes down with shoulder extension and attempts to elevate the chest with scapula adduction (Figure 9–10). The therapist may first need to assist the patient with this elevation, which promotes a SHRC in the rhomboids and posterior deltoid muscles. These muscles are important for upper trunk and upper extremity stability.

Assumption of supine on elbows may initially require assistance by the therapist. Some patients, because of tightness in the structures of the anterior shoulder, may experience pain when initial attempts are made to balance in this position. Although maintenance of supine on elbows may be difficult at first, AI and RS with manual contacts on the scapula, can be used to improve stability in the posture (Figure 9–11). Holding of this supine-on-elbows position with the scapula adducted even further in shortened ranges will help to strengthen the proximal muscles isometrically.

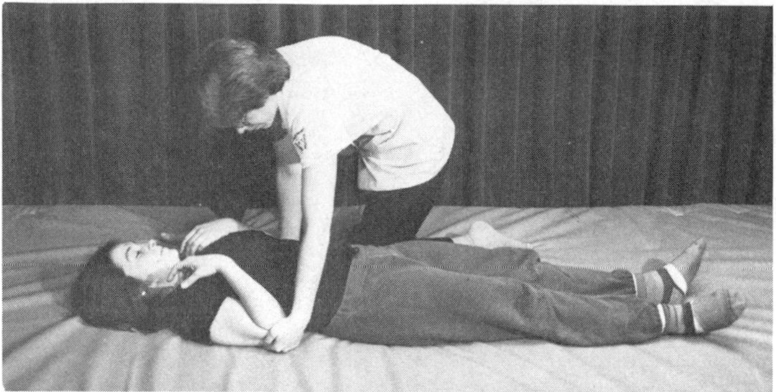

A. Supine: bilateral shoulder extension and elbow flexion.
T. Holding the position.
E. MC elbows.

FIGURE 9–10

Sidelying. Sidelying activities are preliminary to rolling. In sidelying, upper trunk rotation is strengthened in both directions with the techniques of SRH and RC. The trunk and scapula motions are combined with shoulder movements. Upper trunk forward rotation and scapula protraction are combined with shoulder flexion to accomplish rolling from supine to prone (Figure 9–12). The rolling movement proceeds through increments of range from sidelying until the patient can initiate rolling from supine. Exaggera-

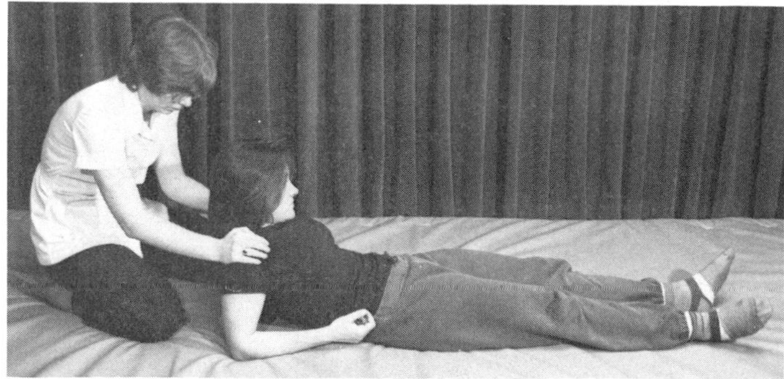

A. Supine on elbows.
T. AI-RS.
E. MC scapulae.

FIGURE 9–11

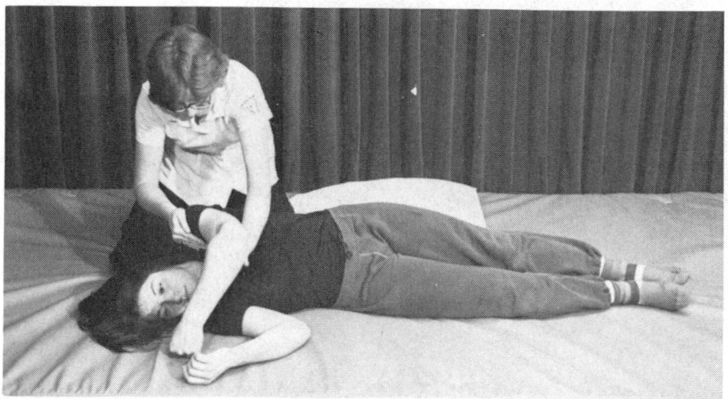

A. Sidelying: UTR, forward movement, pillow under pelvis, shoulder flexion.
T. SRH with RC.
E. MC scapula and pelvis.

FIGURE 9–12

tion of the upper trunk and upper extremity movement causes the lower trunk to follow in the rolling movement. Rolling from supine is first practiced with a pillow under one pelvis and one lower extremity crossed over the other so that the patient has less body weight resistance to overcome. The pillow may be removed and legs uncrossed as the patient becomes proficient in this activity. Cuff weights on the wrist can add momentum to the movement while simultaneously strengthening the shoulder muscles. Although the process is difficult, the patient must learn to disassociate the movements of elbow flexion and shoulder flexion in order to effectively use the arms to gain momentum in rolling. The arms should move bilaterally with the shoulders in flexion, and horizontal adduction and abduction with the elbows maintained in extension. To accomplish the disassociation of elbow and shoulder motion, the patient can practice shoulder flexion to approximately 45 degrees in supine against the resistance of gravity or a cuff weight without allowing the elbow to flex.

Prone Activities. Quadriplegic push-ups are preliminary to assuming prone on elbows. In prone, the patient's hands are positioned near the shoulders, and the elbows are placed near the trunk. The patient protracts the scapula and flexes the shoulders in attempting to lift the upper trunk off the mat. As with all activities, the patient may need assistance initially to push up (Figure 9–13). Emphasis is placed on arching the back and on protracting the scapula as much as possible to strengthen the serratus anterior.

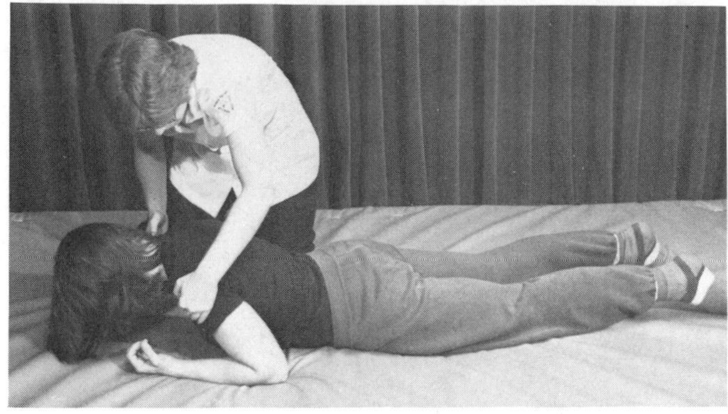

A. Prone: quadriplegic push-ups.
T. Assist position.
E. MC as needed.

FIGURE 9–13

In the prone-on-elbows posture with manual contacts on the scapula, AI and RS will improve isometric strength and stability. Lateral weight shifting is promoted by the technique of SRH through increments of range, which will gradually increase the weight-bearing resistance and improve balance reactions. The anterior-posterior direction of weight shifting is practiced to strengthen the scapula and shoulder muscles needed for independent assumption of the posture. In the prone-on-elbows position repeated arching of the upper trunk is emphasized for purposes of strengthening the muscles that will be used later to lift the pelvis in the long-sitting position (Figure 9–14). Scapula protraction and shoulder flexion are coupled with head and neck flexion to obtain maximum range in this lifting motion. Upper trunk arching should be practiced first in prone on elbows, where the B of S is large and the C of G low, before attempting this movement in the more difficult long-sitting position.

Long Sitting. Maximal assistance usually will be needed by the patient to assume the long-sitting posture during this initial stage because of decreased strength and flexibility. If triceps weakness is present, assistance also may be needed to maintain this position until the patient learns to externally rotate the shoulder to mechanically lock the elbow. Hypotension may be experienced until circulation is regulated. As indicated in the evaluation, mobility in the lower trunk extensors and hamstrings must be sufficient to allow the patient to balance forward in the long-sitting position without requiring upper extremity support. Unsupported balance in long sitting requires that the C of G of the upper trunk be anterior to the hips. Excessive tightness of posterior structures will limit this forward position. However, mobility must be gained with caution. Overstretching can reduce the support provided by both the ligaments and the passive insufficiency of the back extensors and hamstrings, and thus may result in an unstable posture.

The position of the fingers is important if a tenodesis grasp is necessary for the patient's function. The distal finger joints should therefore remain in

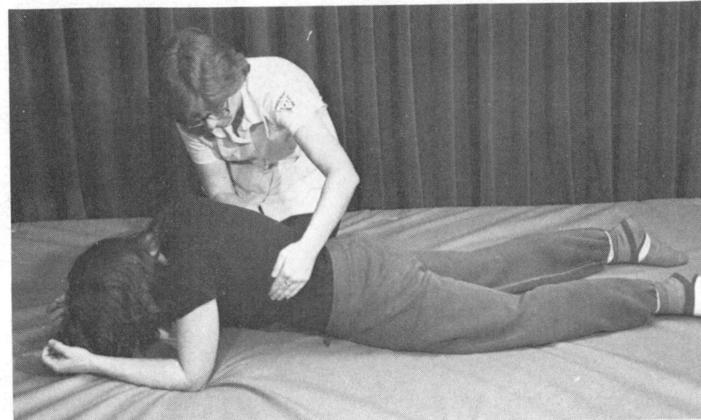

A. Prone on elbows: arching upper trunk.
T. Assist position.
E. MC as needed.

FIGURE 9–14

flexion to prevent overstretching of the flexor tendons when weight bearing occurs on the hands.

In the long-sitting position the upper extremities can be positioned posterior, anterior, and lateral to the trunk to assist with stability in the posture. With the arms in these three different positions, stability and controlled mobility can be promoted by the techniques of RS or AI and SRH through increments of range, respectively. These procedures are begun with the arms posterior to the trunk, a position that results in the largest B of S (Figure 9–15). When the arms are placed anteriorly, the patient can increase balance by hooking both hands under the knees. Balancing "erect" with the hands lateral, at the level of the greater trochanter, decreases the B of S and is therefore the most difficult of the three positions for the quadriplegic patient. To enhance the patient's ability to maintain this posture, the upper trunk and head are flexed to keep the C of G within the B of S. The techniques to promote stability and controlled mobility are appropriate in this posture but are difficult for the patient to perform. Resistance is

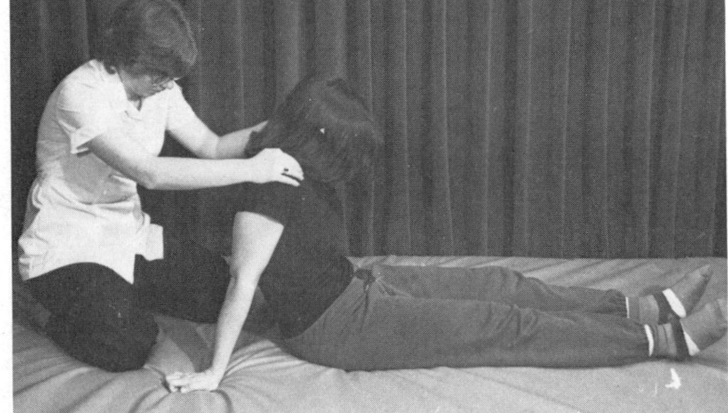

A. Long sitting: shoulders in extension.
T. RS.
E. MC scapula.

FIGURE 9–15

given in the rotatory and lateral directions before being applied in the anterior and posterior plane, where the support is most compromised. During all these procedures in long sitting the patient can learn to balance by substituting head, upper trunk, and upper extremity movements to compensate for the lack of lower trunk control.

■ Middle Progression

At this point in treatment, the patient should no longer require any external orthotic immobilization. No physical activities are contraindicated. Strengthening exercises are continued with the added resistance of pulleys or cuff weights. Endurance and proficiency in wheelchair propulsion and transfer activities should be increasing.

The major goal at this middle stage is to further increase controlled mobility in the discussed postures. This goal is attained when the patient can both shift weight through full range and independently assume the various positions.

Supine. Some patients may achieve the posture of supine on elbows by hooking wrists or thumbs under the hips or in the pants pockets and by flexing the elbows to raise the upper trunk from the mat. By then walking posteriorly on the elbows, the position can be assumed. Stronger patients may be able to extend the shoulders and "walk" the elbows back, without the assistance of the initial elbow flexion.

In supine on elbows, lateral weight shifting can be progressed to unilateral weight bearing. Static-dynamic procedures are practiced to increase the control of the static limb and to enable the patient to move into other postures from this position (Figure 9–16). Control in the static limb is promoted by unilateral balancing in the posture. The weight-bearing arm must be positioned in shoulder hyperextension and scapula retraction to move the B of S under the C of G. To enhance reactions in the supporting limb, the non-weight-bearing dynamic limb moves through increasingly larger ranges. These movements change the C of G and require proximal dynamic stability to counteract the weight shifting.

Both the prone-on-elbows and long-sitting postures can be assumed from supine on elbows. Prone on elbows is gained by first moving into the unilateral supine-on-elbows position just described. The dynamic limb is brought forward across the body and the trunk is allowed to rotate until a midposition is reached. By protracting the scapula on the supporting limb, the upper body can roll to the supine-on-elbows position. To assist the patient with this change in position, the therapist helps the patient to the midline, where stability techniques are applied. This is followed by slow reversal movements through increments of range to improve the patient's upper trunk control and subsequent ability to assume prone on elbows independently.

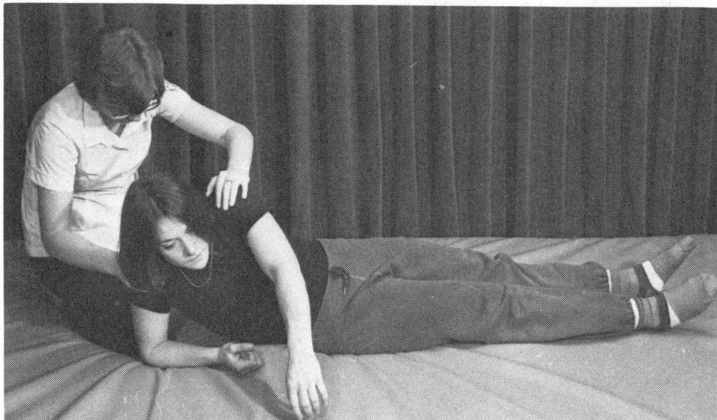

A. Supine on elbows: static-dynamic (midposition).
T. Assist to position.
E. MC as needed.

FIGURE 9–16

The independent assumption of long-sitting is an extremely important goal. Many functional activities such as dressing and transfers are performed in the long-sitting position. The ability to assume this posture unassisted will increase the patient's independence. The method of assuming long sitting can vary greatly among patients and is somewhat dependent on the flexibility of the shoulder and trunk, the strength of the triceps, and the presence of moderate extensor spasticity in the lower extremities. Two means of assumption can be used as a guide, but can be varied according to patient's needs. Both of these methods begin in supine on elbows:

1. Without rotating the lower trunk, the patient turns from a unilateral supine-on-elbows to a prone-on-elbows position and then "walks" on elbows around toward the knees. One arm is then hooked under the knee and by pulling with one arm and pushing with the other, long sitting can be assumed. This can be accomplished without triceps control but does require trunk mobility and some LE spasticity (Figure 9–17).

2. For the patients with triceps control and flexibility of the shoulders, long sitting may be achieved from a static-dynamic supine-on-elbows position by swinging the dynamic limb posteriorly so the shoulder and elbow extend. Weight is transferred onto that limb while the other arm assumes a symmetrical extended position. The patient can then walk on hands up to long sitting. If upper extremity strength is unequal, the weaker arm is positioned posteriorly first so the elbows can be biomechanically locked. The stronger upper extremity will then extend against the resistance of body weight. Patients may find that loops, bed rails, or other assistive devices may be needed to assume long sitting.

Long Sitting. In long sitting, wide-range weight shifting is followed by static-dynamic activities (Figure 9–18). The equilibrium developed during these controlled mobility and static-dynamic activities can be challenged by the therapist by gently disturbing balance, first with arm support then with-

(a)

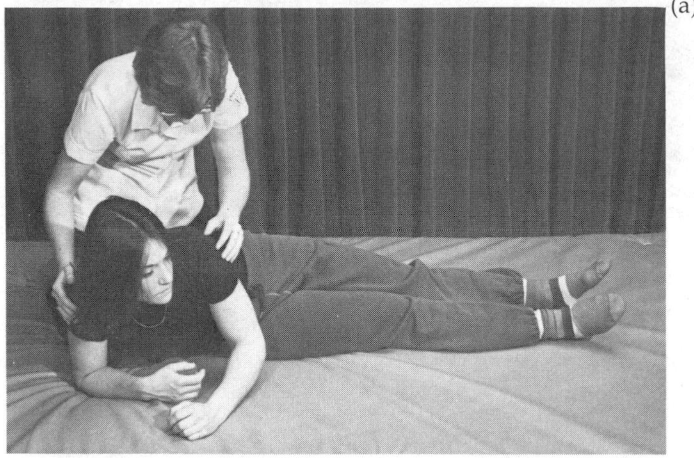

(b)

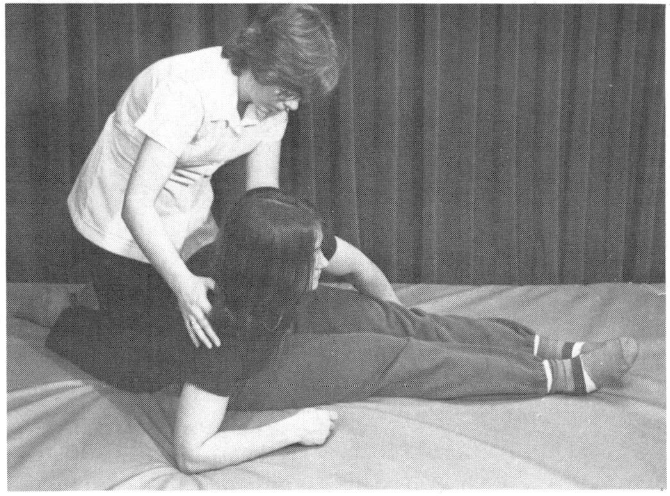

A. Long sitting.
T. Assumption of position.
E. MC as needed.

FIGURE 9–17

out. Quick disturbances of balance in the unsupported position promote fast compensatory movements of the upper extremities to prevent falling. When trunk control is sufficient, one upper extremity can be freed from a supporting position to perform functional activities such as moving the lower extremities in preparation for transfers and dressing. By placing the extended wrist under the knee and flexing the elbow, the patient can reposition the leg.

To transfer independently, the patient must be able to vertically lift the pelvis off the supporting surface and exert control over lower trunk movements while in this elevated posture. With the hands positioned laterally beside the greater trochanter, the patient lifts the trunk by combining the motions of scapula protraction and depression, slight shoulder flexion, and head and upper trunk flexion (Figure 9–19). If necessary, the therapist can

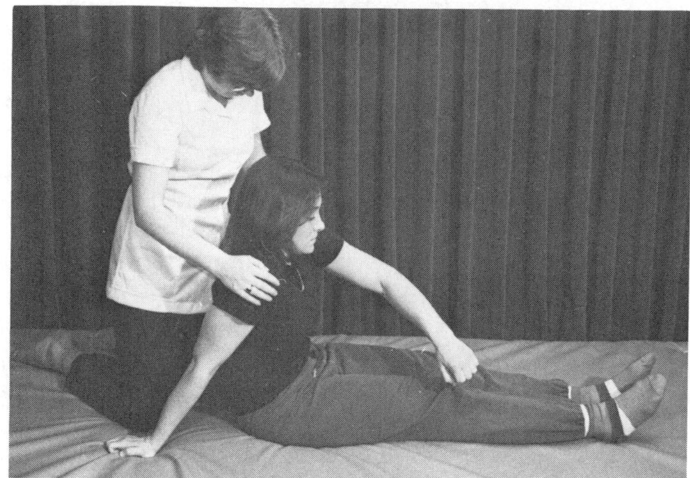

A. Long sitting: static-dynamic.
T. RS.
E. MC scapula.

FIGURE 9–18

assist the assumption of the lift position by elevating the pelvis from the supporting surface. Stability in the lift position is promoted by isometrically resisting at the shoulders, where the patient can feel the resistance applied, and later at the pelvis, where the manual contacts may not be felt. The progression in the placement of manual contacts is an example of leading through the patient's strength. Sensory input is first provided to the areas that are sensitive to touch, and resistance is given to innervated muscles. The goal of the procedure, however, is that the patient begin to maneuver the entire trunk, especially the lower trunk. Therefore, once the patient has experienced the sensory input and can adequately respond, the manual contacts are repositioned on the pelvis. The minimally resistive forces provided by the therapist are compensated for by excessive upper trunk motions. Because tactile sensation may be lacking, the therapist may have to emphasize verbal cues to assist the patient in responding to the resistance.

Controlled mobility or weight shifting follows the stability procedures. In the pelvic lift position, the pelvis is first moved rotationally and laterally,

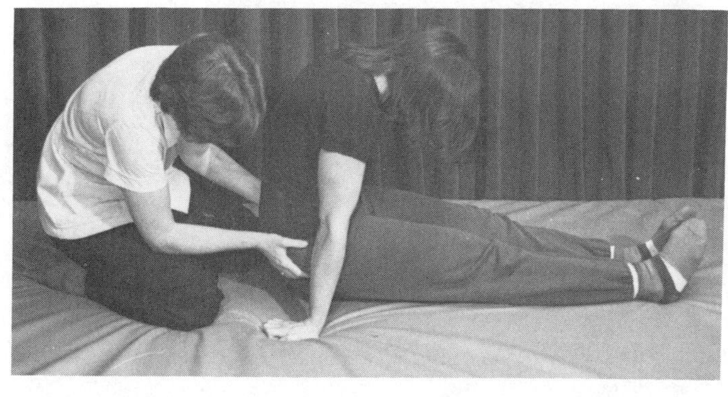

A. Long sitting: lift.
T. Assist to position.
E. MC pelvis.

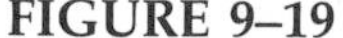

FIGURE 9–19

then in the more difficult anterior-posterior direction. The pelvic movement is first assisted before any resistance is provided.

Prone. Prone activities in this middle stage include weight shifting to unilateral weight bearing in prone on elbows. Resistance may be provided to improve control in the static limb by isometrically resisting maintenance of the posture, then by resisting the dynamic limb with reversal techniques (Figure 9–20). By increasing the excursion of controlled mobility movements, especially in the anterior-posterior direction, the ability to assume prone on elbows is promoted. Arching of the upper trunk in prone on elbows is still incorporated into treatment procedures at this stage. This activity can be made more difficult by increasing the height of the lift, the number of repetitions, and the amount of resistance. Emphasizing this activity and "quadriplegic push-ups" should improve the patient's ability to lift the pelvis in long sitting and ultimately to transfer.

From a static-dynamic position in prone on elbows the patient can move to supine on elbows. The dynamic limb pushes from the supporting surface as the upper trunk rotates until the midline position is reached. The dynamic limb is then hyperextended to support the body in supine on elbows. If the upper trunk rotational motion is exaggerated, the lower trunk will also turn to the supine position.

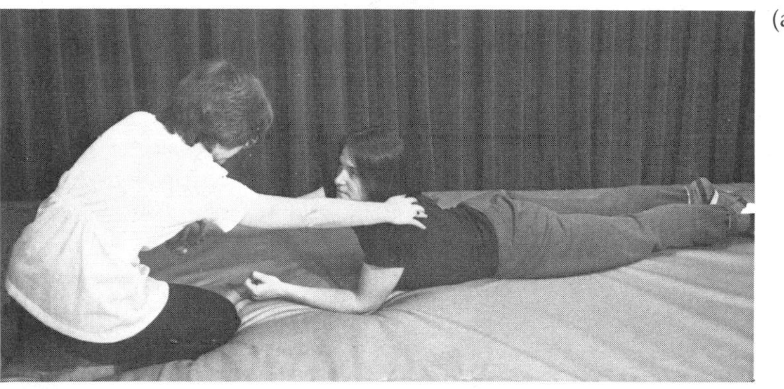

(a)

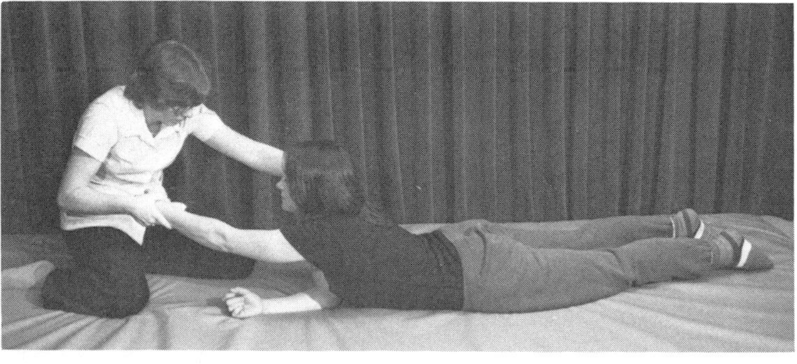

(b)

A. Prone on elbows: static-dynamic.
T. SRH.
E. MC wrist and scapula.

FIGURE 9–20

Advanced Progression

Wheelchair locomotion should be performed independently at this time, but transfers may still require minimal assistance. Transfer activities to the bed, wheelchair, toilet, and car seat should be practiced. Dressing and other ADL are also emphasized.

Long Sitting. Procedures in long sitting will include added resistance to all pelvic motions while in a lift position. If these procedures are successful, the patient should be able to move on the mat in all directions by lifting and not sliding the pelvis. Transfers to surfaces of unequal heights is often required. The height discrepancy with which the patient can cope is partially dependent on the height of the lift the patient can achieve in long sitting. The transfer movement combines a lift followed by a lateral and a posterior rotational motion. A wheelchair cushion placed on the mat is used so that the patient can practice the transfer motions. In long sitting the patient practices moving the lower extremities laterally with his arms and also practices crossing one leg over the other for dressing.

Prone. Prone procedures in this advanced stage include stability and controlled mobility techniques in elbows and knees, or quadruped if the patient has triceps control. Once the patient is assisted into the posture, AI, RS, and SRH through increments of range are performed with manual contacts on the scapulae, and then at the pelvis (Figure 9–21). The purpose of these procedures is not to make these postures functional, but rather to further stress the muscles of the arms and trunk and to use them to enhance the control of the lower trunk movements. The lower trunk motions promoted in these postures are necessary for transfers and have been previously enhanced during sidelying, long sitting, and movements from prone

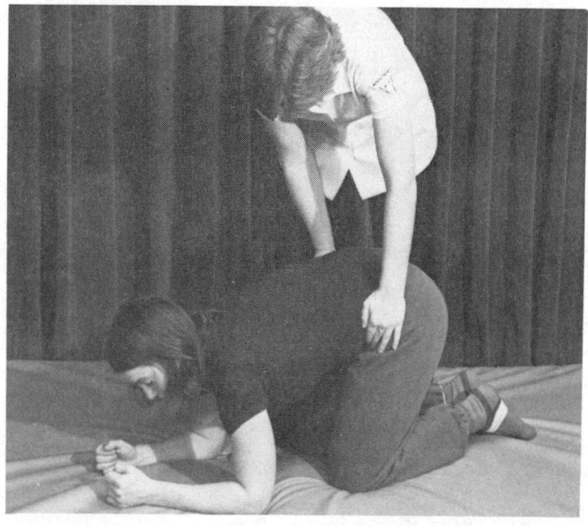

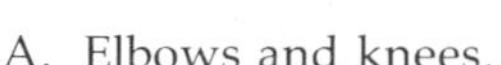

A. Elbows and knees.
T. AI.
E. MC pelvis.

FIGURE 9–21

on elbows to supine on elbows. When manual contacts are positioned on the pelvis, the resistance provided is minimal and additional sensory cues such as verbal input must be provided.

Sitting—Supine. Following a transfer from the wheelchair to a raised mat or to bed, the patient must be able to move from the short sitting to the supine position. In short sitting, stability and controlled mobility procedures are performed to enhance balance in the posture and they follow a sequence that is similar to that performed in long sitting. To move to supine, the lower extremities must be lifted onto the mat. This may be accomplished by placing one arm under one or both lower extremities, followed by a pivoting motion on that elbow and rolling to supine. The patient flexes the lower extremities with the arm that is hooked under the thighs and rotates the trunk around to supine by moving the dynamic limb.

The sequence of procedures presented in the initial, middle, and advanced stages has been designed to enhance the patient's functional ability to transfer, dress, and perform other ADL. These long-range goals have been achieved by progressing through stages of motor control in the sidelying, prone, supine, and sitting positions.

MAT PROCEDURES FOR THE PATIENT WITH PARAPLEGIA

As with the progression of procedures presented for the patient with quadriplegia, the procedures for the patient with paraplegia are divided into three levels. The divisions for the paraplegic patient are determined by level of lesion. Exercises appropriate for patients with the common levels of disability—T_{10}, L_{1-2}, and L_{4-5}—are presented. The progressions are sequential. Many patients, however, are able to perform at more advanced levels than anticipated by the level of lesion. Patients with lower level lesions need procedures that will develop the trunk control required for ambulation in addition to procedures that will strengthen specific lower extremity muscles. Some of the procedures may have to be modified if external trunk support limits trunk and hip flexibility.

■ Initial Procedures for All Paraplegics

These procedures are designed to:

1. Increase the strength of the trunk musculature
2. Improve stability and controlled mobility of the lower trunk
3. Improve ADL

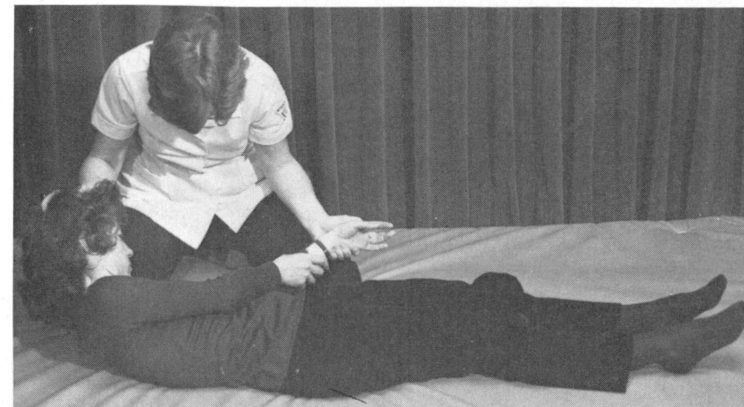

A. Supine chop.
T. SRH with TE.
E. MC head and wrist.

FIGURE 9–22

The patient with a T_{10} lesion is not expected to be a functional ambulator. Many young patients will want to attempt ambulation, however, and it may be appropriate as an exercise. Highly motivated patients with good strength and body proportions may be semifunctional ambulators on flat surfaces.

Strengthening of the trunk musculature is promoted by using overflow from the stronger upper extremity and upper trunk musculature. Abdominals can be strengthened with the upper trunk chopping pattern in supine, long sitting, or short sitting with the technique of TE (11) (Figure 9–22). In long sitting, as the abdominals are resisted through range, the mobility in the low back and hamstring muscles is maintained. The upper trunk lifting pattern performed in supine, sitting, and prone can strengthen the back extensors (Figure 9–23). When performing the trunk patterns in sitting, bal-

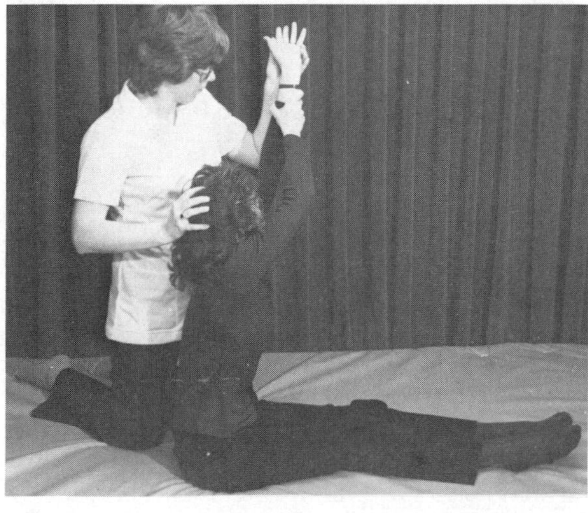

A. Long sitting: lifting pattern.
T. RS.
E. MC head and wrist.

FIGURE 9–23

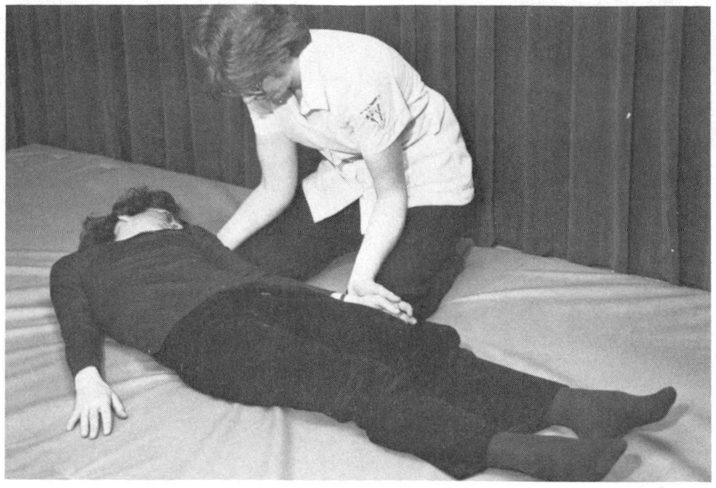

A. Supine: quadratus pattern.
T. TE.
E. MC scapula and arm.

FIGURE 9–24

ance in the posture is promoted. Altering the posture in which the chop and lift are performed will alter the resistance of gravity. The greatest demands are placed on the trunk musculature during the chop in supine and the lift in prone.

The quadratus lumborum and latissimus dorsi can be strengthened by positioning one upper extremity in the shortened range of D_1E and by resisting trunk extension, lateral flexion, and rotation (15). The technique of TE is performed by locking in the arm and upper trunk extensors, and pivoting the lower trunk movement (Figure 9–24). The activity of the hip hikers is enhanced first in this quadratus pattern, which leads from the patient's strength, before promoting hiphiking in supine or in the functional standing position.

Sidelying is another posture in which stability and strengthening of the trunk musculature can be promoted. Overflow from the stronger upper trunk musculature can be enhanced by the techniques of AI, RS, RC, and TE.

Prone procedures may begin with prone on elbows activities to teach the patient how to stabilize and shift weight in a weight-bearing position. Because the upper extremities and upper trunk should be of good to normal strength, the patient should quickly progress to quadruped, where again stability and controlled mobility techniques are applied. Weight shifting through increments of range may be performed in all directions. Lifting one upper extremity will help to improve the balance control in the static limbs and trunk (Figure 9–25). Push-ups in quadruped or in prone will further strengthen the upper extremities that will be needed for ambulation and strenuous wheelchair activities.

Sitting activities may begin with both upper extremities providing trunk support. Arm support is gradually reduced until the patient can balance

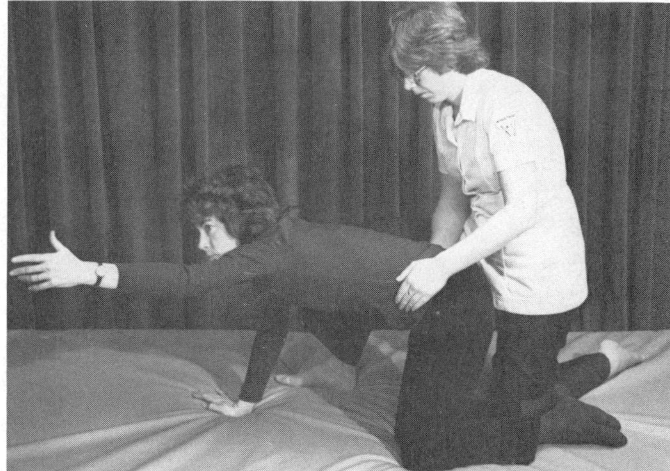

A. Quadruped: static-dynamic.
T. AI.
E. MC pelvis.

FIGURE 9–25

without upper extremity assistance. Because of the larger B of S, long sitting should be easier for the patient than short sitting. Therefore, balance will be improved in the less stressful long-sitting position before progressing to short sitting. As with all postures, the levels of motor control to be attained range from stability through skill. The skill level is the functional goal at which the arms are freed to manipulate the environment and perform ADL.

In long or short sitting, pelvic lifts or elevation may be performed to improve transfer ability. As described under the quadriplegic section, stability and controlled mobility techniques are applied to a lift position with manual contacts on the pelvis. Treatment of the paraplegic patient can include a greater amount of resistance and a wider range of weight shifting. Manual contacts can be positioned on the feet as the patient learns to balance and move the pelvis without the assistance of the proximal tactile input. The patient learns to move the lower extremities by moving the trunk. As the procedure is made more difficult by the distal placement of manual contacts, the stability and controlled mobility techniques may need to be repeated.

Standing procedures are initiated in the parallel bars with the arms assisting with support anteriorly, posteriorly, and then laterally to the hips. Stability techniques using manual contacts on the scapulae, scapula-pelvis, and pelvis will enhance maintenance of the standing posture (Figure 9–26). Weight shifting through increments of range in all directions will promote balance. One upper extremity can be lifted, then both can be raised as the patient attempts to maintain the balance point without assistance. With the upper extremities on the parallel bars, the patient lifts the lower extremities from the floor while stability and controlled mobility techniques are applied at the pelvis (Figure 9–27). Once lower trunk control is established by the preceding procedures, the patient is ready to begin walking with assistance as necessary. After ambulating with the support of parallel bars, the patient

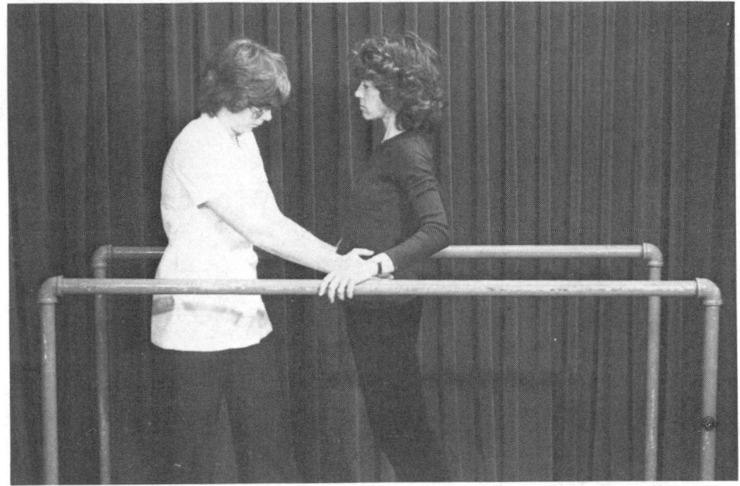

A. Standing in parallel bars.
T. RS.
E. MC pelvis.

FIGURE 9–26

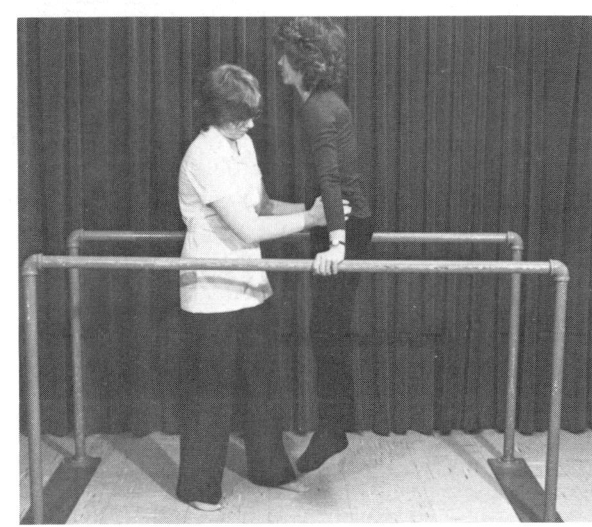

A. Standing in parallel bars: LE lifted.
T. RS.
E. MC scapulae.

FIGURE 9–27

progresses to one forearm crutch and one parallel bar, then to both forearm crutches. After support from the assistive devices has been reduced, stability and controlled mobility procedures can be repeated to enhance balance and confidence. A patient with this level of lesion may be capable of performing a swing to or swing through gait. If ambulation is to be functional, falling and coming to standing from prone also are practiced.

Other functional activities that may be achieved at this level include transferring independently to a car, maneuvering the wheelchair in and out of the car, and independent dressing.

Selected Procedures for a High Lumbar Lesion

The patient with an L_{1-2} level of injury should be able to perform all the procedures in the initial progression. All the trunk muscles are innervated and partial innervation of the hip flexors and quadriceps is present. Procedures at this level are selected to further strengthen the lower trunk and innervated lower extremity muscles. Ambulation should be more functional and a four-point gait pattern possible.

In sidelying, lower trunk rotation is performed with the strengthening technique of TE to increase the activity of the lower abdominals and back extensors. In this gravity-eliminated position, forward pelvic rotation is coupled with manually resisted hip flexion and knee extension (Figure 9–28).

In long sitting, lower trunk control is further challenged by resisting movements with manual contacts on the ankles. Push-up blocks may be used to simulate the upper extremity control required during crutch walking (11) (Figure 9–29). The patient must be able to get into the wheelchair from

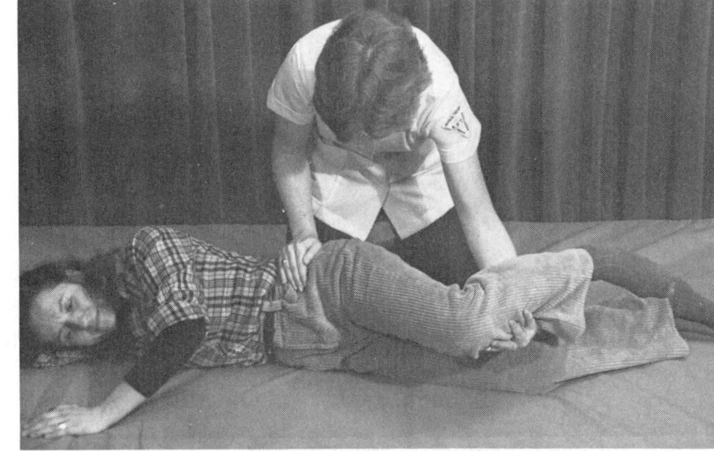

A. Sidelying: lower trunk forward rotation hip flexion.
T. TE.
E. MC pelvis and thigh.

FIGURE 9–28

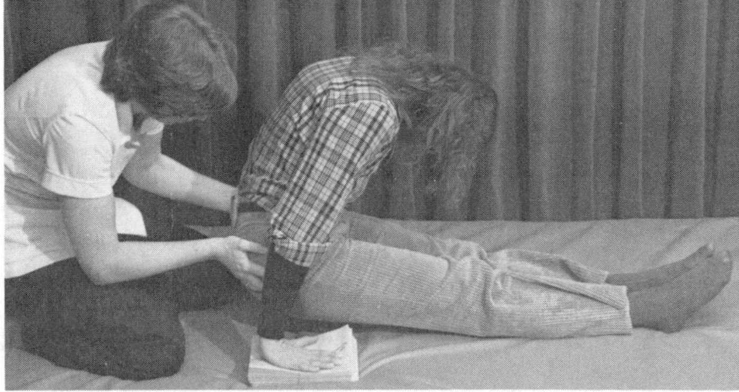

A. Long sitting: lift with push-up blocks.
T. RS.
E. MC pelvis.

FIGURE 9–29

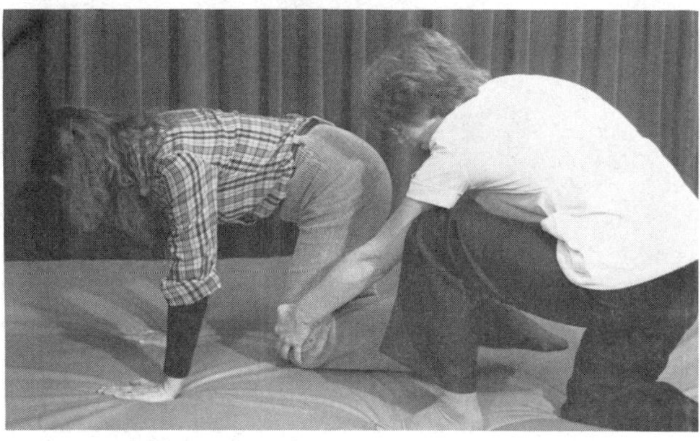

A. Quadruped: D_1F knee flexion.
T. TE.
E. MC thigh and foot.

FIGURE 9–30

the floor. In long sitting, lifting movements are practiced to assist the movement into the wheelchair.

Quadruped is also appropriate at this stage. Lower trunk stability and controlled mobility procedures will improve abdominal and hip flexor control. If the patient can maintain a unilateral weight-bearing position, the hip flexors of the dynamic limb can be resisted in a gravity-assisted position (Figure 9–30).

Ambulation activities in the parallel bars emphasize lower trunk rotation and hip flexion in preparation for a four-point gait. Because ambulation is a functional goal, more of the treatment session is now devoted to this activity.

■ Selected Procedures for a Low Lumbar Lesion

The patient with a low lumbar lesion, L_{4-5}, will have innervation of more lower extremity muscles than the previously described patients. The patient may have a combination of upper motor neuron and lower motor neuron dysfunction, depending on the site of the lesion (16). The evaluation may reveal motor and sensory loss that is indicative of a specific level of injury or of a more spotty nerve lesion.

Specific patterns can be used to enhance overflow from stronger to weaker muscles. A treatment plan similar to that described at the beginning of this chapter for strengthening upper extremity muscles for the quadriplegic patient can be designed. The innervated muscles and their grades of strength are first arranged into the patterns in which they optimally function—for example, the iliopsoas and anterior tibial are most active in D_1F, the gluteus maximus and posterior tibial in D_2E (11). The activity of the knee musculature will depend on the movement at the knee.

After assessing which muscles need to be strengthened and which can be used for overflow, the therapist can design the treatment program. Because motor and sensory loss is variable, general treatment guidelines rather than specific examples will be presented in this section.

Stages of Motor Control

Mobility—To Initiate Movement.

A. The diagonal pattern in which the weakened muscle optimally contracts is determined. To optimize overflow from other muscles, resistance to trunk and bilateral patterns is appropriate. During unilateral patterns, overflow occurs primarily from within the limb. A mass movement pattern is usually chosen to enhance activity, unless specific weaknesses indicate the use of another combination. A gravity-assisted or eliminated posture may be necessary so that manual resistance can be applied. The range of initiation and of emphasis is determined by the muscle composition and its function. A weakened muscle that is primarily tonic should neither be kept in the lengthened range for a prolonged period of time nor resisted maximally. A primarily phasic muscle may respond favorably to repeated quick stretch in lengthened ranges. To illustrate these principles, a weakened gluteus medius should be initially exercised in the supine position, where gravity will not resist the movement. A trunk extensor pattern or BS D_1E may be used to enhance overflow from the trunk muscles and the contralateral limb to the weakened muscle (15). Application of a unilateral D_1E with knee extension pattern may be appropriate if the quadriceps is of sufficient strength to increase gluteus medius activity. Because the gluteus medius functions as a postural extensor, the shortened range of the movement would be emphasized during beginning treatment sessions (17).

T. The techniques at the mobility stage should be chosen to emphasize the initiation of movement. HRAM or RC with repeated stretches in the lengthened range may accomplish that goal. Tonic and phasic muscles may respond differently. The gluteus medius, for example, may respond best to HRAM because in this technique the muscle contraction is initiated in the shortened range and the lengthened range is not maintained. If, however, HRAM does not produce the desired initiation of movement, repeated stretches in the lengthened range may be the only way to elicit a contraction. The order of the techniques should be reversed when a primarily phasic muscle is the focus of treatment. RC may be more appropriate with phasic muscles as both the lengthened range and the quick stretches are facilitatory to the muscle.

E. Sensory input is used to augment the initiation of the muscle contraction. Depending on the areas of intact sensory function, vibration, icing, tapping, and light touch may be indicated in addition to the quick stretch and resistance already mentioned.

Stability.

A. The tonic holding stage of stability is most critical for those muscles acting as postural extensors. To accomplish tonic holding, the posture is altered so that gravity is eliminated or assisting the contraction before it is used as a resistive force. Cocontraction follows tonic holding. The posture may be altered to add body weight as a resistive force and place a tonic muscle on prolonged stretch. The shortened range of the D_1E pattern, for example, would put the gluteus medius in the range at which tonic holding is best enhanced. Cocontraction may be promoted in the weight-bearing postures of bridging, quadruped, modified plantigrade and standing. In these postures, weight bearing and stretch combine to produce cocontraction.

T. SHRC will best facilitate tonic holding and AI and RS will lead to cocontraction.

E. Approximation, brushing, vibration, and maintained manual contacts may be chosen to enhance isometric contractions.

Controlled Mobility.

A. The same weight-bearing postures used to enhance the stability level of control may be appropriate to improve controlled mobility in the posture. Weight shifting occurs initially through a small arc of range that is gradually increased as balance and control are gained. Movements in the postures may be chosen to promote functional patterns such as the pelvic motions needed during ambulation. During static-dynamic activities, one limb is lifted from the supporting surface and is free to move in any direction. The remaining weight-bearing limbs support the body weight and maintain the C of G within the B of S. As the dynamic limb moves through greater ranges and is resisted, the challenge to the static or stabilizing limbs is increased.

T. SR or SRH through increments of range is most appropriate to enhance weight shifting. Eccentric control needed during ambulation may be promoted with AR. When static-dynamic activities are first performed, the focus of treatment may be on increasing the static control of the stabilizing limbs with AI and RS. Later, when proximal dynamic stability is the goal, the techniques of SR or SRH may be added to the dynamic limb.

E. Manual contacts can be placed directly on the body part that needs control. With stretch and resistance, manual contacts may also be applied to the dynamic limb to directly strengthen that limb or indirectly enhance proximal dynamic stability of the static limbs. Additional sensory inputs of vibration, approximation, quick stretch, and icing applied to either the static or dynamic limbs may enhance the controlled movements desired at this stage.

Skill.

A. Ambulation is the functional movement emphasized with these patients. The proper timing and sequencing of movement is essential. Unilateral leg patterns performed in sitting, supine, or prone may be used to improve the timing of movement. Control of advanced functional patterns are a goal at this stage. Deliberate ambulation can be promoted in all directions: forward, backward, sideward, and in a diagonal direction. Braiding may enhance lower trunk rotation. Ascending and descending stairs are also included.

T. RP will enhance ambulation activities. During unilateral patterns, NT will improve the proper sequencing of movement and AR the eccentric control needed during free movement.

E. Sensory input is progressively withdrawn during this stage because it is no longer needed for control.

Strengthening. The need for strengthening procedures is determined by assessment of the patient's ability to perform certain movements and also by the results of an MMT and other strength and functional evaluations. Strengthening procedures are used throughout the course of rehabilitation to reinforce motor control.

A. The postures chosen are those having a large B of S and low C of G so that the patient's effort and attention can be focused on the movement. The combinations of patterns are selected to optimize overflow from stronger areas. Other considerations are similar to those discussed in the mobility stage.

T. The application of the strengthening techniques of RC or TE will enhance the performance of a movement pattern or the activity of a specific muscle.

E. Vibration, icing, appropriate manual contacts, visual and verbal cues, and any other input that would further activate muscles are appropriate.

In conclusion, in addition to therapeutic exercise, the physical therapist may be called upon to order all necessary equipment, perform a home assessment, and to suggest appropriate environmental changes.

The physical therapist is only one important member of the rehabilitation team, however. Under the management of the physician, other health professionals are primarily responsible for bowel and bladder training, maintenance of skin integrity, assistance with ADL, fabrications of orthotic devices, and for helping the patient to adjust to the abrupt, traumatic, and permanent change in life style, as well as to cope with the tremendous financial burden that can result from the disability.

REFERENCES

1. Bitter J: Introduction to Rehabilitation. St Louis, CV Mosby, 1979
2. Pierce DS, Nickel VH: The Total Care of Spinal Cord Injuries. Boston, Little, Brown & Co, 1977
3. Frownfelter DL: Chest Physical Therapy and Pulmonary Rehabilitation. Chicago, Year Book Medical, 1978
4. Chusid JG, McDonald JJ: Correlative Neuroanatomy and Functional Neurology, ed 17. Los Altos, CA, Lange Medical, 1979
5. Schoening HA: Neurogenic bowel and bladder. In Krusen FH, Kottke FJ, Ellwood PM(eds): Handbook of Physical Medicine and Rehabilitation. Philadelphia, WB Saunders Co, 1965
6. Bishop B: Neurophysiology of spasticity: Classical concepts. Phys Ther 57:371–376, 1977
7. Jacobs EM, Denault PM: Neurology for Nurses. Springfield, IL, Charles C Thomas, 1964
8. Goodhart RS, Shills ME(eds): Modern Nutrition in Health and Disease, ed 6. Philadelphia, Lea and Febiger, 1980
9. Stewart TD: Psychotherapy and physical therapy common grounds. Phys Ther 57:279–283, 1977
10. Trombly CA, Scott AD: Occupational Therapy for Physical Dysfunction. Baltimore, Wilkins & Wilkins, 1977
11. Knott M, Voss DE: Proprioceptive Neuromuscular Facilitation, ed 2. New York, Harper & Row, 1968
12. Portney LG, Sullivan PE: EMG Analysis of Ipsilateral and Contralateral Shoulder and Elbow Muscles during the Performance of PNF Patterns. Read at the Annual Conference of the Society for Behavioral Kinesiology, Boston, 1979
13. Sullivan PE, Portney LG: Electromyographic activity of shoulder muscles during unilateral upper extremity proprioceptive neuromuscular facilitation patterns. Phys Ther 60:283–288, 1980

14. Long C, Lawton EB: Functional significance of spinal cord lesion level. Arch Phys Med Rehabil 36:249–255, 1955

15. Knott M: Proprioceptive neuromuscular facilitation. Unpublished notes from Vallejo, CA, 1970

16. Pryse-Phillips W, Murray TJ: Essential Neurology. Garden City, NY, Medical Examination Publishing Co, 1978

17. Stockmeyer SA: Analysis of procedures to improve motor control. Unpublished notes from Boston University PT 710, 1979

PART III

TREATMENT OF PATIENTS WITH SELECTED ORTHOPEDIC DISABILITIES

chapter 10

Shoulder

INTRODUCTION

Shoulder disability can result from disease, inflammation, or injury to both contractile and noncontractile tissues of the shoulder complex. The affected structures may include joints, ligaments, capsules, bursae, tendons, and muscles. Humeral fractures, prolonged immobilization, referred pain from thoracic or cervical conditions, hemiplegia, and quadriplegia are some conditions that may result in secondary shoulder dysfunction (1–5). A careful evaluation will help to determine the exact etiology and actual structures involved.

EVALUATION

An evaluation of shoulder dysfunction will usually include, but is not limited to, the areas of assessment that are mentioned and discussed within this section.

History. Knowledge of the onset of the disability will help the therapist to determine which tissues are involved. The patient may relate a twisting or pulling injury affecting the rotator cuff, or a fall resulting in a tearing or snapping of tissues that may have affected, for example, the biceps tendon. In contrast, the onset may be idiopathic with a gradual or acute occurrence of symptoms. Immobilization or surgery may have been indicated if the joint integrity was disrupted. Reports of limitations in ADL are indicative of functional loss of range and strength.

Observation. The observation of gait and other activities, such as sitting and disrobing, will indicate the extent to which the upper extremity automatically participates during such movements.

Pain. Pain is a common symptom accompanying shoulder dysfunction. Careful questioning, observation, and examination will help to determine the exact origin (2–4). The localization of pain may implicate one specific area of involvement, such as the biceps tendon; the patient's description of more generalized pain may be indicative of involvement of the entire glenohumeral area. Pain may be present when the patient is at rest, it may be aggravated by specific movements such as external rotation, or it may occur when objects are lifted and the result is a traction force to the joint. The extent to which pain interferes with daily functioning should be assessed.

Sensation. Sensory testing along dermatomal levels may indicate cervical involvement, a more distal nerve impingement, or compression, as may occur in the case of thoracic outlet syndrome (4,6). Areas of hypersensitivity and localized inflammation may be common.

ROM. Range of motion of the cervical area is performed to rule out any involvement of this region (4,8). The duplication of shoulder pain upon movements of the head and neck may indicate a dysfunction of cervical origin. Osteokinematic and arthrokinematic motions of all the joints in the shoulder girdle should be evaluated, since they all function in harmony to produce full shoulder motion (2,3,7–9). Anatomical ranges are assessed both actively and passively to detect causes of limitation and the ability of muscle(s) to move a limb through an arc of movement. Pain on any motion should be noted.

Strength. Muscle strength can be evaluated both in the classical test positions and with the shoulder in a neutral pain-free position. If an isometric contraction elicits pain, contractile tissues are implicated (3).

During the evaluation of both ROM and muscle strength, the quality of movement should be noted. The scapula, for example, may frequently rotate upwardly at the initiation of shoulder flexion, rather than perform its normal stabilizing function before moving to complement the humeral motion (10,11). Lateral flexion of the trunk often may be substituted for shoulder motion. These two abnormalities of movement are commonly seen with capsular tightness at the glenohumeral joint or with weakness of the rotator cuff musculature.

Medical History. Shoulder pain and dysfunction can be referred or can be caused by medical conditions distant from the shoulder, such as cardiac, pulmonary, or gall bladder involvement (12).

SPECIAL TREATMENT CONSIDERATIONS

The myotome corresponds with the dermatome to the shoulder (13). The similar sensory and motor innervation by C_5 may make the use of various pain relieving modalities such as transcutaneous nerve stimulation and brushing more effective (14–15).

Normal shoulder function depends both on full joint mobility and the inherent muscular stability. Mobility implies full pain-free range at the four joints forming the shoulder girdle. Stability is provided by the scapula and rotator cuff musculature. Initial treatment procedures will emphasize these two aspects of control as preliminary stages to the dynamic stability needed for skilled function.

The shoulder ranges that are most commonly limited are external rotation, abduction, and flexion (4), which are component movements of D_2F (16). To promote passive and active range movement into the D_2F pattern is the ultimate goal of treatment. Before progressing to the D_2F pattern, all stages of motor control should initially be promoted in the D_1F pattern for the following reasons:

- The D_1F pattern requires movement into two of the usually limited motions, external rotation and flexion. However, the ranges of these movements which occur in D_1F are less than the more complete range that occurs in D_2F.
- Because the shoulder is adducting during D_1F, there may be less tendency for the greater tubercle to abut the acromium. In order for complete shoulder flexion to occur during D_2F, the humerus rotates externally and the humeral head must be maintained in a proper position in the glenoid fossa. Dysfunction of the rotator cuff musculature may result in both reduced external rotation and humeral depression (4,9,11), and make D_2F a difficult movement to accomplish. Activity of the rotator cuff is therefore initiated in D_1F before advancing to D_2F.

Following an anterior shoulder dislocation, which is either conservatively or surgically treated, the shoulder movements of abduction and external rotation are usually contraindicated (5). For these patients, then, movement into D_2F usually does not proceed beyond 90 degrees of shoulder flexion so that the involved structures are not overstressed.

TREATMENT PLAN

Treatment is divided into two stages. The initial stage emphasizes the first three levels of motor control: mobility, stability, and controlled mobility, while the advanced stage stresses procedures appropriate for the skill level of control (17).

Initial Stage

The goals of the initial stage are to:

1. Decrease pain
2. Increase ROM—the mobility level of control
3. Promote stability and controlled mobility in weight-bearing postures

Decrease Pain. The assessment of the cause of pain will help the therapist determine the appropriate means to relieve that pain. Various thermal modalities may be indicated for their beneficial physiological effects. As mentioned earlier, both TNS and brushing may be effective in decreasing pain and may be applied prior to or in conjunction with other therapeutic procedures. Pain may result both in a generalized increase in tension and in localized splinting of the musculature around the shoulder. Deep-breathing exercises and other stimuli such as neutral warmth may be appropriately used at the beginning of treatment to promote generalized relaxation (18).

An indirect approach to reduce localized splinting may prove effective if direct attention to the parts results in an increased perception of pain (19). Indirect procedures include resistance to contralateral upper extremity motions (Figure 10–1) and resisted isometric contractions of the involved limb with manual contacts positioned distally on the forearm or hand (Figure 10–2). These procedures will facilitate isometric contractions of the involved shoulder muscles without having the patient focus on those areas (20). The alternating isometric contractions caused by these indirect procedures may result in a localized increase in circulation. The tendency to hold the scapula elevated can be reduced by the relaxation techniques of RS and HR applied to scapula patterns, which will also indirectly promote isometric contractions of the shoulder musculature (Figure 10–3).

Increase ROM—the Mobility Level of Control. When generalized tension and local splinting have been reduced, mobility of the involved struc-

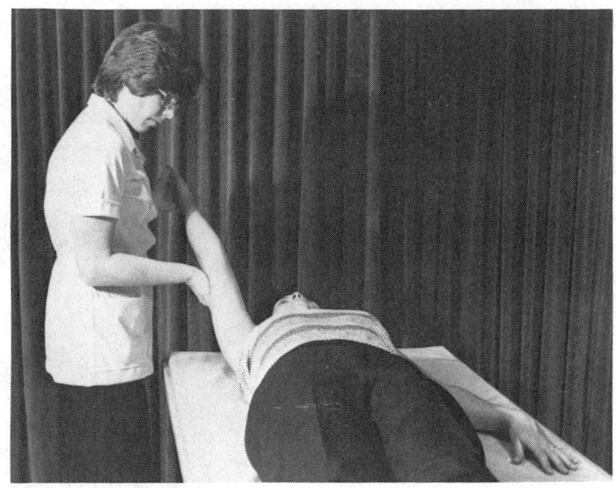

A. Supine: D_2F uninvolved extemity (R).
T. SRH.
E. MC arm and hand.

FIGURE 10–1

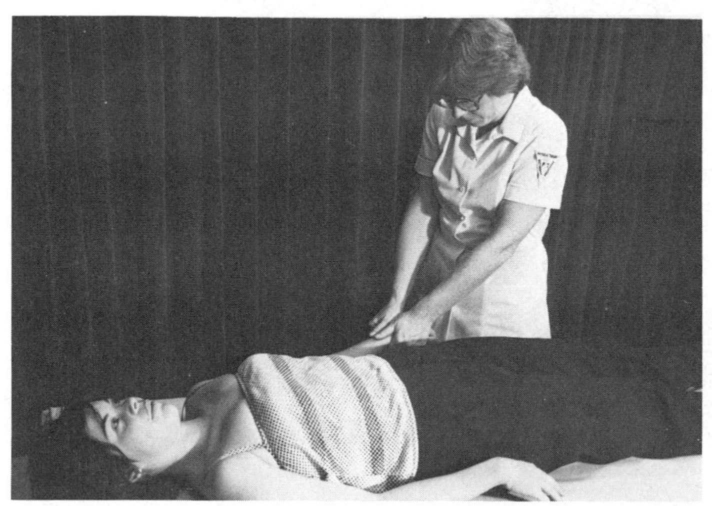

A. Supine: D_1E involved limb (L).
T. RS.
E. MC forearm.

FIGURE 10–2

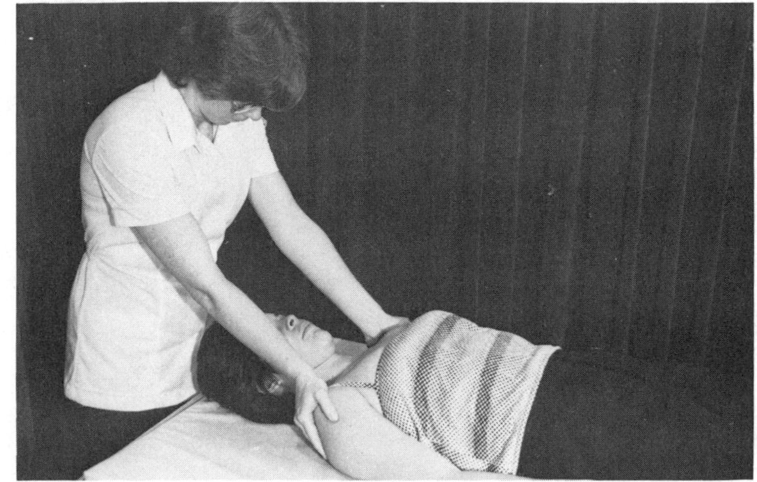

A. Supine: scapula movements.
T. RS.
E. MC scapula.

FIGURE 10–3

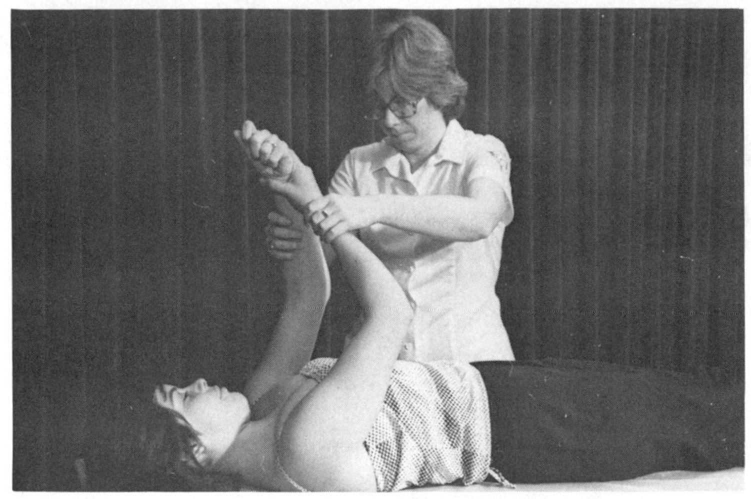

A. Supine: reverse chop.
T. HR.
E. MC forearms.

FIGURE 10–4

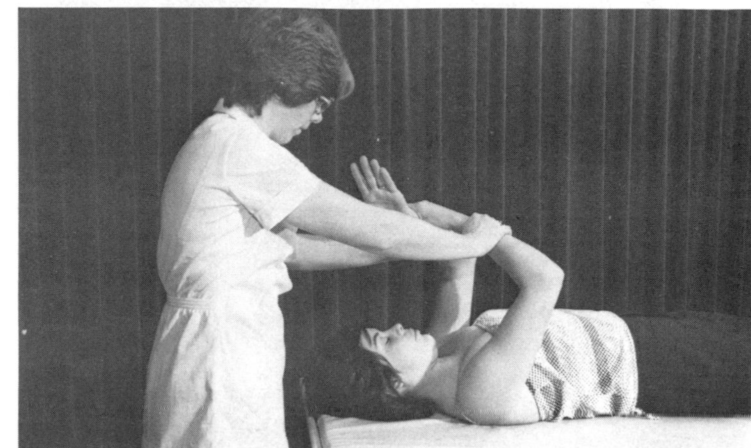

A. Supine: D_1 thrust assisted.
T. RS.
E. MC forearms.

FIGURE 10–5

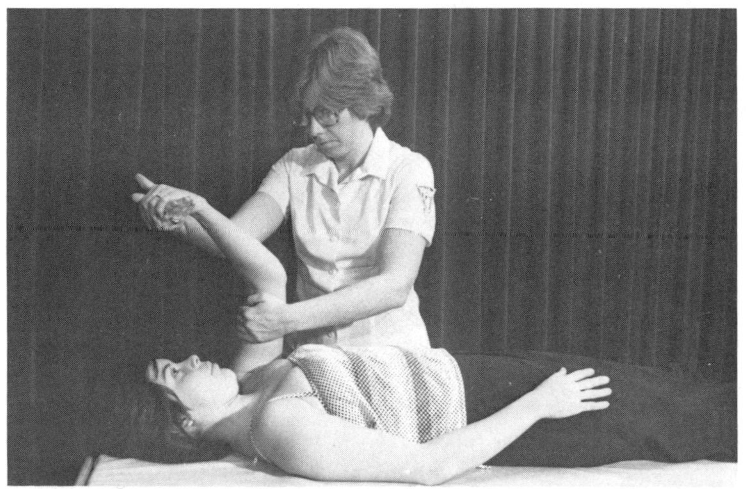

A. Supine: unilateral D_1F.
T. HR.
E. MC arm and hand.

FIGURE 10–6

tures can be initiated. Full range of shoulder motion depends on both muscle relaxation and free movement at all the joints. Joint mobilization of all hypomobile movements may be employed to increase range of the noncontractile structures. To improve arthrokinematic movement, appropriate tractions, glides, and spins are incorporated into the total treatment plan until complete pain-free joint range has been accomplished. A thorough description of the mobilization procedures are included in texts that deal with this specific aspect of treatment (2,3,8).

In conjunction with mobility of the noncontractile joint structures, full ROM of the contractile tissues of the shoulder joint may be achieved by the following procedures. The muscular mobility of the involved limb can first be promoted in the D_1F pattern with these activities: a reverse chop, a D_1 thrust with assistance of the uninvolved upper extremity, or a unilateral D_1F pattern. When pain interferes with movement, the reverse of the chop (Figure 10–4) or an assisted D_1 thrust (Figure 10–5) should precede a unilateral pattern (Figure 10–6). The patient will be better able to control the movement of the involved extremity with the uninvolved limb in either of these two activities. The relaxation techniques of RS and HR can be applied to these activities and may be most effective when pain is a factor (16). Muscular tension is gradually increased with both RS and HR and no joint motion occurs during the resisted phase of these techniques. After range has been increased in the D_1F pattern, full shoulder movement can be promoted in the D_2F pattern. D_2F can be initiated with a lifting (Figure 10–7) pattern that progresses to a unilateral D_2F pattern [Figures 10–8(a) and 10–8(b)] when assistance from the uninvolved extremity is no longer necessary. The relaxation technique of CR can be used with unilateral patterns to increase ROM, but only when increased muscle tension or rotational movements do not cause pain (16, 21).

To reiterate, the preceding procedures have been directed toward the goals of decreasing pain and increasing ROM. The relaxation techniques of RS, HR, and CR have been combined with movements in the D_1F then D_2F patterns.

Promote Stability and Controlled Mobility in Weight-Bearing Postures. Procedures to increase stability and controlled mobility can be overlapped with those just described for mobility. While range is being gained with mobility procedures, appropriate techniques can be initiated in weight-bearing postures to increase the activity of the scapula and shoulder muscles needed for stabilization in that gained range (22). The postures to be used in this sequence of activities are selected for their ability to gradually increase the amount of weight borne through the shoulder, and the range of shoulder movements. Progressing from the easiest to most difficult activities, the sequence of postures in which these two factors can be manipulated are: 1) sitting with upper extremity support or standing in the parallel bars, 2) modified plantigrade or prone on elbows, and 3) quadruped. The activity, technique, and element which make up the procedure can be combined in

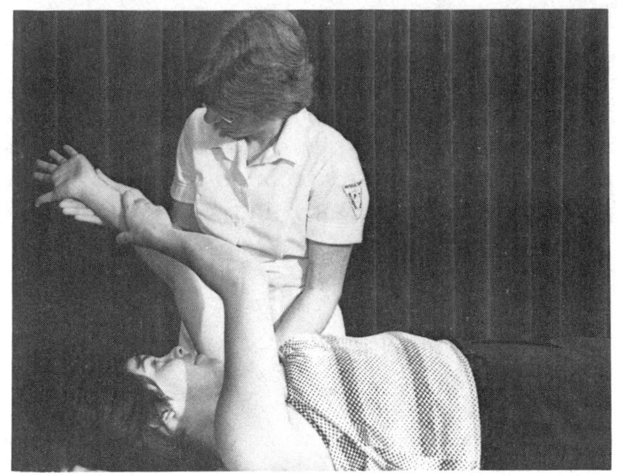

A. Supine: lifting.
T. HR.
E. MC scapula and forearm.

FIGURE 10–7

(a)

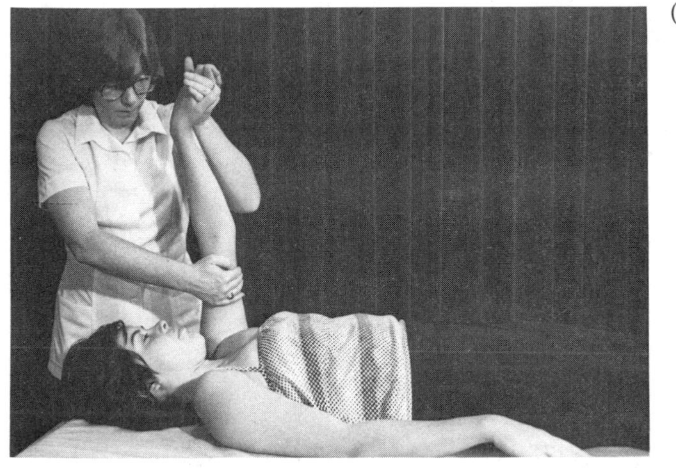

(b)

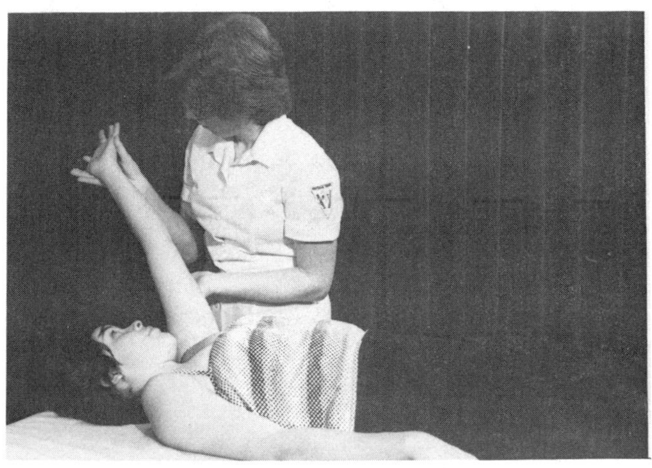

A. Supine: unilateral D_2F.
T. CR.
E. MC arm and hand.

FIGURE 10–8

many ways to gradually improve proximal control. As already discussed, the activity will progress toward increased weight bearing and shoulder motion; the techniques of AI or RS will promote stability followed by SRH through increments of range to improve controlled mobility. Manual contacts can be placed either directly or indirectly on the involved segment, and joint approximation may be applied to facilitate proximal muscular activity. Other elements such as brushing, vibration, or ice may improve the desired muscular contraction.

Sitting or Standing. The following specific procedures are sequenced in an appropriate order for the sitting or standing postures. When sitting or standing with arm support, the shoulder is positioned in the frequently pain-free range of neutral extension. Isometric contractions are promoted with the stability techniques of AI and RS. Activity of the rotator cuff musculature may be best emphasized with the technique of RS because of the rotational component inherent in that technique. Manual contacts can be positioned on the head and uninvolved shoulder as an indirect approach, or on both shoulders when a more direct approach is tolerated (Figure 10–9). Controlled mobility in sitting is gained by rocking through increments of range. The rocking movement will promote an increase in the proximal range of motion and in the amount of weight bearing on the involved shoulder. The direction of rocking can be anterior-posterior, lateral, and diagonal. These various directions will alter the movements at the shoulder and thus the muscular participation in the movement.

Modified Plantigrade. The next activity is modified plantigrade. The range of motion at the shoulder is 45–60 degrees of flexion, and compared to sitting or standing this activity is characterized by a greater amount of weight bearing through the upper extremity. The techniques of AI and RS

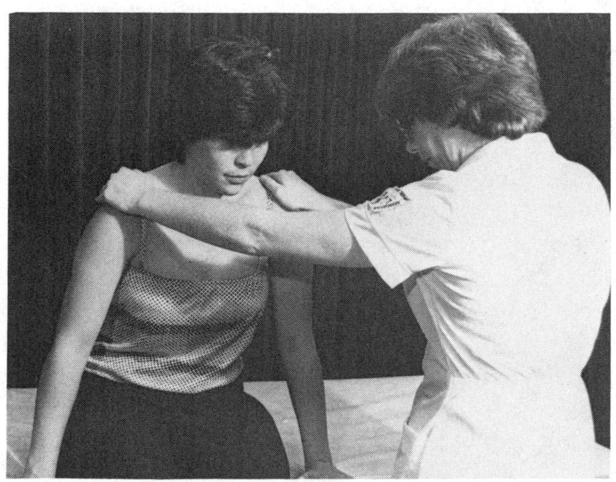

A. Sitting with arm support.
T. RS.
E. MC scapula.

FIGURE 10–9

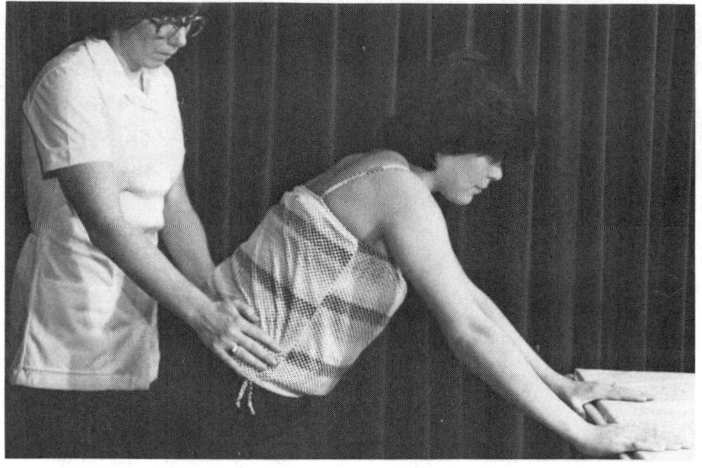

A. Modified plantigrade.
T. SRH.
E. MC pelvis.

FIGURE 10–10

are reapplied in this posture to improve the stability control of the proximal muscles in this increased range of shoulder flexion. Controlled mobility rocking motions should be performed first in the direction that promotes D_1 movements of the involved upper extremity, then in the D_2 direction (Figure 10–10). During the stability and controlled mobility procedures, manual contacts can be positioned on the scapula, the scapula and pelvis, or on both hips. When tolerated, static-dynamic activities in modified plantigrade will further increase the stability around the involved weight-bearing shoulder. To further enhance stability during the static-dynamic activities, one manual contact is positioned on the involved shoulder and applies approximation while the therapist's other arm resists the patient's dynamic limb. Because rocking in modified plantigrade is easy to perform and control, it is an excellent exercise to incorporate into a home program.

Quadruped. The most stressful of the weight-bearing postures for the shoulder is quadruped. An increased amount of weight bearing occurs through the upper extremity, compared to either the sitting or modified plantigrade postures. Control can be developed in the proximal scapula and shoulder muscles at about 90 degrees. The stability technique of RS with manual contacts on different proximal areas will improve isometric control. The controlled mobility technique of SRH will enhance the proximal dynamic stability in the 90-degree range. The therapist's manual contacts may be varied to alter the stress on the shoulder. To further improve this proximal control, static-dynamic activities can be used to increase the resistance of weight bearing on the involved limb (Figure 10–11). As more movement is performed by the dynamic uninvolved limb, a greater amount of dynamic stability is required of the involved static weight-bearing extremity promoting increased control. Movement within the 90-degree arc of range is fre-

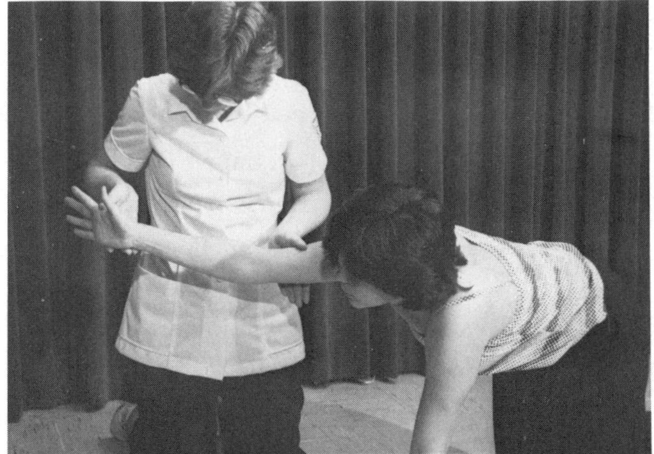

A. Quadruped: D_2F uninvolved limb (R).
T. Resisted movement.
E. MC arm and wrist.

FIGURE 10–11

quently problematic during skilled functional activities such as dressing or combing hair. Many patients substitute a scapula elevation for normal glenohumeral rhythm or use the contralateral limb to assist either concentric or eccentric movement at 90 degrees of flexion. In gravity-resisted positions such as sitting, the lever arm of the upper extremity is the longest at 90 degrees of shoulder flexion or abduction. Therefore, the greatest amount of activity of the scapula and rotator cuff and other shoulder muscles may be required in this range. The dynamic stability of these proximal muscles is essential for the normal timing of skilled movement through range and can be developed as stability and rocking or controlled mobility and static-dynamic procedures are performed in quadruped.

The overlapping of treatment procedures discussed in Chapter 6 can be clearly demonstrated during the progressions within the three postures of sitting, modified plantigrade, and quadruped. Within each posture, the techniques should be sequenced to promote the stages of motor control. When the patient has progressed to the more difficult technique of SRH in modified plantigrade, for example, initial stability control can be developed in quadruped, which is a more stressful posture for the upper extremity. As more advanced control is promoted in quadruped—such as controlled mobility and static-dynamic activities—the patient may be ready to begin initial procedures to develop the skill level of motor control.

In summary, the focus of the initial stage of treatment is to: 1) maintain or increase the **mobility** of all joints of the shoulder girdle by appropriately applying specific and general joint mobilizations and by improving the extendability of the contractile tissues with relaxation techniques; and 2) promote the **stability, controlled mobility,** and **static-dynamic** levels of control in postures that increase both weight bearing resistance and the range of shoulder motion.

Advanced Stage

The advanced stage of treatment for a patient with shoulder dysfunction has been designed to promote the following goals:

- Normal timing of skilled movement
- Dynamic strength of proximal muscles
- Normal functional combinations of movements

The normal timing of movement requires proximal musculature to provide dynamic stability while the distal segment moves in the environment to perform skilled activities (16,17). During the initial stage of treatment, dynamic stability was developed in weight-bearing postures with an approximation force facilitating proximal muscle activity. This proximal control is now used in functional, nonweight-bearing, skilled activities. The transition to this advanced level of control may be difficult for patients who still initiate movement proximally. Some patients—for example, those with a humeral fracture—may not be able to tolerate the compression forces of the weight-bearing postures previously described (22). For these patients, stability and controlled mobility levels of control are promoted in conjunction with extremity patterns until the most advanced normal timing techniques can be coupled with skilled movements.

Skilled activities include trunk, bilateral, and unilateral extremity patterns. This sequence of activities is the same as that used in the mobility stage of control: patterns involving both extremities are used before unilateral patterns. The focus in this advanced stage, however, is on controlled movement through range, and not on the attainment of ROM. For the shoulder muscles, trunk patterns produce the least amount of activity, whereas unilateral patterns demand the most control (23). Following the diagonal progression previously described, the involved limb will first perform movement in D_1 before progressing to D_2. The D_1 pattern of the involved limb can be promoted by the trunk combinations of a reverse chop and an assisted D_1 thrust (Figure 10–12). D_2F is inherent in the lifting pattern. When direct assistance from the contralateral limb is no longer required, the activity can progress from the trunk patterns just described to bilateral combinations. The bilateral combinations of patterns can be varied to facilitate all the proximal muscles of the involved limb. The bilateral patterns include symmetrical (Figure 10–13), reciprocal (Figure 10–14), asymmetrical and cross-diagonal (22,24). The combinations are chosen to promote the D_1F then the D_2F patterns activating at the scapula the serratus anterior and trapezius, and at the shoulder the anterior and middle portions of deltoid, respectively.

Techniques applied to the trunk and bilateral patterns will enhance different aspects of control. Stability or isometric control can be increased with the techniques of AI or RS. Although stability has been promoted in weight-bearing postures during the initial stage of treatment, isometric control in nonweight-bearing skill level activities may need to be improved. Con-

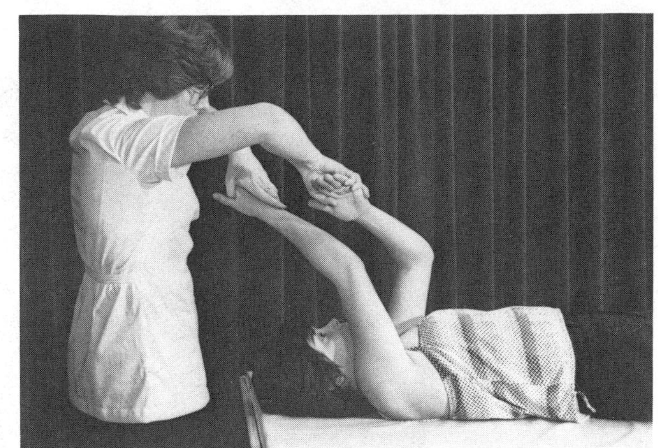

A. BS D_1 thrust.
T. TE.
E. MC wrists.

FIGURE 10–12

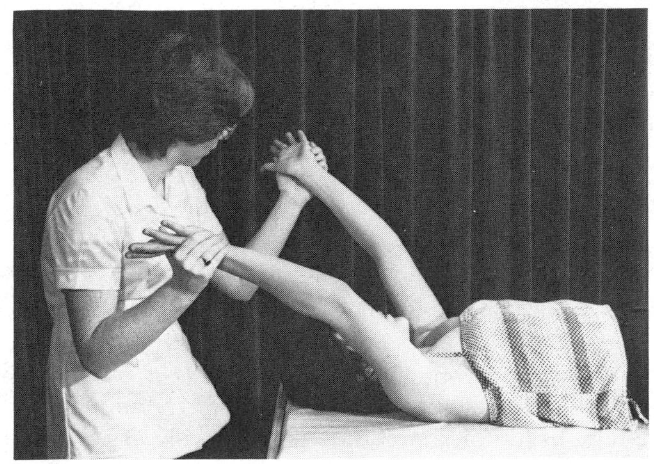

A. Supine: BS D_2F.
T. TE.
E. MC wrists.

FIGURE 10–13

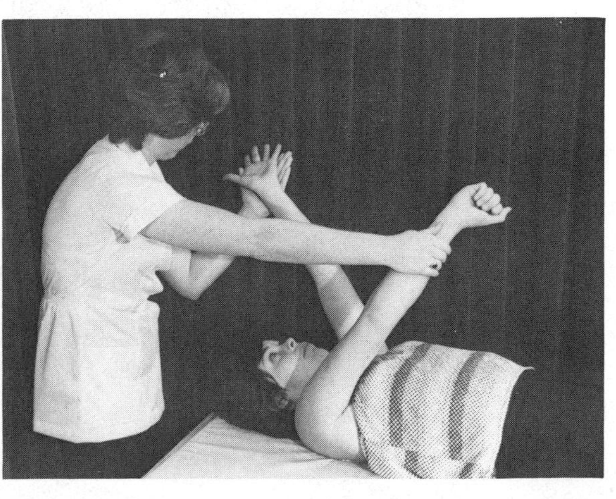

A. Supine: BR D_2.
T. TE.
E. MC wrists.

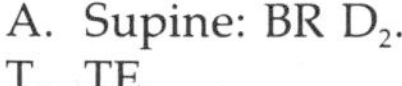

FIGURE 10–14

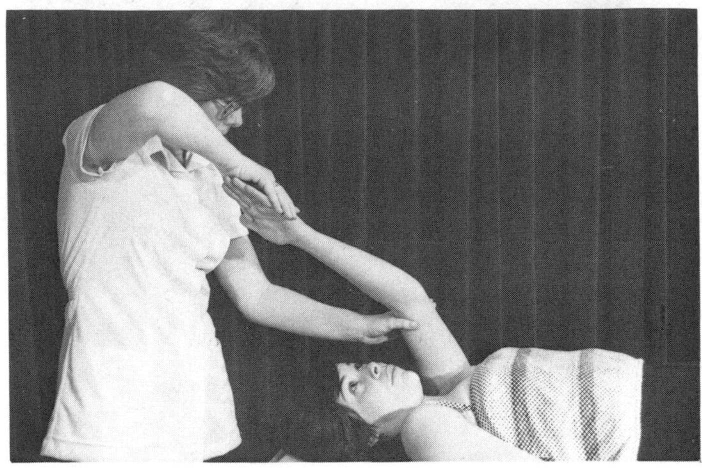

A. Supine: D_1 thrust.
T. SRH.
E. MC arm and hand.

FIGURE 10–15

trolled movement through the range is promoted by the technique of SRH. During the application of this technique weakness may be noted in a certain part of the range. If this occurs, the strengthening techniques of RC or TE would be appropriate.

Unilateral patterns may be the most difficult for the patient to perform, but because both manual contacts are positioned on the limb, the therapist will have optimal control of the movement pattern. As in the trunk and bilateral patterns, the techniques used in the unilateral patterns can promote stability, controlled mobility, and strengthening. In addition, techniques that promote eccentric control and normal timing can be easily applied to unilateral patterns. The elbow component can be varied by remaining straight, flexing, or extending during the pattern. These variations will change the amount of activity in the proximal muscles and will vary the ov-

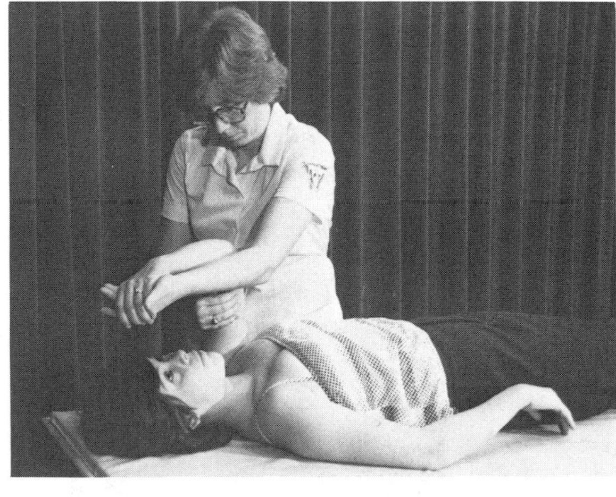

A. Supine: D_1F with elbow flexing.
T. TE.
E. MC arm and hand.

FIGURE 10–16

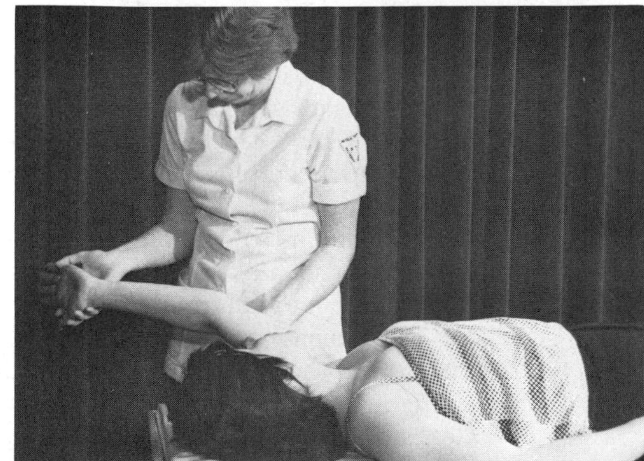

A. Supine: D_2F.
T. SRH.
E. MC arm and hand.

FIGURE 10–17

erflow activity from the more distal muscles (25) (Figures 10–15, 10–16, and 10–17). By performing the many possible combinations of patterns with the appropriate techniques, advanced skilled function and the most normal control can be promoted.

Trunk, bilateral, and unilateral patterns can be performed in supine and sitting. The supine position has the advantage of being a stable posture, so that all efforts can be directed toward the desired movement. In sitting, gravity will resist upward motions through full range and thereby alter the required muscular forces. The scapula may be less restricted by the supporting surface in sitting than in supine (Figure 10–18).

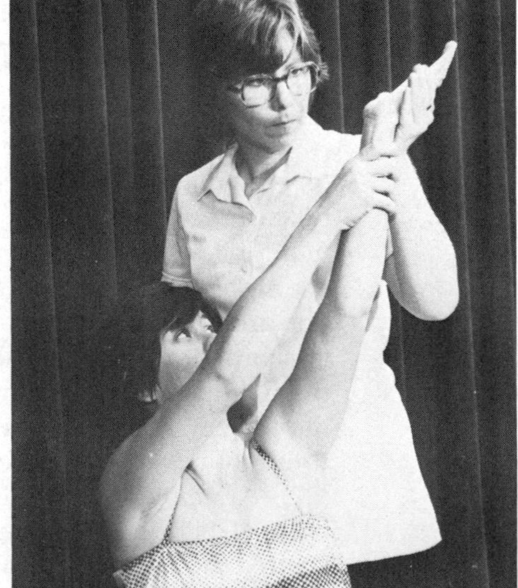

A. Sitting: lift.
T. SRH.
E. MC head and wrist.

FIGURE 10–18

Although prone is not an appropriate posture for bilateral patterns, unilateral patterns can be effectively performed. In this position, the hyperextension and internal rotation of the shoulder, important for some functional activities such as reaching behind the back, can be increased. Because manual contacts can be placed directly on the scapula, scapula control can be specifically emphasized during unilateral patterns in prone.

The elements of traction and approximation may be applied to the extremity patterns to enhance flexor or extensor musculature (16). Other sensory inputs such as vibration or icing may be indicated to promote specific aspects of motor control (see Chapter 5).

The ultimate goal for most patients with shoulder disability is the normal timing of skilled movements performed with sufficient range and strength to be functional. The procedures during the initial and advanced stages of treatment are all directed toward this goal.

HOME EXERCISE PROGRAM

The home exercise program should be designed to follow the sequence of motor control emphasized during treatment. The initial treatment focuses on increasing ROM. Appropriate home exercises for patients at this stage of recovery may include active scapula movements with the arm maintained in a relaxed position or supported with the other upper arm. Codman's exercises or other passive movements at the shoulder joint may also be effective in maintaining range.

The next phase of treatment promotes the stability and controlled mobility stages of control with the shoulder in increasing amounts of flexion. The easiest posture in which these can be accomplished at home is modified plantigrade with a table or back of a couch for support. Quadruped may be used as a progression if the patient's age and general physical condition allow him to attempt this position.

The advanced phase of treatment is aimed at developing the skill level of function. Trunk patterns may be easily performed at home and resisted by cuff weights, a pully, or weights placed in the hand. Cane exercises simulate bilateral patterns. Unilateral D_1 or D_2 patterns performed actively through range, rotation around a shoulder wheel, or climbing a finger ladder are skilled activities and as such are the most difficult movements for the patient to accomplish. Such exercises therefore should not be incorporated into a home program until the advanced stage of treatment. If such movements are performed before proximal control is developed, the substitute motions of scapula elevation or lateral trunk bending may be reinforced (22). Attempts by the patient to eliminate these abnormal motions by externally stabilizing the shoulder with the uninvolved upper extremity will only reduce the normal scapulohumeral rhythm.

Thermal applications for muscle relaxation, pain reduction, or enhancement of muscular activity that are effective during treatment may be applied by the patient preceding or following home exercise.

REFERENCES

1. Salter RB: Textbook of Disorders and Injuries of the Musculoskeletal System. Baltimore, Williams & Wilkins, 1970
2. Kaltenborn FM: Manual Therapy of the Extremity Joints, ed 2. Oslo, Olaf Norlis Bokhandel, 1976
3. Cyriax J: Textbooks of Orthopaedic Medicine. London, Cassell, 1970–1971
4. Cailliet R: Shoulder Pain. Philadelphia, F.A. Davis, Co, 1966
5. Quigley TB: Common musculoskeletal problems. In Srauss RH (ed): Sports Medicine and Physiology. Philadelphia, WB Saunders, 1979
6. Rosse C: The arm, forearm, and wrist. In Rosse C and Clawson DK(eds): The Musculoskeletal System in Health and Disease. New York, Harper & Row, 1980
7. Maitland GD: Peripheral Manipulation, ed 2. Boston, Butterworth, 1977
8. Mennell JMcM: Joint Pain: Diagnosis and Treatment Using Manipulative Techniques. Boston, Little, Brown & Co, 1964
9. Basmajian JV: Muscles Alive, ed 3. Baltimore, Williams & Wilkins, 1974
10. Inman VT, Saunders JB, Abbott LC: Observations on the function of the shoulder joint. J Bone Joint Surg 26:1, 1944
11. Brunnstrom S: Clinical Kinesiology. Philadelphia, FA Davis, 1962
12. Inman VT, Saunders JB: Referred pain from skeletal structures. J Nerv Ment Dis, 660, 1944
13. Chusid JG, McDonald JJ: Correlative Neuroanatomy, ed 17. Los Altos, CA, Lange Medical, 1979
14. Mannheimer JS: Electrode placements for transcutaneous electrical nerve stimulation. Phys Ther 58:1455–1462, 1978
15. Stockmeyer SA: Procedures for improvement of motor control. Unpublished notes from Boston University, PT 710, 1979
16. Knott M, Voss DE: Proprioceptive Neuromuscular Facilitation, ed 2. New York, Harper & Row, 1968
17. Stockmeyer SA: An interpretation of the approach of Rood to the treatment of neuromuscular dysfunction. Amer J Phys Med 46:950–956, 1966

18. Rood M: The use of sensory receptors to activate, facilitate, and inhibit motor response, automatic and somatic, in developmental sequence. In Sattely C(ed): Approaches to the Treatment of Patients with Neuromuscular Dysfunction. Dubuque, IA, WM C Brown, 1962
19. Voss DE, Knott M: The application of neuromuscular facilitation in the treatment of shoulder disabilities. Phys Ther Rev 33:10:536–541, 1953
20. Portney LG, Sullivan PE: EMG Analysis of Ipsilateral and Contralateral Shoulder and Elbow Muscles during the Performance of PNF Patterns. Read at the Annual Conference of the Society for Behavioral Kinesiology, Boston, 1979
21. Markos P: Ipsilateral and contralateral effects of PNF techniques on hip motion and EMG activity. 59:1366–1373, 1979
22. Voss DE: Therapeutic exercise. Unpublished notes from Northwestern University, 1974
23. Francis N: EMG Analysis of Unilateral and Bilateral PNF Patterns. Thesis. Boston, MA, Boston University Sargent College of Allied Health Professions, 1980
24. Knott M: Proprioceptive neuromuscular facilitation. Unpublished notes from Vallejo, CA, 1970
25. Sullivan PE, Portney LG: EMG activity of shoulder muscles during unilateral upper extremity PNF patterns. Phys Ther 60:283–288, 1980

chapter 11

Knee

INTRODUCTION

Disabilities of varying etiology can affect both the contractile and noncontractile structures of the knee. Knee problems can affect a wide age range of patients. Athletic injuries occur primarily in younger patients, while arthritic conditions are common in an older age group. The severity of the disability and the involvement of supporting structures will determine whether a surgical or conservative medical approach is indicated (1).

Nonsurgical conditions that are frequently referred for physical therapy include: 1) ligamentous and capsular sprain or stretch, 2) slight disruption of the meniscus, 3) chondromalacia, and 4) some arthritic conditions. Postsurgical referrals may be made for those patients with repair of ligamentous or capsular tears or avulsions, medial or lateral menisectomy, partial or complete patellectomy, "shaving" the undersurface of the patella, arthrotomy, partial or complete joint replacement, or relocation of the quadriceps tendon or other tendon relocations (1–3). Prior to surgery many of these patients are referred to therapy to improve quadriceps function.

Knee disability can also occur in patients who have had a fracture of the distal femur, the tibial plateau, or the shaft of the tibia. Knee function may be affected not only by fractures, but also by any condition that results in prolonged immobilization of the lower extremity.

GENERAL CONSIDERATIONS

Of major concern throughout the entire rehabilitative process of any knee problem is the maintenance or improvement of quadriceps control. The quadriceps, like most muscles, are composed of both tonic and phasic extrafusal muscle fibers (4). The tonic or slow twitch fibers have a low threshold to stimulation and do not easily fatigue (5–6). After prolonged immobilization however, these fibers tend to atrophy resulting in an inability of the quadriceps to sustain an isometric contraction in the shortened range (7). The initial focus of treatment in such cases is to enhance the isometric activity by facilitating a shortened held resisted contraction (SHRC) (8–9). Additional sensory input such as brushing or vibration may be appropriate to enhance the contraction (see Chapter 5). Prolonged stretch and heavy resistance to a quadriceps muscle that is unable to sustain a SHRC may result in inhibition (8, 10). Consequently, activities that incorporate these inhibitory elements should not be used as part of these initial procedures. As quadriceps control is gained, these two inhibitory factors can be gradually introduced into treatment.

As more people become involved in athletics, the incidence of chondromalacia may increase (11). Malalignment of the foot and ankle during standing, walking, or running may produce abnormal forces at the knee (12). Wedges or inserts in the shoe may be indicated, especially when abnormal wearing of the sole of the shoe or sneaker is noted. Malalignment and an imbalance in muscle pull may cause the patella to shift laterally during knee extension and may result in arthritic changes in the patellofemoral joint. Resisted movement through range may aggravate this condition. Increased control of the vastus medialis is usually indicated, and can be promoted by resisted isometric contractions in the shortened range of knee extension (13–14). With the knee maintained in extension, external rotation of the hip may increase the angle of pull of the vastus medialis. Once the balance between medial and lateral forces has been established, a neutral position of the patella during knee extension should result.

Patients who have undergone surgical repair of ligamentous and capsular structures may require prolonged immobilization. Tonic control of the quadriceps is therefore an important goal in initial treatment sessions. The introduction into treatment of procedures emphasizing increases in ROM depends on the extent of damage and degree of repair. Rotational motions of the knee are not indicated during the first stages of treatment following most ligamentous repairs. In addition to guarding against rotation, the patient should avoid medial-lateral stress following collateral ligament repair, and anterior-posterior forces following cruciate ligament or posterior capsular surgery. These movements may unduly stress already damaged structures (15–16).

EVALUATION

The specific evaluative tools used by the therapist will depend on the patient's condition at the time of referral. The following may be included:

History. The description of the problem may be obtained from both the medical record and from the patient. The disability may have been caused by a traumatic incident or may have had a gradually evolving course. If surgical repair was undertaken, the exact nature of the surgery is noted. The therapist should be aware of occupational and recreational activities, particularly repetitive stressful movements such as jogging. The extent to which ADL is limited is evaluated both by questioning and observation.

Sensation. A sensory evaluation should determine the presence of any pain or sensory loss. Pain may be localized to one area or may be diffuse. On palpation, the involved structures may be sensitive to touch or pressure. Pain in the knee can be referred from the hip. The presence of knee discomfort with no other positive findings in that area indicates that a careful evaluation of hip function should be included (2).

Range of Motion. Both passive and active hip, knee, and ankle ranges are compared with the uninvolved limb. Malalignment, laxity, or tightness at the hip and ankle joints may be the cause of the knee problem (17). If the limb has been immobilized, the involvement of these joints is possible. Passive range of the knee joint includes: patella mobility in a cephalocaudal and medial-lateral direction; movement of the tibia on the femur both ventrally and dorsally; mobility of the proximal talofibular joint. Tightness or laxity of ligamentous and capsular structures can be evaluated by these articulations. The Q angle should be calculated to determine the relationship of the tibia to the femur (18). Limitations in contractile and noncontractile structures can be differentiated by assessing both the arthrokinematic and passive and active osteokinematic motions (19–20).

Girth Measurements. The circumference of the leg can be measured at the knee and at various proximal and distal points to assess the presence of edema and atrophy.

Strength. The strength of the knee musculature can be assessed in many ways. Of major concern is the control of the quadriceps. Isometric holding in the shortened range is an indication of tonic holding. The lag that is frequently found may be due to decreased patella mobility or a lack of ability to activate a sufficient number of motor units to sustain the contraction in the shortened range. The strength of the quadriceps can also be assessed by the ability to maintain a weight-bearing position. Moving a mechanical device through range indicates tension development. Functional strength includes eccentric ability and the development of tension at a fast enough speed to walk at a normal pace or to run. The hamstring muscles may be weak but are often not as involved as the quadriceps. Assessment of the hamstrings is similar to that of the quadriceps. Strength in the lengthened range, however, is functionally more critical for hamstrings and must be evaluated.

Gait Evaluation. When the patient's condition allows, a gait evaluation is performed. Previously assessed problems such as a lack of ROM, pain, or reduced motor control may become evident in weight bearing, joint compression, or in free movement of the limb. Ascending and particularly descending stairs may be problematic.

Functional Activities. Assessment of ADL may reveal limitations in dressing, for example, in donning socks or shoes. The patient may also demonstrate difficulty with sitting, standing, or more strenuous activities.

TREATMENT PLAN

The application of various physical agent modalities to provide neutral warmth, heat, or cold may be appropriate. Depending on the desired physiological effects, modalities may be used preceding, during, or following exercise.

Pain is frequently a factor during initial treatments, especially in postsurgical patients. Elements such as prolonged ice may cause an anesthetic effect, while others, such as brushing, neutral warmth, and transcutaneous nerve stimulation (TNS) may be used to block the pain cycle (21). Procedures are always performed within the patient's pain tolerance to prevent further trauma to the tissues. An increase in pain is usually indicative of an increase in stress to either the inert or contractile tissues. If the pain threshold has been altered by the use of various modalities or other sensory input, extra caution must be taken during ROM and strengthening procedures to prevent trauma.

The exercise procedures are divided into three stages: initial, middle, and advanced. The goals presented at the beginning of each level indicate the focus of each progression.

Initial Stage

Procedures at this level will be directed primarily toward caring for the patient who has just undergone surgery. The goals of the initial stage are to:

- Facilitate quadriceps control so that a straight leg raise (SLR) can be performed
- Strengthen the trunk, upper extremities, and uninvolved lower extremity as needed
- Promote ambulation with appropriate weight bearing and use of assistive devices
- Increase ROM

Postsurgical pain and joint effusion may result in reflexive inhibition to the quadriceps (22). To promote quadriceps activity initially, an indirect approach that will facilitate overflow from intact, uninvolved areas to the quadriceps may be the most appropriate treatment. Quadriceps activity may be promoted indirectly by resistance to: the trunk patterns of a chop (Figure 11–1) or lift (23–25), an extensor pattern of the uninvolved lower extremity

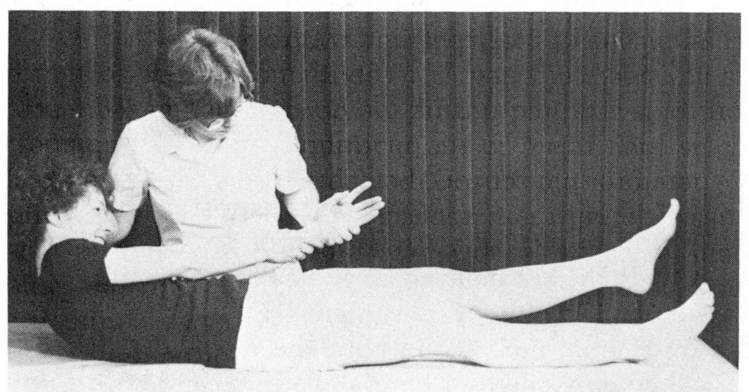

A. Supine: chop.
T. Holding in shortened range.
E. MC head and wrist.

FIGURE 11–1

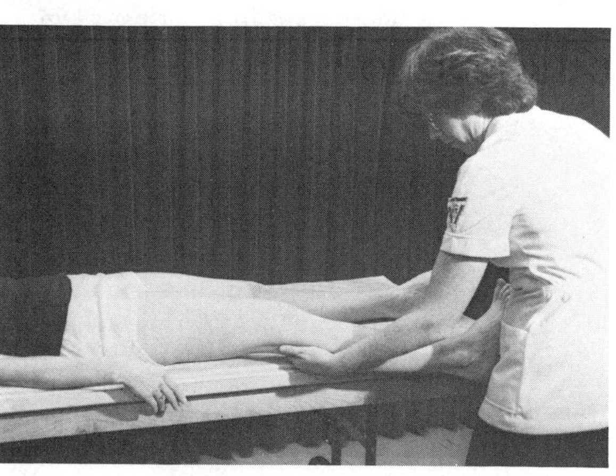

A. Supine: D_1E with knee extension.
T. Holding in shortened range.
E. MC thigh and foot.

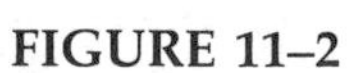

FIGURE 11–2

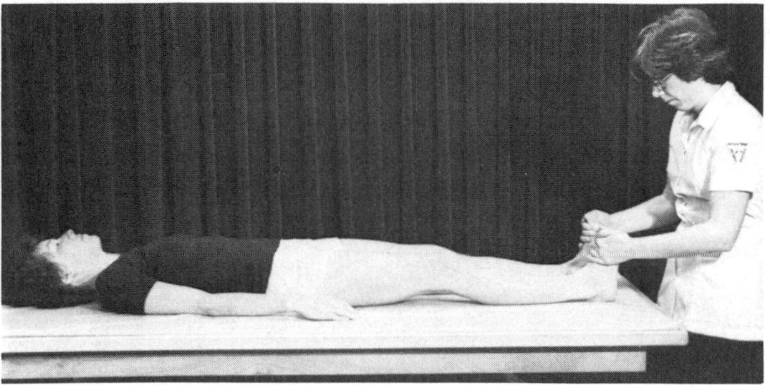

A. Supine: bilateral dorsiflexion.
E. MC dorsum of feet.

FIGURE 11–3

(26) (Figure 11–2), or bilateral dorsi (Figure 11–3) or plantar flexion. Resistance to these patterns will also strengthen the trunk and other extremities. As an adjunct to treatment, biofeedback may be effectively used to assist the patient in gaining voluntary control of the knee extensors.

A more direct approach can be initiated once the patient has experienced the sensation of the quadriceps contraction. Quadriceps setting exercises and active terminal extension will directly promote muscular activity and help to develop the control needed to perform an SLR (27). If the patient is able to maintain the knee in extension with a minimal lag during an SLR, quadriceps control is generally sufficient to begin assisted ambulation.

When the trauma of surgery has decreased, treatment may be directed at further improving quadriceps control and increasing ROM. The type of surgery performed will dictate the most immediate goal. In the case of some total knee replacements, for example, ROM may be the most critical factor initially. Following ligamentous repair, quadriceps control is usually the primary goal, and increases in ROM are delayed until healing occurs and the structures can cope with the stress of joint movement (16).

Full ROM depends on normal mobility in both the noncontractile and contractile tissue (19,20). Free movement of the patella in a caudal direction is needed for full passive range into knee flexion and in a cephalo direction for active terminal extension. Traction, dorsal-ventral glides, and rotational motions are progressively applied to the knee to promote full mobility of the noncontractile tissues. To promote full range in the contractile tissues, the techniques of HR, RS, and CR may be effective (26,28). Attention can be given simultaneously to increasing ROM and to improving quadriceps control. As already stated, heavy resistance and prolonged stretch may increase inhibitory influences to the quadriceps and therefore should be avoided during any procedures to increase ROM if quadriceps facilitation is desired. A technique which can facilitate quadriceps while increasing mobility of the hamstrings is a preferable treatment choice. To achieve this mobility into extension, HR can be applied directly to the agonistic quadriceps with minimal to moderate resistance (23). Through the neurophysiological mechanism of reciprocal inhibition, elongation of the hamstrings may be achieved.

The gradual buildup of resistance to a submaximal contraction will improve the tonic holding ability of the quadriceps in the shortened range but should not result in residual inhibitory influences to that muscle (Figure 11–4). If the application of HR to the quadriceps is not successful, an alternative way to increase the ROM into knee extension is to apply HR directly to the hamstrings with moderate to maximal resistance. This resistance will elicit a maximal contraction, which is usually followed by maximal relaxation. The maximal contraction of the hamstrings may also result, however, in reciprocal inhibition of the quadriceps. Although this latter means of applying the technique may be effective in increasing extendability of the hamstrings, the inhibitory influence to the quadriceps is not consistent with the equally important goal of improving quadriceps control.

Increasing movement into knee flexion is also a goal of treatment and is promoted following the increasing of range into extension and the enhancement of quadriceps control. To increase the mobility of the range-limiting quadriceps and therefore increase knee flexion, the technique of choice is HR applied directly to the hamstrings. By reciprocally inhibiting the quadriceps, the range of knee flexion can be increased. Direct maximal resistance to the tight quadriceps with the HR technique should be avoided. As range into flexion is gained, the combination of prolonged stretch and heavy manual resistance to a weakened muscle that functions as an extensor may result in a predominance of inhibitory influences. While elongation of the quadriceps is certainly necessary for movement into knee flexion, excessive inhibitory influences may decrease the ability of the quadriceps to subsequently contract. Quadriceps control is an important consideration throughout all stages of treatment. Because of the inhibitory influences, extendability of the quadriceps, whenever possible, should be promoted by resisting the hamstrings. HR applied to the hamstrings in this manner may produce the desired increases in range with minimal detrimental effects to the knee extensors.

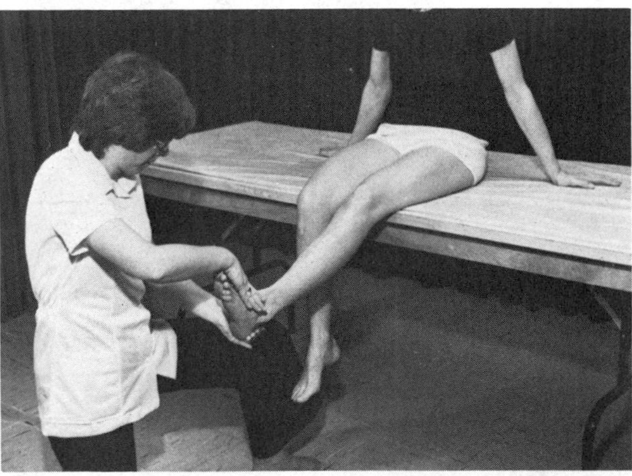

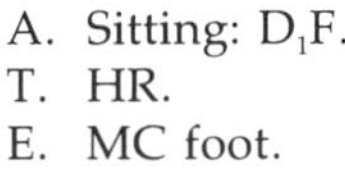

A. Sitting: D_1F.
T. HR.
E. MC foot.

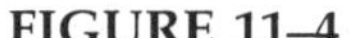

FIGURE 11–4

To summarize, in order to increase range into extension, HR is best applied with minimal to moderate resistance to the agonistic quadriceps. To increase range into flexion, the same amount of resistance is best applied to the agonistic hamstrings. The technique of CR can be used but may not be appropriate during this initial stage if the patient has pain. The fast increase of muscular tension and the rotatory movement occurring at the knee during CR may only aggravate the pain and result in splinting around the joint.

The mobility relaxation techniques are most frequently applied to a unilateral lower extremity pattern either in supine or in sitting. The unilateral pattern allows the therapist to have more effective control of joint movement, because both manual contacts are placed on the involved limb. However, trunk or bilateral patterns can be used advantageously to produce overflow to the involved limb to indirectly increase ROM or to enhance muscular contractions.

In summary, the goals that can be promoted during the initial stage of treatment include: 1) indirect activation of the quadriceps if voluntary control is lacking; 2) direct quadriceps activation with the focus on tonic holding; and 3) increased knee ROM. The goal of improved function of the trunk and uninvolved extremities has also been met by many of the procedures to indirectly activate the quadriceps such as the chopping and lifting patterns and unilateral lower extremity patterns on the uninvolved limb. The treatment described in this initial section is directed toward postsurgical patients. The specific procedures appropriate for each patient will depend on the surgery performed and the indications for exercise.

Middle Stage

At this stage most postsurgical patients have achieved full passive motion into extension and knee flexion to at least 90 degrees. Quadriceps strength has improved to a grade of fair throughout most of the available range, although many patients may still lack complete active terminal extension. For

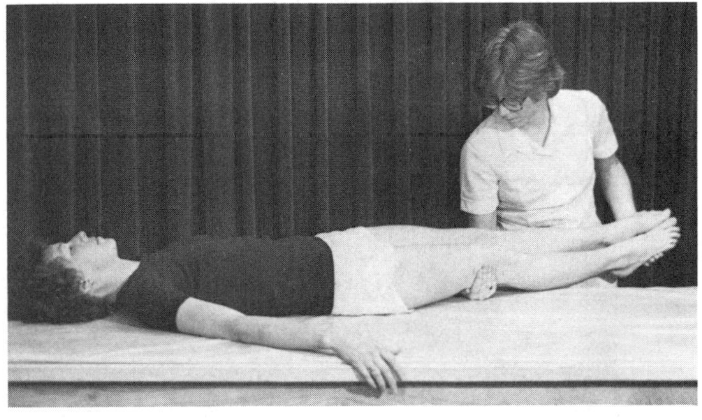

A. Supine: lower trunk extension.
E. MC thighs and feet.

FIGURE 11–5

many nonsurgical patients, treatment may begin at this stage. The nonsurgical diagnoses may include chondromalacia, dislocated patella, strain or sprain of the knee, or immobilization due to other conditions. Because specific exercises are indicated and contraindicated with each diagnosis, treatment procedures must be specifically developed for each patient.

The goals of the middle stage are to:

- Increase quadriceps isometric control specifically in the shortened range and improve isometric and isotonic control of both the quadriceps and hamstrings throughout range
- Further increase ROM
- Increase power, strength, and endurance of the quadriceps and hamstrings

Isometric control in the shortened range of knee extension is emphasized for all patients, and for some may be the only type of exercise indicated. Although many activities in this stage may be similar to those in the initial stage, the focus here is more on direct rather than indirect activation of the quadriceps, with a progressive increase in the amount of resistance. To enhance isometric quadriceps activity, lower trunk (Figure 11–5) and bilateral patterns (Figure 11–6) can be used to increase the amount of overflow (23–24). As already mentioned, unilateral patterns (Figure 11–7) will create the most support for the limb, but will reduce overflow from other areas. When performed with the knee straight, all these lower extremity combinations can improve isometric control of the quadriceps. If activity in the vastus medialis is a specific goal, as it is for patients with chondromalacia or lateral dislocation of the patella, then the D_1F or D_2E patterns should be emphasized (28). The strengthening techniques of RC and TE may be applied to all these activities. Resistance to the hip flexor phase of the pattern may need to be reduced if an increase in the patient's lumbar lordosis results. During the performance of the extensor patterns, overflow from the gluteus maximus in D_2E and the gluteus medius in D_1E may occur. Isometric control

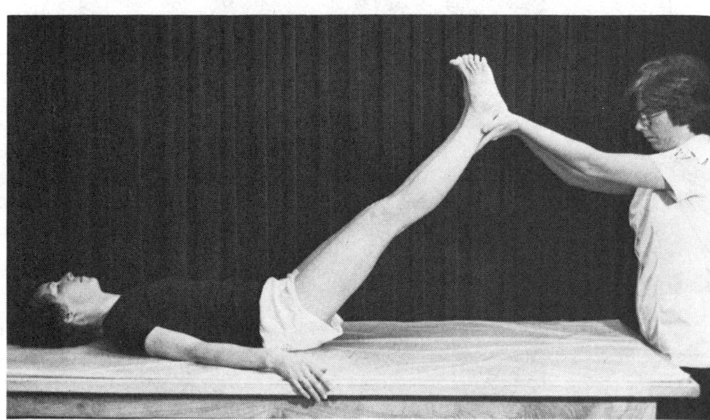

A. Supine: BS D_1F.
E. MC feet.

FIGURE 11–6

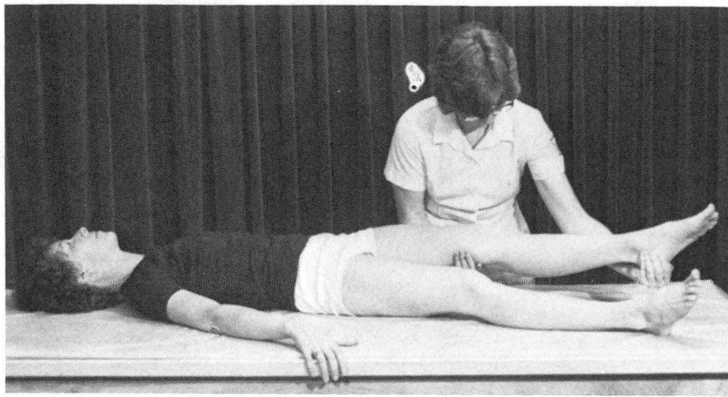

A. Supine: D_2E.
E. MC thigh and foot.

FIGURE 11–7

of the quadriceps in the shortened range can also be promoted in the weight-bearing postures of modified plantigrade and standing, when the patient can tolerate the compression force and the resistance of weight bearing. Manual resistance applied to the pelvis by means of AI and RS will increase the difficulty of the activity by challenging the quadriceps to maintain the knee in extension against the proximally applied force (Figure 11–8). An increase in body-weight resistance is achieved by weight shifting over the involved limb and is further increased during static-dynamic activities.

The next phase of treatment occurs when resistance through range is tolerated. The strengthening techniques of SRH, RC, and TE can be applied to mass flexor and extensor patterns. Lower trunk patterns performed in supine will promote overflow from the trunk and uninvolved lower extremity. Bilateral patterns emphasizing knee control are most easily performed in sitting and in prone.

In prone, gravity assists knee extension. Strengthening of the quadriceps with bilateral patterns in prone would be appropriate when the quadriceps strength is less than a fair grade. Because the hip is maintained in

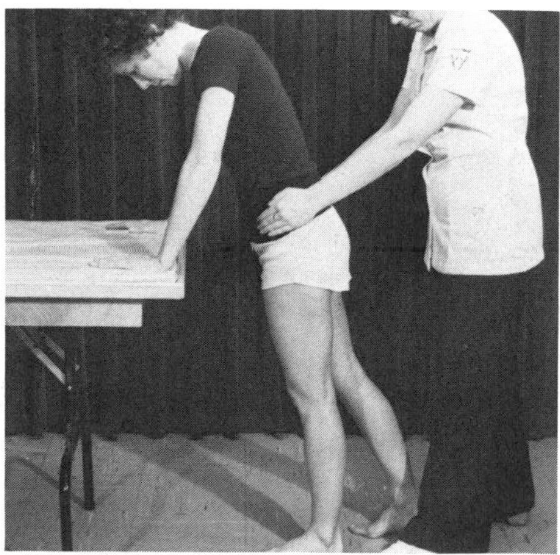

A. Modified plantigrade.
T. RS.
E. MC pelvis.

FIGURE 11–8

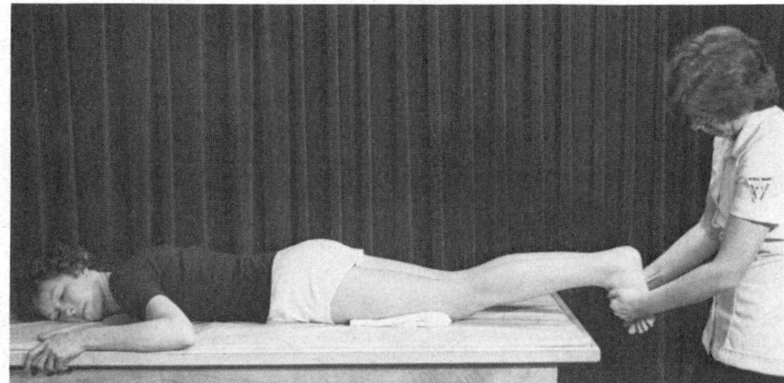

A. Prone: BA knee extension.
E. MC feet.

FIGURE 11–9

extension, the rectus femoris does not become actively insufficient and is able to assist with knee extension (Figure 11–9). Movement into knee flexion may be limited by passive insufficiency of the rectus femoris and active insufficiency of the hamstrings (29). The contraction of the hamstrings against gravity can be resisted through the full range of knee flexion with various strengthening techniques (Figure 11–10). However, control of the hamstrings in the lengthened range is most important for gait activities (30–31). Excessive resistance applied in the shortened range of knee flexion can result in cramping. HR may be used to increase range into knee flexion. RC will increase either quadriceps or hamstring activity and AR will promote concentric-eccentric control of either muscle group.

In sitting, the hip is maintained in flexion and the result is active insufficiency of the rectus femoris during knee extension. Full knee extension may be reduced by passive insufficiency of the hamstrings in this posture. All combinations of bilateral patterns can be performed in sitting. The patterns selected will depend on the patient's normal pattern of reinforcement. Some normal subjects, for example, reinforce most strongly with symmetri-

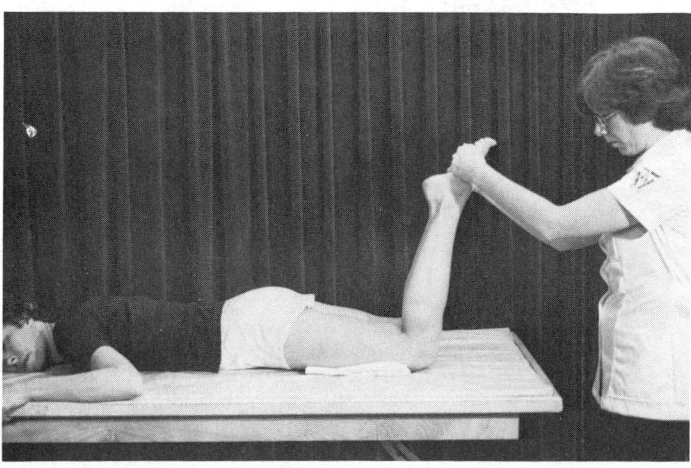

A. Prone: BA knee flexion.
E. MC feet.

FIGURE 11–10

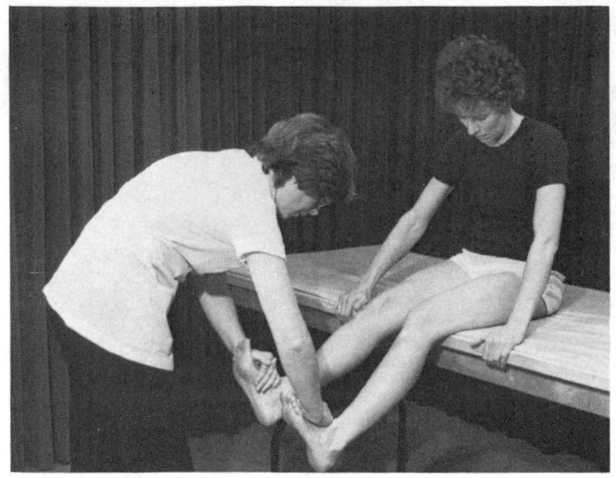

A. Sitting: BS D_1F.
T. TE.
E. MC feet

FIGURE 11–11

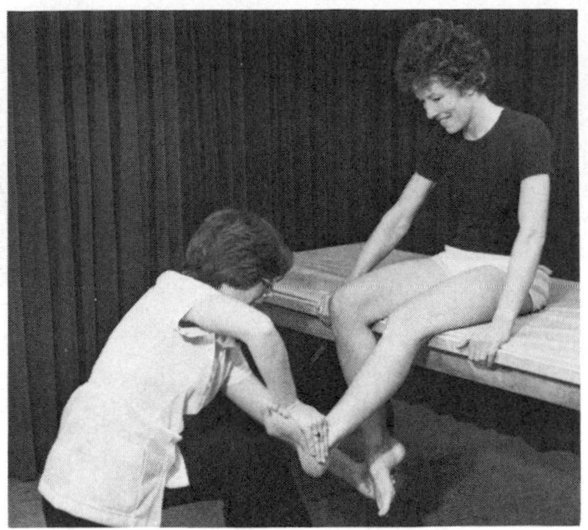

A. Sitting: BR D_2.
T. TE.
E. MC feet.

FIGURE 11–12

cal patterns, while others use reciprocal patterns. Therefore, during treatment symmetrical D_1 or D_2F patterns (Figure 11–11) would be the most appropriate choice for the former group, and reciprocal diagonal (Figure 11–12) patterns for the latter group. If bilateral imbalances of strength exist, the strongest contralateral movement is used for overflow. The techniques applied to these patterns would first emphasize strengthening of the quadriceps in the shortened range of knee extension. Resistance would then be applied through gradual increments of range until resistance through full range of knee extension can be accomplished. Strengthening techniques may also be applied to knee flexor movements if hamstring weakness is present.

Following slow controlled movements through range, quick reversal motions with minimal resistance can be used to emphasize phasic control.

Advanced Stage

At this stage the patient has good strength of the quadriceps and hamstrings and little difficulty with terminal extension. Complete ROM into flexion still may be lacking. Pain is usually not a factor. The goals of the advanced stage are to:

- Promote normal functional ability
- Improve eccentric control of the quadriceps
- Promote advanced stages of motor control

The procedures suggested for this stage incorporate knee flexion into most of the activities. Therefore these procedures probably would not be indicated for patients with patellofemoral disorders (32).

The progression of activities at this stage is designed to further improve quadriceps control by gradually increasing and combining: 1) the amount of weight bearing on the involved limb, 2) the prolonged stretch on the quadriceps, and 3) the amount of body weight borne directly on the quadriceps tendon. All three factors tend to increase the inhibitory influences to the quadriceps (10). By altering the postures of the developmental sequence and the movements performed in those postures, these inhibitory influences can be gradually increased. The goal of this phase of the treatment is to improve the quadriceps control while maintaining functional ability. The quadriceps should then be able to cope with difficult activities such as descending stairs.

The postures discussed in this section are sequenced according to the progressive difficulty of demands placed upon the quadriceps. At this point in the treatment program, standing and modified plantigrade have already been incorporated to improve quadriceps activity in the shortened range of knee extension. An increase in body-weight resistance was achieved earlier by lateral weight shifting and unilateral weight bearing. In the advanced stage of treatment, weight bearing on a partially flexed knee is added to the activity. When the body-weight resistance is increased, the cocontraction around the knee becomes more difficult to maintain with the quadriceps on a slight stretch (Figure 11–13).

When the structures around the knee can cope with the stress of weight bearing, the bridging posture is another activity that can be used to vary two possible inhibitory influences to the quadriceps. The angle of the knee can be altered, beginning with the knees near full extension and then increasing the angle of knee flexion. The amount of weight bearing through

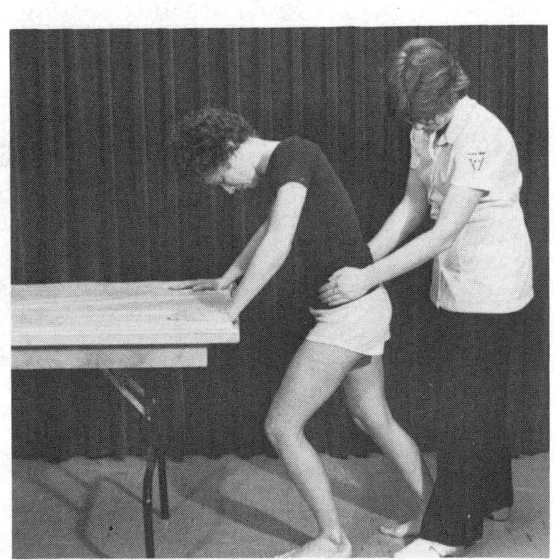

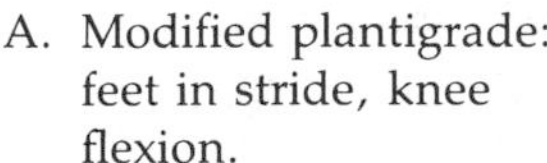

A. Modified plantigrade: feet in stride, knee flexion.
T. SRH.
E. MC pelvis.

FIGURE 11–13

the lower extremity is increased in this posture by lateral weight shifting and by progressing to unilateral, static-dynamic activities. The inhibitory influence of weight bearing on the quadriceps tendon is not a factor in the bridging posture. The activity can be made more difficult by decreasing the B of S and by raising the C of G; the techniques and elements can all be varied to change the stress of the posture. To illustrate, the techniques may begin with AI and RS with manual contacts on the pelvis. Stability is thus promoted in the musculature around the knee, an important factor for patients who have deficient ligamentous stability. Controlled mobility techniques include SRH to the movements of pelvic rotation and lateral shifting, which will further improve the muscular stability around the knee. The technique of AR will promote concentric-eccentric control of the hip and knee extensors as the hips are slowly lowered to the supporting surface. The manual contacts are first positioned on the pelvis, then moved distally to the knees, where stability and controlled mobility techniques are repeated. When the manual contacts are positioned on the ankles, the activity of the knee musculature may be increased. Isometric resistance can be applied at either the knees or ankles in a symmetrical or reciprocal fashion to further enhance knee stability (Figure 11–14).

To increase the difficulty of the bridging activity, the C of G can be raised and B of S decreased, so that the patient is weight bearing on elbows or on hands. In either of these modified positions the progression of techniques and elements, including manual contacts, can be repeated. Quickly alternating weight bearing on the lower extremities with the knees near full extension will simulate the fast bursts of muscular activity that are needed for walking and running. In this bridging position there is less weight bearing than in the upright postures. The more advanced procedures just described are appropriate for patients returning to strenuous activities, but may not be suitable for an older or sedentary population.

Half-kneeling with the involved leg placed anteriorly results in 90 degrees of knee flexion (Figure 11–15). As with bridging, weight bearing on

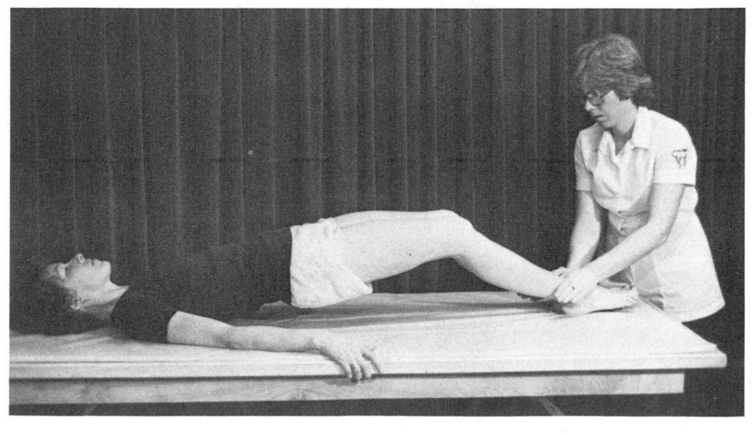

A. Bridging: knees near full extension.
E. MC ankles.

FIGURE 11–14

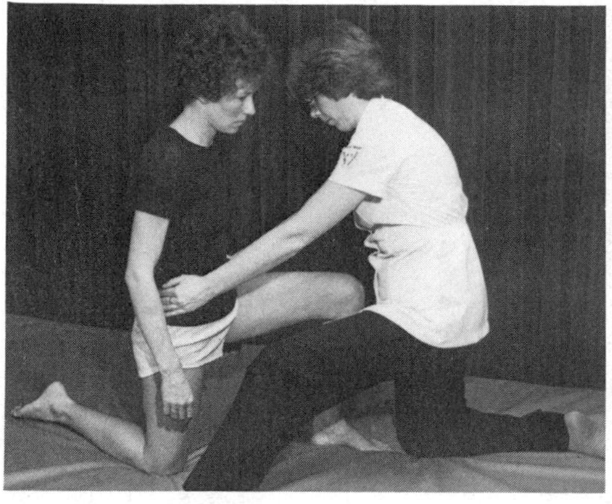

A. Half-kneeling.
T. RS.
E. MC pelvis.

FIGURE 11–15

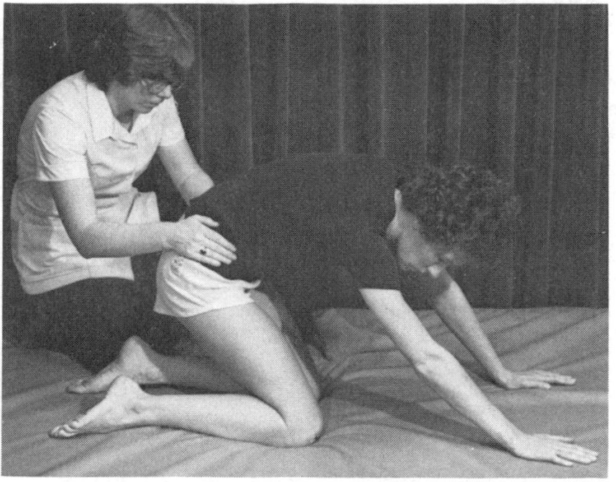

A. Quadruped: rocking.
T. SRH.
E. MC pelvis.

FIGURE 11–16

the quadriceps tendon is not a factor. The controlled mobility techniques of SR can be used to alter the amount of knee flexion and also to vary the amount of weight bearing on the involved limb.

The quadruped posture incorporates all three inhibitory influences. The knee is flexed to 90 degrees and can be further flexed by rocking movements performed in a posterior direction; weight bearing occurs on the quadriceps tendon; body-weight resistance can be accentuated by weight shifting on to the affected knee and dynamic movements of the unaffected limb. The techniques applied to the posture can begin with RS to the pelvis for enhancement of muscular stability around the knee. SRH superimposed on rocking motions, will improve both isotonic control as well as functional range of motion (Figure 11–16). Static-dynamic activities can be performed to improve both the dynamic unilateral control of the involved limb or to increase the stability demands of the involved limb when it is performing in a static weight-bearing fashion. Resistance can be applied to the dynamic limb either manually (Figure 11–17) or mechanically with pulleys or weighted cuffs. Following procedures in quadruped, resisted terminal extension exercises may need to be repeated if the many inhibitory influences produced by the activities in quadruped have temporarily reduced quadriceps control. For many patients, terminal extension exercises must be incorporated in all stages of rehabilitation.

Kneeling is even more strenuous than quadruped for the knee extensors. The increased amount of weight borne on the quadriceps tendon in this posture will increase the inhibitory influences to that muscle. As in the

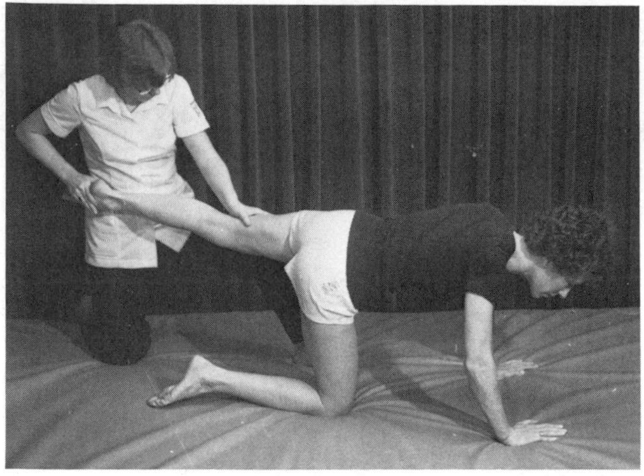

A. Quadruped: D_1E involved limb.
T. SRH.
E. MC thigh and foot.

FIGURE 11–17

other postures, the application of techniques should begin with RS to enhance stability, then should progress to SRH to promote isotonic-concentric control. Concentric-eccentric contractions of the quadriceps can be achieved with the technique of AR. This technique is performed through gradual increments of range approaching the heelsitting position, in which the quadriceps are in a very lengthened position (Figure 11–18). The quadriceps appear to be more active in kneeling procedures than in the previous bridging and quadruped postures (33). Therefore the increased eccentric control promoted in kneeling is considered preliminary to the control needed to descend stairs. A pillow placed under the knees will make this weight bearing posture more tolerable for patients who might complain of pain.

Half-kneeling with the involved limb posterior is a progression from kneeling. More weight bearing occurs on the supporting limb than in the previous postures; thus rocking in half-kneeling is very difficult and may not be possible for some patients.

Procedures discussed to this point for the treatment of patients with knee disability have emphasized first isometric then isotonic control using

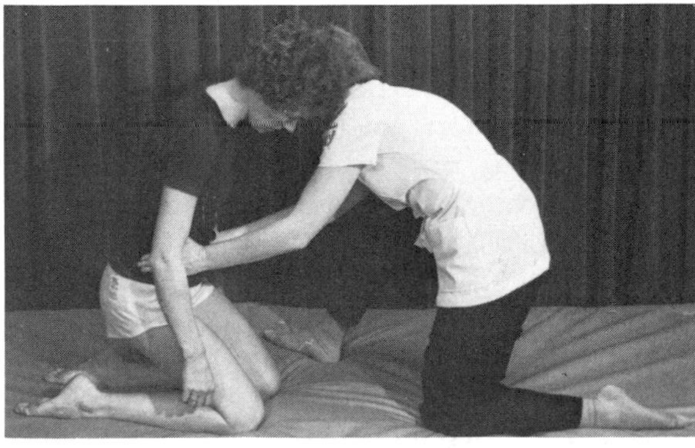

A. Kneeling.
T. AR.
E. MC pelvis.

FIGURE 11–18

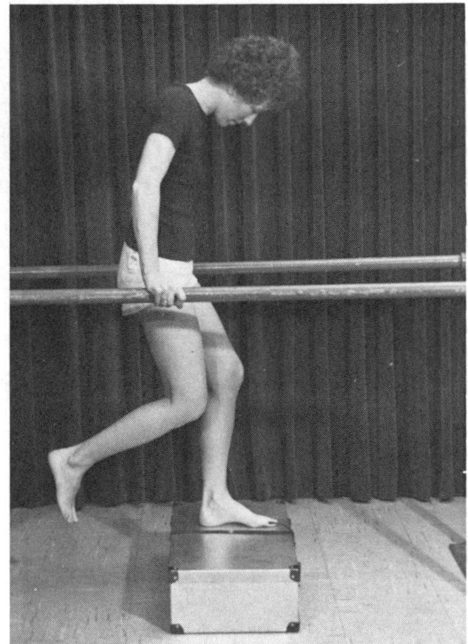

A. Running up and down curb in parallel bars.
T. Fast concentric-eccentric contractions.

FIGURE 11–19

the stability techniques of SHRC, AI and RS, the strengthening techniques of RC and TE, and the controlled mobility techniques of SRH and AR in various postures. The treatment has incorporated procedures designed to improve strength and to enhance control so inhibitory influences that normally affect the quadriceps do not become the prevailing factor. For many patients this control will be sufficient for their functional needs. For patients who are going to return to strenuous athletic events, procedures to improve the timing of quadriceps activity are necessary. Although fast bursts of activity can be promoted by some mechanical devices (34), to simulate the control needed for most athletic endeavors and to emphasize a specificity of training, timing exercises performed in weight-bearing postures are important.

Fast alternating weight bearing, such as running in place, can be done in standing or the patient can practice jumping up and down a small curb. Parallel bars may be used initially for support if necessary (Figure 11–19). Quick changes in weight bearing in the bridging posture were mentioned earlier. In full plantigrade, running in place will further challenge the timing of quadriceps activity because the angle of knee flexion is increased (Figure 11–20). However, in this plantigrade position an excessive amount of knee flexion should be avoided because it may simulate the squat thrusting exercises that can overstress the knee.

These last procedures are strenuous as they require normal quadriceps strength, completely free range, good eccentric control, and the ability to produce fast bursts of quadriceps activity. Sideward, backward, and rotational movements may be added to further simulate the control needed for the specific athletic event. The high degree of control needed to perform

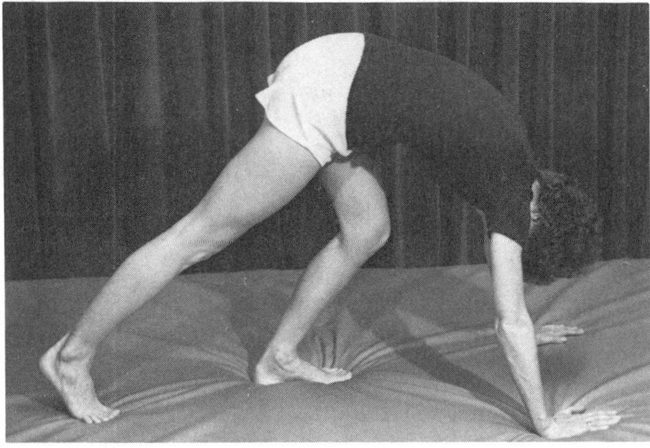

A. Plantigrade: running in place.
T. concentric-eccentric contractions.

FIGURE 11–20

these last exercises make them the culmination of most physical therapy treatments and should be attempted only toward the end of rehabilitation.

To summarize, the sequence of procedures for the rehabilitation of a patient with knee disability has been to:

1. Increase quadriceps control by first emphasizing tonic holding in the shortened range and by progressing to resistance through range
2. Increase ROM using relaxation techniques and joint mobilization
3. Gradually increase the stress on the quadriceps by balancing the influences of weight bearing and prolonged stretch
4. Strengthen the hamstrings
5. Improve stability, controlled mobility, and skill levels of control

The use of physical agents and resistive equipment may be incorporated as needed into the entire treatment plan. Only certain aspects of this sequence may be appropriate for patients with various disabilities. Because there are many causes of knee dysfunction and each patient reacts differently to the same disability, treatment should be individualized depending on the evaluation, goals, and specific problem and asset lists.

REFERENCES

1. Salter RB: Textbook of Disorders and Injuries of the Musculoskeletal System. Baltimore, Williams & Wilkins Co., 1970
2. Brashear HR, Raney RB: Shand's Handbook of Orthopaedic Surgery, ed 9. St Louis, CV Mosby Co, 1978

3. Helfet AJ: Disorders of the Knee. Philadelphia, JB Lippincott Co, 1963
4. Johnson MA, Pulgar J, Weightman D, et al: Data on the distribution of fibre types in thirty-six human muscles: An autopsy study. J Neurol Sci 18:111–129, 1973
5. Henneman E: Peripheral mechanisms involved in the control of muscle. In Mountcastle VB(ed): Medical Physiology, ed 13. St Louis, CV Mosby Co, 1974, vol 1
6. Milner-Brown HS, Stein RB, Yemm R: The orderly recruitment of human motor units during voluntary isometric contractions. J Physiol 230:359–370, 1973
7. Edstrom L: Selective atrophy of red muscle fibers in the quadriceps in long-standing knee-joint dysfunction injuries to the anterior cruciate ligament. J Neurol Sci 11:551–558, 1970
8. Stockmeyer SA: An interpretation of the approach of Rood to the treatment of neuromuscular dysfunction. Amer J Phys Med 46:950–956, 1966
9. Lawrence MS: Strengthening the quadriceps: Progressively prolonged isometric tension method. Phys Ther Rev 36:658–661, 1956
10. Stockmeyer SA: Procedures for improvement of motor control. Unpublished notes from Boston University PT 710, 1978
11. DeHaven KE, Colan WE, Mayer PJ: Chondromalacia in Athletes: Clinical Presentation and Conservative Management. Read at the American Orthopaedic Society Sports Medicine Annual Meeting, San Diego, 1977
12. Davies GJ, Larsen R: Examining the knee. The Physician and Sports Medicine 6:49–67, 1978
13. Lieb FJ, Perry J: Quadriceps function: An anatomical and mechanical study using amputated limbs. J Bone Joint Surg 50:1535–1548, 1968
14. Pevsner DN, Johnson JRG, Blazina ME: The patellofemoral joint and its implications in the rehabilitation of the knee. 59:869–874, 1979
15. Walsh WM: Rotary instabilities. Phys Ther 60:1633–1639, 1980
16. Malone T, Blackburn TA, Wallace LA: Knee rehabilitation. Phys Ther 60:1602–1610, 1980
17. Cailliet R: Knee Pain and Disability. Philadelphia, FA Davis Co, 1973
18. Duchenne GB: Physiology of Motion, Kaplan EB(trans). Philadelphia, WB Saunders Co, 1959
19. Cyriax J: Textbooks of Orthopedic Medicine. London, Cassell, 1970–1971
20. Kaltenborn FM: Manual Therapy of the Extremity Joints, ed 2. Oslo, Olaf Norlis Bokhandel, 1976
21. Mannheimer IS: Electrode placements for transcutaneous electrical nerve stimulation. Phys Ther 58:1455–1462, 1978

22. DeAndrade JR, Grant C, Dixon A: Joint distension and reflex muscle inhibition in the knee. J Bone Joint Surg 47-A:313–322, 1965
23. Knott M: Proprioceptive neuromuscular facilitation. Unpublished notes from Vallejo, CA, 1970
24. Voss DE: Therapeutic exercise. Unpublished notes from Northwestern University, 1974
25. Michaels J: Exercise Overflow: An Electromyographic Investigation. Thesis. Boston, MA, Boston University Sargent College of Allied Health Professions, 1978
26. Markos P: Ipsilateral and contralateral effects of proprioceptive neuromuscular facilitation techniques on hip motion and electromyographic activity. Phys Ther 59:1366–1373, 1979
27. Leach RE, Stryker WS, Zohn DA: A comparative study of isometric and isotonic quadriceps programs. J Bone Joint Surg 47-A:1421–1426, 1965
28. Knott M, Voss DE: Proprioceptive Neuromuscular Facilitation, ed 2. New York, Harper & Row, 1968
29. O'Connell AL, Gardner EB: Understanding the Scientific Bases of Human Movement. Baltimore, Williams & Wilkins Co, 1972
30. Saunders JB, Inman VT, Eberhart HD: The major determinators in normal and pathological gait. J Bone Joint Surg 35-A:543–558, 1953
31. Murray MP: Gait as a total pattern of movement. AM J Phys Med 46:290–333, 1967
32. Ficat RP, Hungerford DS: Disorders of the Patellofemoral Joint. Baltimore, Williams & Wilkins Co, 1977
33. Sullivan PE, Markos PD: Comparison of Quadriceps Activity in Kneeling and Bridging Postures. Pilot Study. Boston University, Sargent College of Allied Health Professions, 1980
34. Moffroid MT, Whipple RH: Specificity of speed of exercise. Phys Ther 50:1692–1700, 1970

chapter 12

Low Back

INTRODUCTION

Low back pain is a common complaint of patients. The severity of the disability can range from an acute disabling problem to a chronic, mild discomfort. The primary structures that are usually affected are the joints, ligaments, disc, and capsule. Damage to any of these may affect the nerve roots or spinal cord, and may lead to secondary muscle spasm, tightness, or weakness. A pain-spasm cycle may also occur as a result of direct injury to the back muscles. Because of the many variables, low back dysfunction can be very difficult to evaluate adequately and treat successfully (1–4).

EVALUATION

A careful evaluation can assist the therapist in determining some of the underlying causes of pain. Differentiation between primary and secondary symptoms is not always easy, and in many instances an evaluation may not uncover the exact cause of the disability. A physical therapy evaluation should cover or include the history of the problem, sensory factors, strength, palpation, ROM, and posture and body mechanics.

History. A careful history delineating the onset of the problem will aid the therapist in localizing the cause(s) of the patient's pain. The patient may relate one of the following:

- A fall on slippery ground or from a ladder: A compression fracture or other internal derangement may result from an injury of this type and may require a proper medical evaluation. The sacroiliac joint is commonly traumatized by a fall and should be assessed for normal mobility.
- Lifting a heavy object: Muscle strain and spasm with localized pain often accompany such trauma. A description by the patient of "locking" of the back may be indicative of damaged joint structures.
- A twisting motion followed by acute pain: This rotary movement is commonly associated with muscular or joint involvement (1, 5–8).
- Chronic pain: This may be the chief complaint without any specific precipitating trauma.

Continual lifting or reaching with improper body mechanics can be expected to affect both joint and muscle tissue over time. A description of the patient's occupational and recreational activities and other types of physical stress should be included in a complete history. Standing or sitting for prolonged periods can be detrimental to the low back area and should be noted (9).

Determining the patient's ability to relax is important. The autonomic nervous system influences the body's general reactions to stimuli (10). Evaluation and periodic reevaluation of blood pressure, pulse, depth of respiration, and temperature of distal segments can provide the therapist with information pertaining to the patient's autonomic function and anxiety level (11).

Sensation. Sensory testing along the dermatomes of the lower trunk and lower extremities may help to determine specific nerve root involvement (12). Pain or paresthesias should be carefully noted including: type, location, occurrence, duration, and any predisposing aggravating factors (13).

Strength Assessment. In addition to the dermatomal evaluation, results of a specific myotomal strength evaluation may also indicate a nerve root involvement. The strength of the trunk musculature, specifically of the lower trunk, can be assessed with a manual muscle test in conjunction with active ROM and postural evaluations. A complete evaluation of muscle strength may not be possible if pain is a factor.

Palpation. Manual probing of the low back area can be used to localize trigger points or uneven degrees of muscular tension in one area. Palpation of joint structures may indicate unevenness or malalignment of vertebral bodies.

ROM. SLR has been the traditional means of assessing the presence of pressure on the sciatic nerve (5). Toe-touching in long sitting will produce the same traction force on the nerve while allowing the therapist to evaluate the flexibility of the low back muscles. Gross ROM of trunk movements—flexion, extension, lateral bending, and rotation—may reproduce the symptoms and help to localize the painful area. These motions have been classically evaluated by having the upper trunk move on the lower trunk (1). Limitations of the low back extensors and quadratus lumborum may be more specifically evaluated by moving the lower trunk on the stabilized upper trunk. This assessment can be conducted in supine by passively moving the lower trunk into flexion and rotation to both the left and right sides and by noting the amount of pelvic elevation from the plinth (14) (Figure 12–1). A ROM test may reveal tightness of the hip flexors (Figure 12–2). This tightness may contribute to the forward pelvic tilt observable during the postural

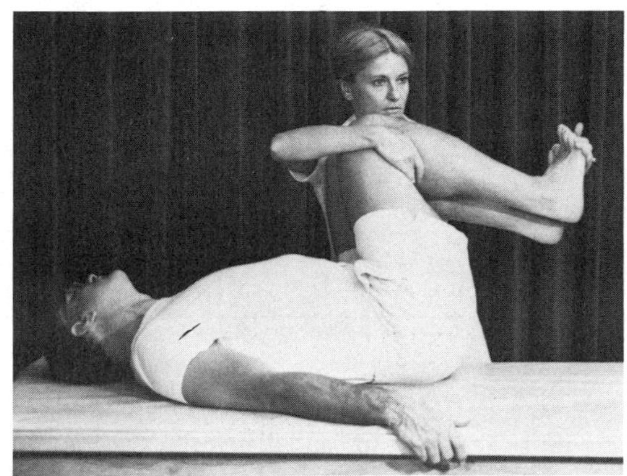

A. Supine: lower trunk flexion and rotation.

FIGURE 12–1

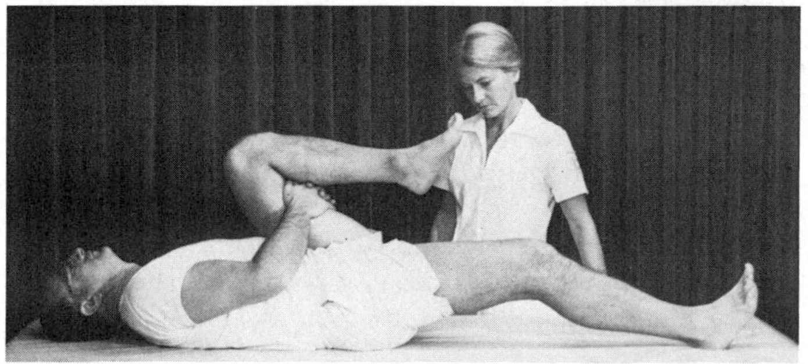

A. Thomas test: unilateral leg extension.

FIGURE 12–2

evaluation (15). The performance of specific vertebral joint ROM assessments will determine local areas of hyper- or hypomobility and may be used to pinpoint the painful area (16).

Posture and Body Mechanics. Cervical, thoracic, and lumbar spinal regions should be examined for the presence of increased or decreased anterior, posterior, or lateral curvatures. Any structural abnormalities should be consistent with the findings from the ROM and strength evaluations. Symmetry can be determined through assessment of leg length measurements and the bilateral equality of bony landmarks (6,7,15). Whenever feasible, the evaluation of body mechanics during lifting, reaching, and movement in general should simulate the patient's employment and recreational demands. When possible, a gait evaluation should be conducted since it may reveal dynamic postural abnormalities such as reduced trunk counterrotation and decreased heel strike.

All the gathered information should be matched with the patient's symptoms to determine areas of consistency or inconsistency. Any discrepancy among the evaluative findings may be indicative of a nonstructural cause of back pain (17).

In summary, evaluative findings may include paresthesia, areas of muscle spasm, pain at rest or during movement, specific or generalized decreases in muscle strength, decreased ROM of combined movements or in specific vertebral joints, postural abnormalities, bilateral asymmetry, poor body mechanics, and occupational body stress. An attempt should be made to differentiate primary and secondary signs and both contractile and noncontractile tissue involvement.

TOTAL TREATMENT PLAN

A conceptual basis of treatment is a necessary part of the total treatment process. In this chapter the sequence of procedures is designed to initially reduce anxiety and sympathetic responses, to promote mobility or normal ROM, to enhance stability around the lower trunk, and to strengthen the muscles that are most frequently weak. This plan is organized to increase the patient's functional capabilities.

Many controversies exist regarding the most beneficial treatments for patients with low back problems. The reason that a variety of plans have been formulated can be related to the many mechanisms of injury, the tissues involved, and the variability of patient symptoms. The diagnosis and resultant symptoms will indicate to the therapist whether trunk flexion, extension, rotation or no movements are indicated during treatment. In keeping with the general context of this book, these various philosophies will not be addressed. Instead the treatment will focus on alleviating the problems that seem to be present in most patients with low back disability. Specific trunk motions, as mentioned, may be incorporated into treatment when appropriate.

ROM, which is generally limited in the lower trunk extensors and hip flexors, may detrimentally affect the function of the lower trunk and pelvis. The extendability of the hamstrings may also be limited, but because of the posterior origin on the pelvis, they contribute to its proper positioning. Excessive tightness of any muscle group should be corrected. However, the normal adaptive shortening of the hamstrings that commonly occurs may not necessarily contribute to the symptoms associated with low back dysfunction. For this reason, no specific procedures have been included in the following section to increase the length of the hamstring muscles.

Once the primary cause of the back pain has been established, the treatment plan can be directed toward alleviating that problem. The initial focus of treatment is to alter any external biomechanical causes of the disability. This may include the addition of shoe lifts to correct an existing leg length discrepancy, improvement of body mechanics, and alteration of postural stresses. Various physical agents may be indicated to decrease pain, reduce muscle spasm, and increase local areas of circulation. Joint mobilization is indicated if specific areas of joint hypomobility exist.

The treatment presented in this chapter focuses primarily on therapeutic exercise. The goals of treatment and the procedures suggested to reach those goals are only a segment of the total rehabilitation process. Goals appropriate at the acute stage preliminary to the mobility stage of control include:

1. Promote homeostasis of the autonomic nervous system (ANS)
2. Promote generalized relaxation and reduce localized muscle spasm

The patient in the acute, painful stage may have symptoms that reflect an imbalance in the ANS. Acute pain, a generalized increase in tension, and an oversensitivity to stimuli may all be associated with predominance of the sympathetic division (18). An increase in parasympathetic influences may lead to a balance or homeostasis of the ANS. Procedures or sensory inputs that may be considered parasympathetic in nature include deep breathing, maintained pressure over the abdomen, neutral warmth, slow stroking down the posterior primary rami (PPR) located deep to the paravertebral muscles, and a slightly inverted tilt position of the entire body to stimulate the carotid sinuses (19–20). Traditional treatment incorporates some of these stimuli in a modified form. For example, treatment frequently begins with the patient lying prone with a pillow under the abdomen, a hot pack on the low back, and the patient covered with a blanket. The stimuli automatically included in this procedure are a slight head-down position, maintained pressure on the abdomen, and neutral warmth. While many patients respond favorably to the application of hot packs, others complain of increased posttreatment pain. This increased discomfort can be attributed to a rebound effect that results in intensification of the original pain. Prolonged applications of ice, although often effective in producing relaxation, many produce a similar rebound effect (19–20). When the patient reacts adversely to extremes of temperature, these thermal applications are not appropriate and more neutral temperatures should be applied (19–21).

Massage often follows the application of thermal stimuli. Although massage traditionally applied appears to be an effective relaxant, the beneficial results might be enhanced by the inclusion of caudally directed effleurage strokes (22–24). Therefore, with slight modification of traditional treatment, stimuli directed at promoting generalized relaxation can be easily incorporated into the initial treatment procedures. If the prone posture cannot be tolerated, the sidelying position is an appropriate alternative.

Jacobsen's relaxation exercises have been found empirically to be effective (25). The gradual increase and relaxation of muscle tension that results from the application of this technique can be incorporated into treatment both to promote general relaxation and to decrease localized muscle spasm. For patients with pain and spasm in a specific area, muscle contraction is sequenced to follow an indirect to direct approach (14,26). Isometric contractions followed by conscious relaxation or a modified hold-relax technique against minimal resistance can be performed first by those segments distant to the painful area before this technique is applied to the muscles of the involved area. In general, isometric contractions of unilateral extremity patterns with the limb positioned in the shortened range of the pattern will activate the trunk musculature. To emphasize upper trunk activity, the proximal-manual contact can be positioned on the scapula. Because positioning of the proximal hand on the pelvis for lower trunk activation is not practical in the supine posture, contractions of unilateral lower extremity patterns in this position are best elicited with both of the therapist's hands on the limb.

As a means of illustrating the indirect to direct approach, a sequence of procedures will be outlined for a patient with spasm in the *left* lumbar region. With the patient supine, treatment would begin on the nonpainful *right* side, with a contraction of the muscles in the upper trunk antagonistic to those in spasm. The right upper abdominals can be activated by resisting the D_2E pattern of the right upper extremity in the shortened range (Figure 12–3). If this procedure does not elicit pain, the next procedure can be directed at either the right upper trunk extensors or the right lower abdominals. Right upper trunk extensors may be activated with a D_2F pattern of the right upper extremity (Figure 12–4); the right lower abdominals with D_1F (Figure 12–5) of the right lower extremity; and the right lateral trunk flexors by D_1E of the upper right extremity (Figure 12–6). The last goal of the indirect progression would be to activate the right lower back extensors with contraction of the D_1E pattern of the right lower extremity (Figure 12–7). Contractions of muscles on the involved side follow the same sequence just described for the uninvolved side. All these patterns are resisted in the

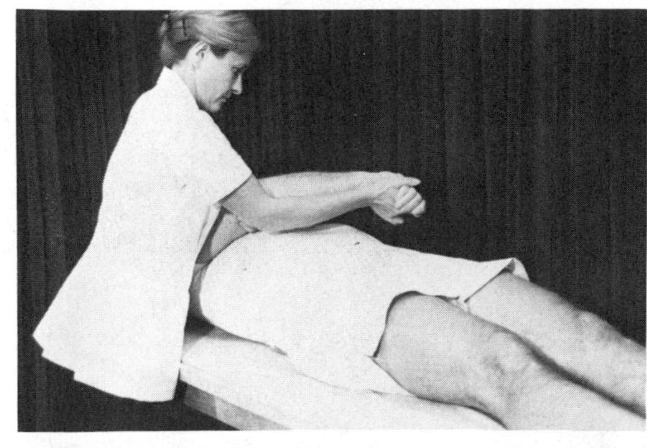

A. Supine: UE D_2E, SE (shortened range of emphasis).
T. HR (modified).
E. MC arm and hand.

FIGURE 12–3

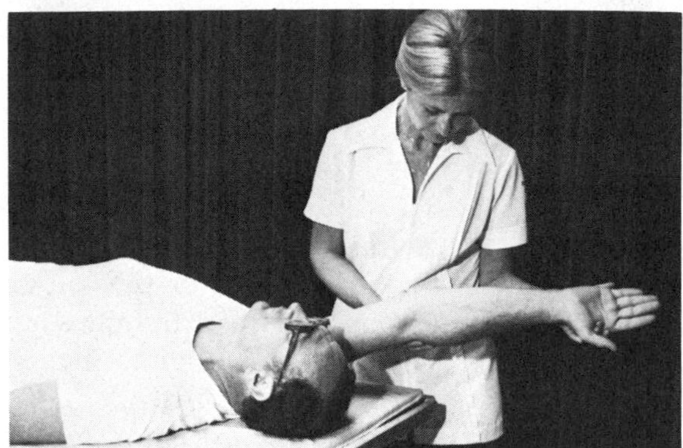

A. Supine: UE, D_2F, SE.
T. HR (modified).
E. MC arm and hand.

FIGURE 12–4

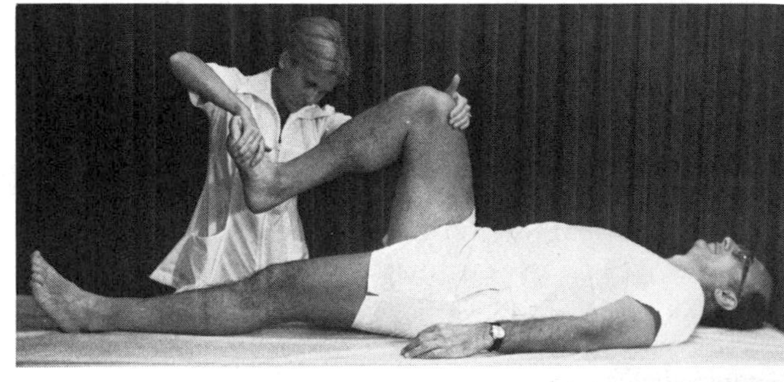

A. Supine: LE D_1F SE.
T. HR (modified).
E. MC thigh and foot.

FIGURE 12–5

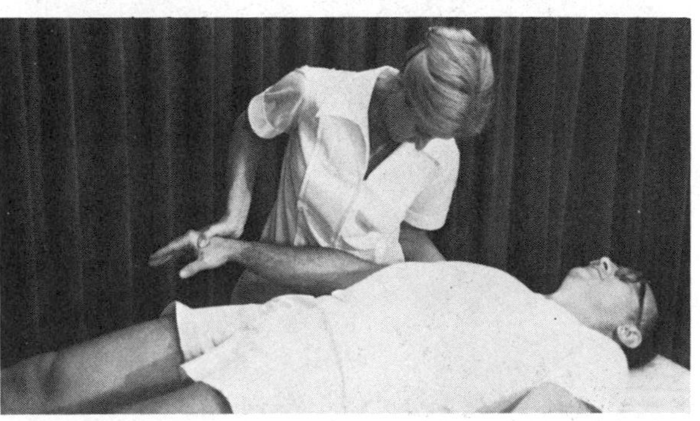

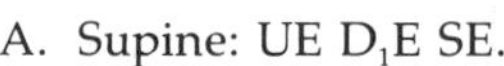

A. Supine: UE D_1E SE.
T. HR (modified).
E. MC arm and hand.

FIGURE 12–6

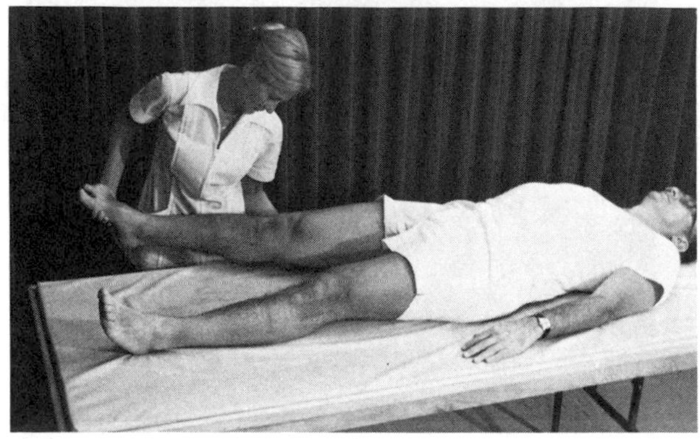

A. Supine: LE D_1E.
T. HR (modified).
E. MC thigh and foot.

FIGURE 12–7

shortened range. Direct contraction of the involved left low back extensors with D_1E of the left leg would be the final activity of the sequence (Figure 12–8). All these procedures should be aimed at teaching the patient how to contract and relax gradually.

Incorporated into this program of isometric exercises are progressive movements of the extremities against minimal resistance. Like the isometric progression, the isotonic movements should begin with the contralateral upper extremity. Bilateral upper extremity patterns would be followed by unilateral lower extremity movements on the uninvolved and then on the involved side. This gradual progression of isometric then isotonic exercises may enable the patient to move slowly without increasing pain (27).

Chronic Stage

Procedures at this stage of treatment are geared toward the patient who is not hampered by acute debilitating pain, even though some discomfort may interfere with normal movement. The patient may have proceeded through

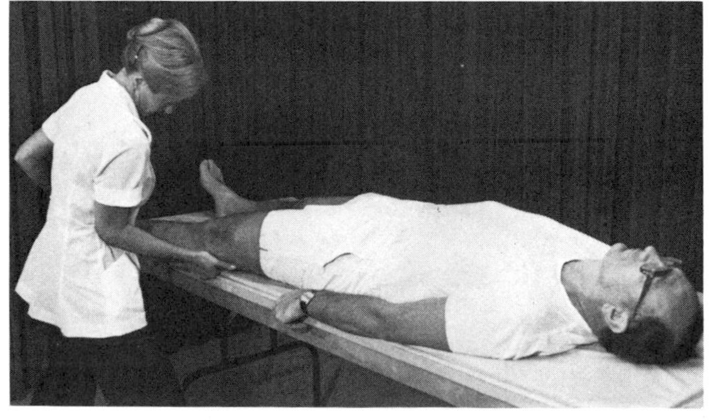

A. Supine: LE D_1E SE.
T. HR (modified).
E. MC thigh and foot.

FIGURE 12–8

the acute stage, or because of a less stressful injury may begin treatment at this stage. The goals of the chronic stage are to:

- Increase ROM of low back and hips.
- Increase strength of lower abdominals and other weakened muscles.
- Improve trunk cocontraction.
- Promote movement through range.
- Improve body mechanics.

Increase ROM. Muscular tightness in patients with low back pain is often present in the low back extensors and the hip flexors (15). This combination of tightness may contribute to the commonly found increased lordotic posture. Specific procedures can increase ROM in these two areas and other procedures, to be described later, will help to make this range functional.

Hip flexor tightness may be equal bilaterally or may be more limited on one side. The lengthened range of the D_1 flexor pattern (Figure 12–9) will put the iliopsoas on stretch and the lengthened range of the D_2 flexor pattern (Figure 12–10) will stretch the tensor fascia lata. HR to either the agonistic hip extensor or the antagonistic hip flexor will promote an increase in ROM. If contraction of the tight antagonist results in an anterior pelvic tilt or increases pain, HR to the hip extensor may be used to reciprocally inhibit the tight flexor. The patient can be positioned for either of these procedures with the other lower extremity flexed on the plinth to maintain a posterior pelvic tilt. Range into the normal excursion of hip hyperextension can be best promoted in sidelying, with the contralateral unexercising lower extremity flexed toward the chest (Figure 12–11).

Increased ROM of the low back extensors can be accomplished by the lower trunk flexion with rotation patterns that incorporate movement of

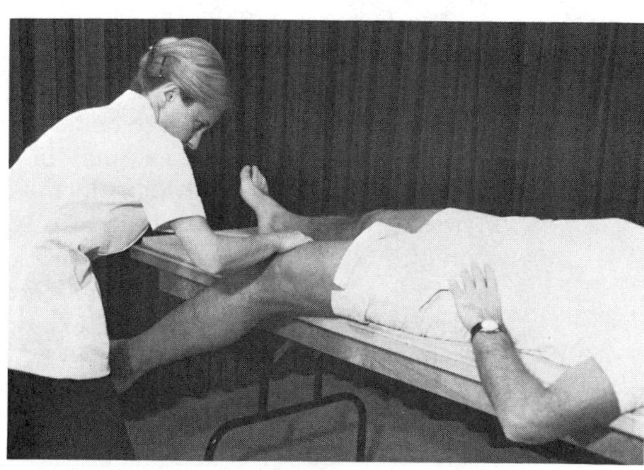

A. Supine: LE D_1F LE (lengthened range of emphasis).
T. HR to antagonist.
E. MC thigh and foot.

FIGURE 12–9

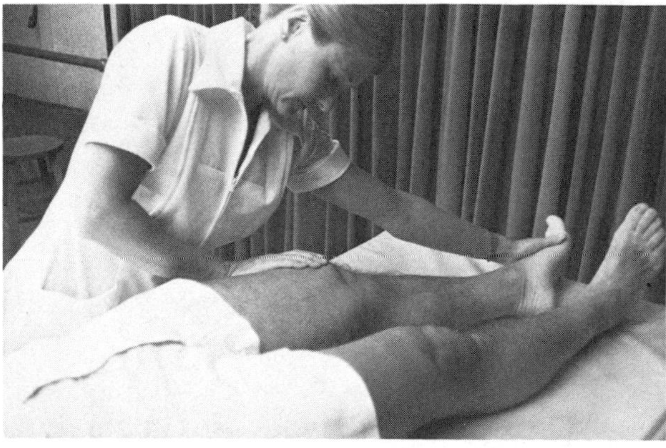

A. Supine: LE D_2F LE.
T. HR to antagonist.
E. MC thigh and foot.

FIGURE 12–10

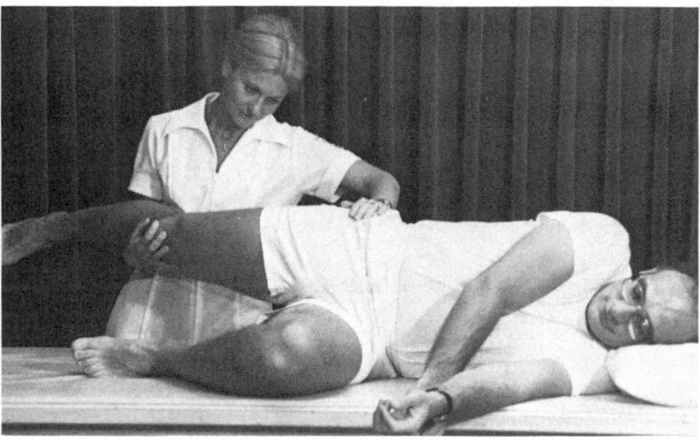

A. Sidelying: uppermost LE in hyperextension.
T. Holding shortened range.
E. MC thigh and foot.

FIGURE 12–11

both legs simultaneously. These patterns can specifically increase range in the low back without the confounding effects of other normally tight muscles such as the hamstrings. The patient is passively moved to the shortened range of the lower trunk flexor pattern where HR of the total flexor pattern is performed. HR applied to the agonistic flexor pattern empirically has been found to be more effective in increasing range than contraction of the antagonistic back extensor muscles (Figure 12–12). Although contraction of abdominals might produce better results, the therapist should be aware that the hip flexors, which also may be tight, are being facilitated. In a long-sitting position, the relaxation techniques of HR and RS may be used to increase ROM in the low back area. Chopping with manual contacts directly on the trunk or on the head and wrist is an effective activity to combine with long sitting (Figure 12–13). However, increases in ROM in this posture can be the result of increased extendability of either or both the hamstrings or low back extensors (28).

Strengthen Trunk Musculature. The main focus of treatment is to strengthen the lower abdominals (29–30) and the low back extensors. Cocontraction around the lower trunk in standing while maintaining the pelvis in a neutral position or in a posterior pelvic tilt is the major goal. The sequence of activities will begin with postures that have a large B of S and a low C of G, and that progress to postures with less biomechanical support. The techniques should first emphasize isometric contractions, progressing to isotonic movements only when the isometric contractions can be performed without pain.

The following procedures are sequenced according to the difficulty of the activity, which is determined by the amount of stretch applied to the hip flexors. The greater the stretch, the more difficult it will be for the patient to maintain the proper lower trunk position.

The supine hooklying posture and the lower trunk rotation (LTR) activity can be effectively used to strengthen the lower abdominals. In hooklying, the lower trunk may be easily maintained in a posterior pelvic tilt or neutral position. If the patient has both weakness in the lower abdominals and tightness in the hip flexors a complete supine position may cause an anterior pelvic tilt and thus should be avoided. In hooklying, the techniques of AI and RS, with manual contacts on the knees, will activate the lower

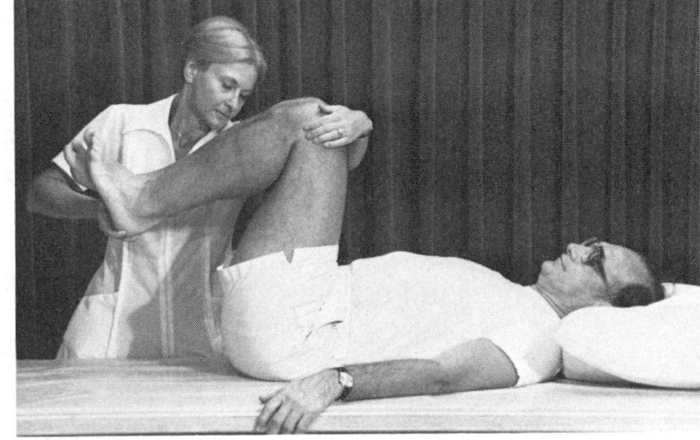

A. Supine: LTF with rotation, knee flexion.
T. HR.
E. MC thigh and foot.

FIGURE 12–12

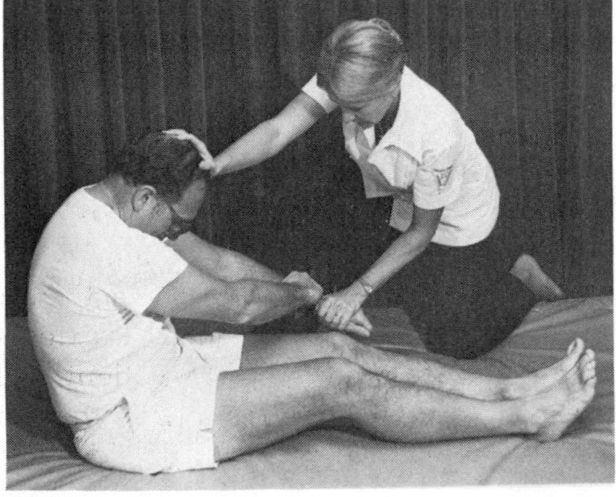

A. Long sitting with chop.
T. RS.
E. MC head and wrist.

FIGURE 12–13

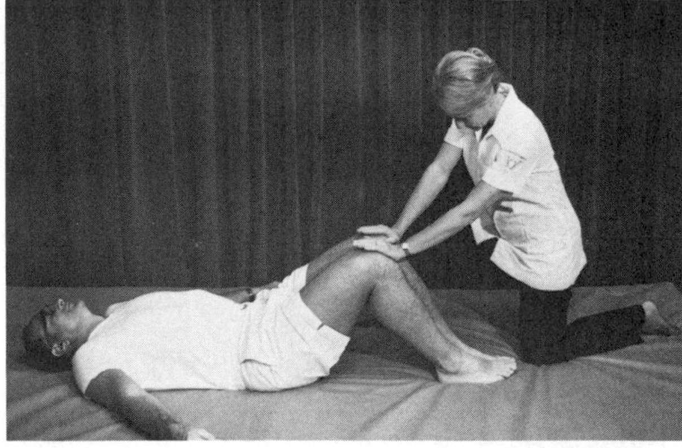

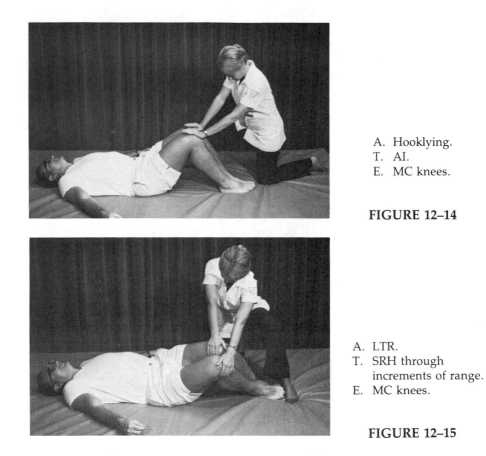

A. Hooklying.
T. AI.
E. MC knees.

FIGURE 12–14

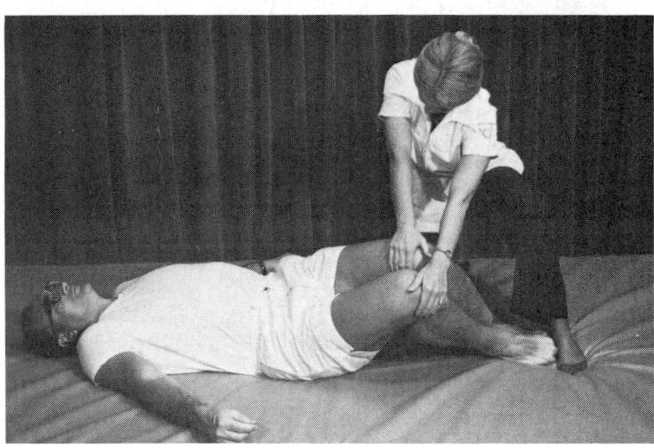

A. LTR.
T. SRH through increments of range.
E. MC knees.

FIGURE 12–15

abdominals and the lumbar back extensors (Figure 12–14). The techniques should be applied with the knees together. This position leads to greater activity of the trunk musculature than when the knees are separated. Of the two techniques, AI will produce a greater amount of muscular activity on alternate sides of the trunk, but RS will facilitate cocontraction around the lower trunk (32). During these procedures the patient's low back should be monitored to ensure that a posterior pelvic tilt is maintained. Lower trunk rotational movements through increments of range follow the isometric procedures (Figure 12–15). This activity can be effective in activating all the lower trunk muscles and in increasing the general mobility of the lower trunk area (33). Strengthening techniques such as RC superimposed on the movement can further enhance the activity of the lower trunk musculature, and are appropriate when movement does not cause pain.

All the lower trunk patterns are very effective in activating both the lower abdominals (Figure 12–16) and the lower back extensors (Figure 12–17). If movement through range is difficult for the patient, these patterns can be performed isometrically by passively positioning the extremities in the shortened range of the pattern, and asking for a "hold." If the patterns

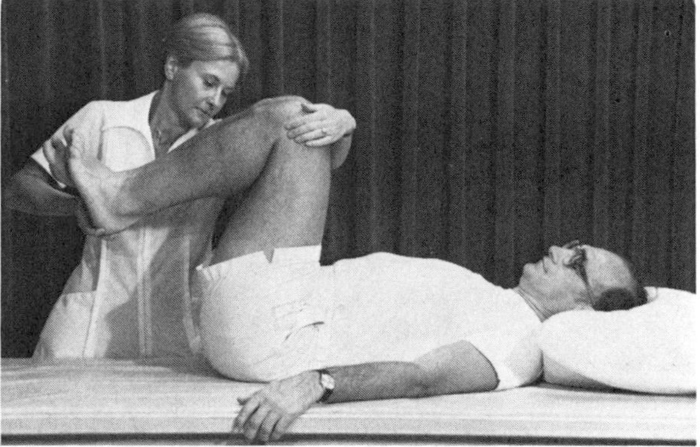

A. LTF with rotation knee flexion.
T. Holding in shortened range.
E. MC thighs and feet.

FIGURE 12–16

can be performed isotonically, movement combinations should be restricted to the mass flexor and mass extensor patterns. Compared to the straight leg patterns, these mass combinations produce the least amount of stress on the low back. The upper trunk patterns of a chop or a lift may be included in supine and also in sitting. Chops and lifts activate the upper trunk musculature most directly, although activity in the lower trunk musculature is also evident (33) (Figures 12–18 and 12–19).

Sidelying is another stable posture in which both isometric and isotonic strengthening of the trunk muscles can be performed. The lower extremities can be positioned in extension so that the shortened range of hip flexion will not be reinforced. This is one of the few postures in which abdominals can be emphasized without activating hip flexors in the shortened range. The technique of RS will increase isometric strength and promote trunk co-contraction (Figure 12–20). When pain does not limit movement, the techniques of SRH and RC are useful to promote isotonic activity of the lower trunk muscles (Figure 12–21).

To evaluate the effectiveness of the previous procedures in both increasing the range of the hip flexors and strengthening the lower abdominals, the angle of hip flexion in the hooklying position can be decreased (Figure 12–22). The techniques of AI and RS applied with manual contacts on the

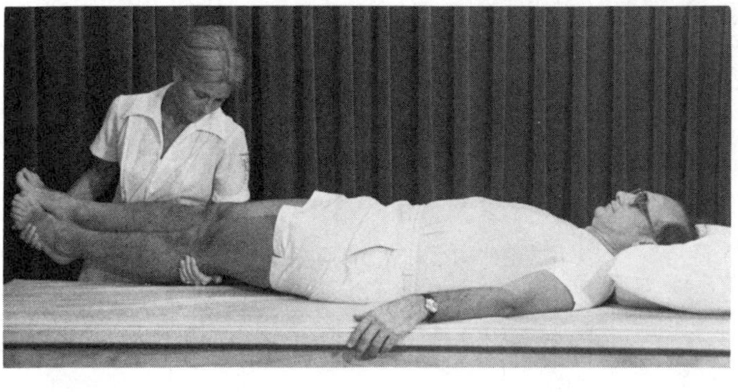

A. LTE with rotation knee extension.
T. Holding in shortened range.
E. MC thighs and feet.

FIGURE 12–17

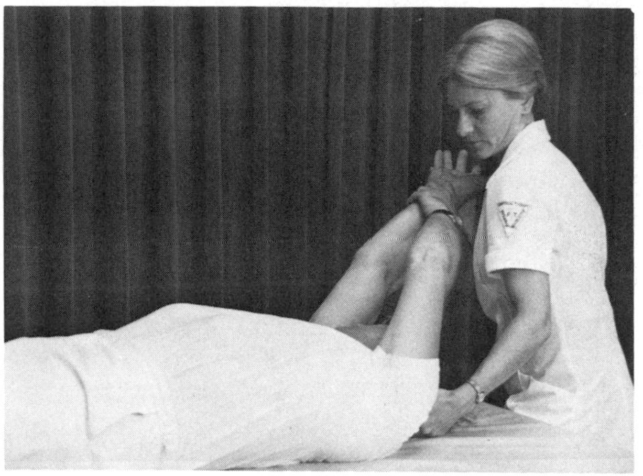

A. Supine: lift.
T. Holding in shortened range.
E. MC head and wrist.

FIGURE 12–18

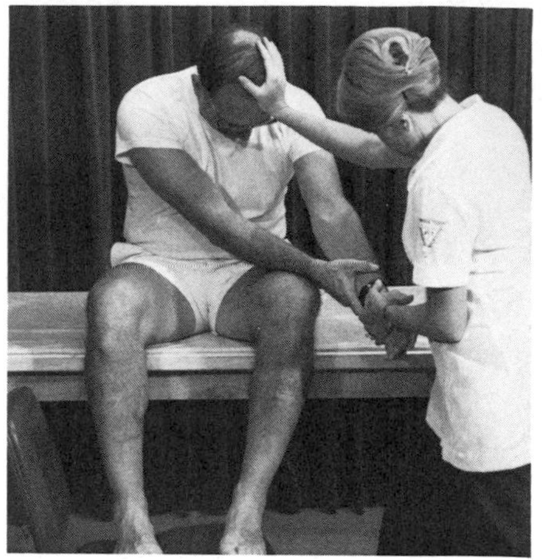

A. Sitting: chop.
T. Holding in shortened range.
E. MC head and wrist.

FIGURE 12–19

knees can be repeated in this position. If a posterior pelvic tilt can be maintained when the hips are near full extension, the patient probably has enough flexibility and strength around the hips and lower trunk to progress to bridging.

The position of the low back and hips in the bridging posture is similar to that which occurs in standing. Because bridging increases the stress placed on the low back, an anterior pelvic tilt may result if hip flexor tightness is still present, an indication that the patient is not ready to assume

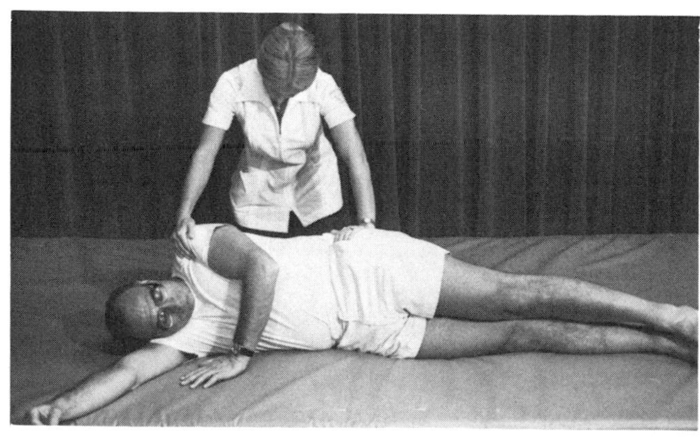

A. Sidelying: lower extremities positioned in extension.
T. RS.
E. MC scapula and pelvis.

FIGURE 12–20

this posture. In bridging, the isometric activity of the low back extensors can be emphasized with the stability techniques of AI and RS (34) (Figure 12–23). The lower trunk and pelvic motions of rotation and lateral shifting in this posture are promoted with the technique of SRH and will enhance the control needed during ambulation. Increased activity of the lower extremity musculature occurs when the feet are positioned further away from the buttocks. The placement of manual contacts can be progressed from the pelvis to the knees to the ankles. Quadriceps activity can be enhanced in bridging, which will improve the patient's body mechanics during ADL motions in standing.

Other postures that can be effectively used in treatment are quadruped and modified plantigrade. The major difference between these two postures for the patient with low back dysfunction is the angle of hip flexion. If a posterior pelvic tilt can be maintained in modified plantigrade, use of the quadruped posture as a preliminary activity to upright postures may not be necessary. In both activities, however, the abdominals support the viscera against the force of gravity and isometrically contract to produce a posterior pelvic tilt or neutral position. The technique of RS with manual contacts on

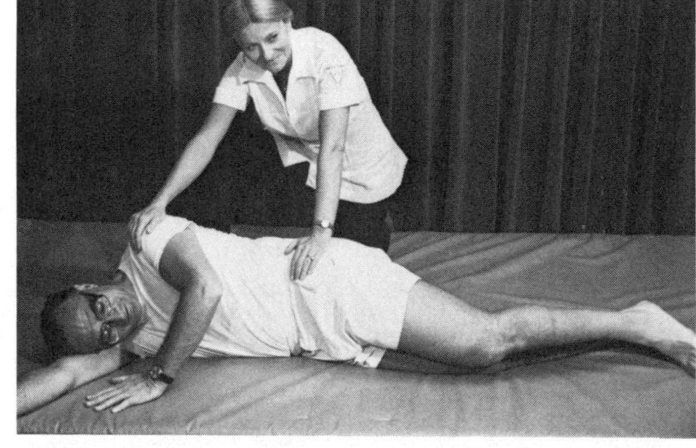

A. Sidelying: lower trunk protraction.
T. SRH.
E. MC scapula and pelvis.

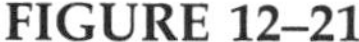

FIGURE 12–21

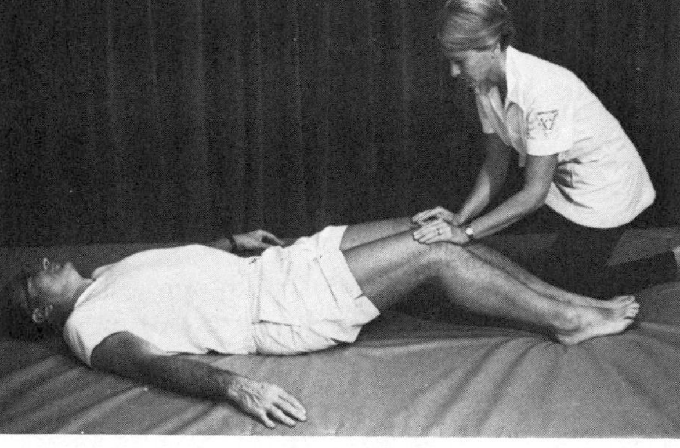

A. Supine: hooklying knees near full extension.
T. RS.
E. MC knees.

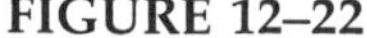

FIGURE 12–22

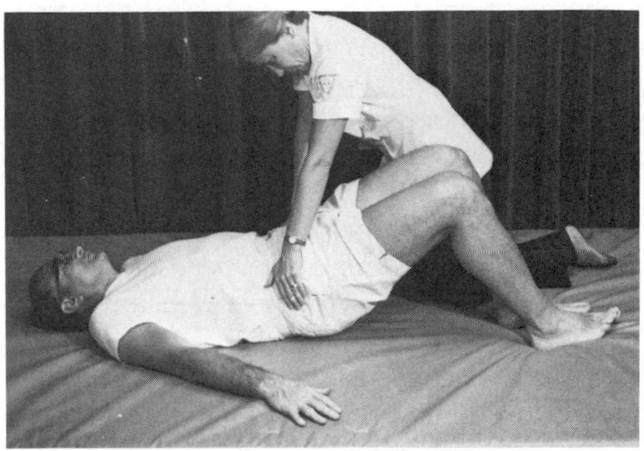

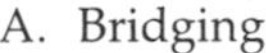

A. Bridging.
T. AI.
E. MC pelvis.

FIGURE 12–23

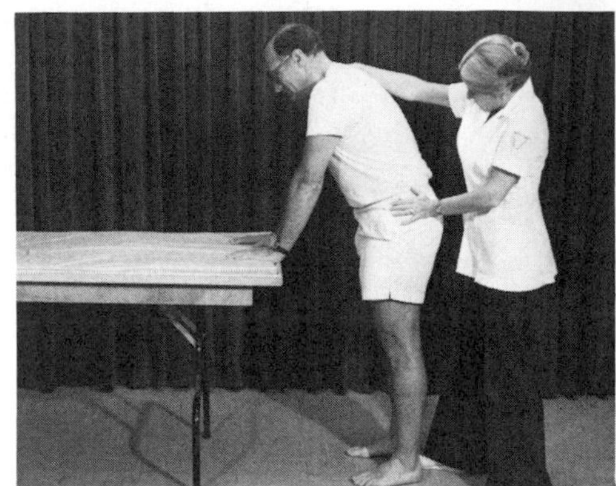

A. Modified plantigrade.
T. RS.
E. MC scapula and pelvis.

FIGURE 12–24

the pelvis, or scapula and pelvis, can further enhance this isometric contraction. In modified plantigrade these techniques are applied with the hip in some flexion (Figure 12–24). The progression is to have the patient stepping closer to the supporting surface while maintaining the lumbar and pelvic tilt position. This movement toward upright should be increased until the proper alignment can be achieved in a fully erect posture.

When mobility in the hip and low back are present the lower abdominals should be able to maintain the proper pelvic alignment. The ability of the patient to stand and ambulate painlessly and with good posture will indicate to the therapist the success of the previous procedures. A functional evaluation of the abdominal and back extensors during more active movements such as reaching, bending, and lifting also should be conducted.

As already mentioned, the patient must be educated in proper body mechanics and back care. ADL are modified to reduce back strain. Modifications may include rolling to sidelying during the assumption of sitting from supine, proper use of pillows while sleeping, alternating feet on a low stool if standing for prolonged periods, and adequate support in sitting postures. Transfer of learning to everyday activities is essential and can be promoted with both instruction and practice in lifting, moving, and reaching for objects.

In summary, the progression of procedures in this chapter has been developed on the basis of the most common clinical findings among patients with low back disability: pain, tightness in the hip flexors and low back extensors, and decreased strength of lower abdominals and low back extensors. Other therapeutic interventions will probably be indicated. These may include joint mobilization, external support (35), TNS, and behavior modification (17). The combination of therapeutic exercise procedures carefully sequenced for each patient coupled with other appropriate interventions should restore the patient to as functional a level as possible.

REFERENCES

1. Cailliet R: Low Back Pain Syndrome, ed 2. Philadelphia, FA Davis Co, 1968
2. Maitland GD: Vertebral Manipulation, ed 3. Woburn, MA, Butterworth, 1973
3. Cyriax JH: Examination of the Spinal Column. Physiother (London) 56:3–7, 1970
4. Salter RB: Textbook of Disorders and Injuries of the Musculoskeletal System. Baltimore, William & Wilkins Co, 1970
5. Shands AR, Raney RB: Handbook of Orthopaedic Surgery, ed 7. St Louis, CV Mosby Co, 1967
6. Cyriax JH: Textbook of Orthopaedic Medicine: Diagnosis of Soft Tissue Lesions. Baltimore, Williams & Wilkins Co, 1967, vol 1
7. Howarth MB, Petrie JG: Injuries of the Spine. Baltimore, Williams & Wilkins Co, 1964
8. McNab I: Backache. Baltimore, Williams & Wilkins Co, 1977
9. Nachemson AL, Elfstrom G: Intravital dynamic pressure measurements in lumbar discs: A study of common movements, maneuvers and exercises. Scand J Rehab Med 2: (suppl 1) 1–40, 1970
10. Youmans WB: The visceral nervous system and skeletal muscle activity. Amer J Phys Med 46:173–188, 1966
11. Chusid JG, McDonald JJ: Correlative Neuroanatomy and Functional Neurology, ed 17. Los Altos, CA, Lange Medical, 1979
12. Hoppenfeld S: Orthopaedic Neurology. Philadelphia, JB Lippincott Co, 1977
13. Mennell J McM: Back Pain. Little, Brown & Co, Boston, 1960
14. Knott M: Proprioceptive Neuromuscular Facilitation, Unpublished notes from Vallejo, CA, 1966
15. Kendall HO, Kendall FP: Posture and Pain. Baltimore, Williams & Wilkins Co, 1952
16. Paris SV: Mobilization of the spine. Phys Ther 59:988–995, 1979
17. Gottlieb HJ, Alperson BL, Koller R, et al: An innovative program for

the restoration of patients with chronic low back pain. Phys Ther 59:996–999, 1979

18. Koizumi K, Brooks C McC: The integration of autonomic system reactions: A discussion of autonomic reflexes, their control and their association with somatic reactions. Reviews of Physiol 67:1–68, 1972

19. Rood M: The use of sensory receptors to activate, facilitate, and inhibit motor response, autonomic and somatic, in developmental sequence. In Sattely C(ed): Approaches to the Treatment of Patients with Neurological Dysfunction. Dubuque, IA, WM C Brown, 1962

20. Stockmeyer SA: Procedures for improvement of motor control. Unpublished notes from Boston University, PT 710, 1979

21. Stockmeyer SA: An interpretation of the approach of Rood to the treatment of neuromuscular dysfunction. Amer J Phys Med 46:950–956, 1966

22. Jacobs M: Massage for the relief of pain: Anatomical and physiological consideration. Phys Ther Rev 40:96–97, 1960

23. Mennell JB: Physical Treatment by Movement, Manipulation and Massage, ed 5. Philadelphia, The Blakiston Co, 1945

24. Tappan FM: Healing Massage Techniques. Reston, VA, Reston Publishing Co, 1978

25. Jacobson E: Progressive Relaxation. Chicago, University of Chicago Press, 1938

26. Voss DE: Proprioceptive neuromuscular facilitation. Amer J Phys Med 46:838–898, 1966

27. Jensen MA: Biomechanics of the lumbar intervertebral disc: A review. Phys Ther 60:765–773, 1980

28. Ray D, Ruiz N, Zigun R: Effects of hold-relax on relaxation of back extensors. Unpublished study, Boston, MA, Boston University Sargent College of Allied Health Professions, 1979

29. Partridge M, Walters C: Participation of the abdominal muscles in various movements of the trunk in man. Phys Ther Rev 39:791:800, 1957

30. Carmen DJ, Blanton PL, Biggs NL: Electromyographic study of the anterolateral abdominal musculature utilizing indwelling electrodes. Amer J Phys Med 51:113–129, 1972

31. Smidt GL, Amundsen LR, Dostal WF: Muscle strength at the trunk. J Orthopaedic Sports Phys Ther 1:165–170, 1980

32. Sullivan PE: Isometric techniques applied in the hooklying position. Pilot study, Boston, MA, Boston University Sargent College of Allied Health Professions, 1980

33. Konecky C: An EMG Study of Abdominals and Back Extensors during Lower Trunk Rotation. Thesis, Boston, MA, Boston University Sargent College of Allied Health Professions, 1980

34. Rich C: EMG Analysis of Trunk Musculature During Isometric Techniques in Bridging. Thesis, Boston, MA, Boston University Sargent College of Allied Health Professions, 1981

35. Von Werssowetz OF: Back braces and supports. Clin Orthop 5:169–183, 1955

Index

(Page numbers printed in italic indicate definition of term)

A

S

T